The Evidence-based Parenting Practitioner's Handbook

Kirsten Asmussen

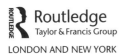
Routledge
Taylor & Francis Group

LONDON AND NEW YORK

First published 2011
by Routledge
2 Park Square, Milton Park, Abingdon, Oxon OX14 4RN

Simultaneously published in the USA and Canada
by Routledge
711 Third Avenue, New York, NY 10017

Routledge is an imprint of the Taylor & Francis Group, an informa business

British Library Cataloguing in Publication Data
A catalogue record for this book is available from the British Library

Library of Congress Cataloging in Publication Data
Asmussen, Kirsten.
The evidence-based parenting practitioner's handbook / Kirsten Asmussen. -- 1st ed.
p. ; cm.
Includes bibliographical references and indexes.
1. Parenting. 2. Evidence-based social work. 3. Developmental psychology. I. Title.
HQ755.8.A76 2011
--dc22
2010048566

ISBN: 978-0-415-60992-0 (hbk)
ISBN: 978-0-415-60993-7 (pbk)
ISBN: 978-0-203-81573-1 (ebk)

Typeset in Baskerville by
Bookcraft Ltd, Stroud, Gloucestershire

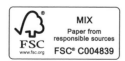

MIX
Paper from
responsible sources
FSC
www.fsc.org
FSC® C004839

Printed and bound in Great Britain by
CPI Antony Rowe, Chippenham, Wiltshire

To R, B & K

The Evidence-based Parenting Practitioner's Handbook

The Evidence-based Parenting Practitioner's Handbook provides a comprehensive overview of the knowledge necessary to effectively deliver evidence-based parenting interventions within community and health settings. Using clear examples of how this knowledge can inform frontline work with parents, this practical handbook includes:

- an overview of the policy context underpinning evidence-based parenting work in the US, UK, Australia and Norway
- a discussion of how a robust evidence base is established and the ways in which practitioners can access information about good-quality research
- an overview of how research in the field of child development has contributed to the development of evidence-based parenting interventions
- an overview of how theories and research in the field of therapeutic practice have contributed to the development of evidence-based parenting interventions
- what research evidence suggests about the role of the practitioner in the delivery of evidence-based support
- outcome-focused methods for establishing the evidence base for new parenting interventions
- outcome-focused methods for commissioning evidence-based parenting services.

Emphasizing the ways in which practitioners can evaluate and translate messages from research into applied work with parents and families, *The Evidence-based Parenting Practitioner's Handbook* is suitable for all those involved in the delivery of evidence-based parenting support, including frontline practitioners, service managers, parenting commissioners, heads of children's services and policy makers.

Kirsten Asmussen is a developmental psychologist with expertise in the parent/child relationship and parenting interventions. She works at the National Academy for Parenting Research where she leads a team of researchers who evaluate the programmes appearing on the Commissioning Toolkit.

"A splendidly thorough account of what is involved in parenting interventions, together with a convincing argument on why proper assessments of efficacy are essential."

Sir Michael Rutter

"Societies benefit when children thrive," Kirsten Asmussen notes, in launching her compelling overview of best practice in equipping parents for their most important role in life. The book encompasses the origins and nature of evidence-based parenting practices, how to improve these practices through evaluation and monitoring, and how to build broad systems for community-wide parenting support. Asmussen's analysis is both scholarly and highly accessible. It is a valuable resource for professionals, program directors, and policy-makers who work to support good parenting and to strengthen families.

John R. Weisz, Ph.D., ABPP
Professor of Psychology, Harvard University

Finally, a clear and comprehensive book that tells the truth to practitioners and policymakers about parenting. You don't have to guess about how to help parents. Good evidence exists and more is on the way. Learn it and use it!

J. Lawrence Aber,
Distinguished Professor of Applied Psychology and
Public Policy at the Steinhardt School of Culture, Education,
and Human Development, New York University

Contents

List of boxes

List of figures

List of tables

Acknowledgments

Countless people have contributed to this book. These individuals include my many mentors, managers, colleagues and friends who have provided me with endless support and enthusiasm. They also include the many parents and children I have had the pleasure of working with over the years who are an ongoing source of inspiration.

There are also a number of people who deserve special mention with respect to the writing of this book. These include Bekah Little, who encouraged me to write it in the first place and Stephen Scott, whose tireless dedication to the National Academy of Parenting Research has made it possible. I would also like to thank my valued colleagues Celia Beckett, Moira Doolan, Megan Ellis, Sajid Humayan and Rosemarie Roberts for their thoughtful comments on various chapters. I would especially like to thank Neda Bebiroglu, Suna Eryigit, Tim Matthews and Katey Weizel for their meticulous work on the glossary and illustrations.

Preface

What is evidence-based parenting support?

During the past century we have learned a great deal about child development. We have discovered much about children's physical, intellectual, social and emotional growth and the systems that best support these processes. While there is still much to learn, we can now make some scientifically informed decisions about how services and policies can improve child outcomes and family life. In the words of Lawrence Steinberg (2001: 16), we now 'know some things'.

One of the things we now know is that parents make a big difference in their children's lives. Research consistently tells us that while a good-quality parenting environment is important at all stages of a child's development, it is especially significant during the first three years of life and then again in early adolescence. These periods are marked by a phase of increased brain cell growth and connectivity, followed by a process of 'synaptic pruning', where the newly formed neural connections are either strengthened or lost. During these times, the quality of children's interactions with their environment influences what connections are made and whether or not children 'use or lose' them. While schools and communities make an important contribution to this process, research consistently tells us that parents play the biggest role in determining their children's wellbeing.

What are the things that parents do to positively influence their children's development? Most people have an implicit understanding of good parenting that goes beyond meeting children's physical needs. This understanding includes the provision of love, safety, educational guidance and economic security. A societal perspective might also define parenting in terms of developmental outcomes that include children's physical and emotional health, socially responsible behavior and the ability to enter the workforce. Within these broad categories, research has now also identified specific parenting behaviors that particularly contribute to these developmental outcomes. These behaviors include 1) giving children a high amount of warmth, praise and affection, 2) utilizing effective disciplinary strategies that set clear limits but are not overly punitive, 3) maintaining high levels of supervision that permit age-appropriate levels of autonomy and 4) providing good-quality opportunities to learn and engage with others.

Research also tells us that most parents are 'good enough' when it comes to providing this support to their children. Most parents understand their children's emotional and physical needs and are able to meet them. There may be times, however, when some parents need more help, and research tells us that some methods are better than others in supporting parents in their parenting role. These methods are 'evidence-based', meaning that they have been proven, *beyond anecdote or chance*, to make a positive difference in the lives of parents and children. This evidence includes findings from rigorously conducted studies that verify the extent to which parenting interventions are beneficial and provide value for money.

Delivering evidence-based parenting interventions involves knowing what this evidence is and understanding how best to use it. This means being aware of the most up-to-date research and using it when making decisions about individual and group work with parents. It also includes steps which a practitioner or agency can take to ensure that everything they do is evidence-based. Evidence-based practice is 'finding out what works, and ensuring that the interventions we and others make in children's lives are as good as they possibly can be' (Lloyd 1999).

Reading this book

This book provides an overview of what those involved in the delivery of parenting support need to know to make sure that their work is evidence-based. While it is not a 'how to' guide describing what to do and how to do it, it does aim to provide those delivering parenting interventions with a solid understanding of why some practices may be better than others. In doing so, it begins with a discussion of the rationale, history and principles underpinning evidence-based practice. This is followed by an examination of the criteria used to establish an evidence base for interventions aimed at parents and children. The book also includes two chapters describing how theories from child development and therapeutic practice have informed the development of evidence-based parenting services. This is followed by an overview of how evaluation and monitoring can be used to establish the evidence base for new parenting interventions. The book concludes with a set of guidelines for developing an area-wide parenting strategy that includes systems for measuring progress towards community-wide change.

Key terms and definitions

Throughout this book, the term parent is used to refer to a child's biological or adoptive father or mother. The terms *intervention, treatment* and *program* are used interchangeably to describe services, involving a beginning, middle and end, which aim to measurably improve outcomes for children by teaching parents new ideas and behaviors. The term *support* is used to describe parenting services more generally. The term *evidence-based* refers to interventions which have demonstrated significant positive results for children or parents through at least one randomized controlled trial. Text boxes appear throughout the book highlighting parenting interventions which are underpinned by one or more randomized controlled trial demonstrating a long-term (over one year) positive effect for children. Additional key terms requiring further definition are highlighted in bold. The definition of all key terms is provided in the glossary at the end of the book.

Foreword

by Professor Stephen Scott
Director, The National Academy for Parenting Research
Professor of Child and Adolescent Mental Health
Institute of Psychiatry, Kings College London

It is both a pleasure and a privilege to write a foreword to this extremely important book, for it essential tool if we are to improve the quality of the parenting that the next generation of children receives.

As Nelson Mandela has said 'there can be no keener revelation of a society's soul than the way in which it treats its children'. Yet, in societies across the world, even well-developed ones, children continue to be treated in ways that place them at risk. At the extreme end, children are abused and neglected by parents in ways that can seriously impede their life chances. At the less extreme end, children are often raised in environments that are mediocre, under-stimulating and in other ways be much improved.

This is no academic matter. In 2007, UNICEF ranked children's wellbeing in the United States and the United Kingdom at the bottom of 21 industrialised countries. These findings were echoed by the UK Children's Society *Good Childhood* Inquiry that also observed that children's lives in Britain have become 'more difficult than in the past' and that 'more young people are anxious and troubled'. Moreover, the report concluded that many of the problems children experience could be avoided through effective interventions and improved parenting environments.

The good news is that these issues have been taken seriously by governments around the world. 2011 has already seen the UK government publish four separate reviews which all emphasise the importance of good parenting: firstly the Munro Review on the future of social work, which is wrestling with the problem of abusive parenting and the most effective way of stopping it; secondly the Allen Review of Early Childhood Intervention, which is trying to maximise children's life chances; thirdly the Field review on poverty, which concludes that better parenting provides a major opportunity to improve the health, wealth and wellbeing of individuals starting life in disadvantaged conditions and fourthly, the Tickell review of early care emphasises the centrality of good quality rearing environment to help children develop their potential.

The sad news, however, is that most parenting services offered to families are often old-fashioned and ineffective. This is not due to any lack of love for children or malicious intent, but it is nonetheless a shocking state of affairs. A leading reason for this lack of effective services is simply that those in power are unaware the effective parenting interventions exist: perhaps because we all have relationships and have a feeling about what does and doesn't work in the area of bringing up children or perhaps because some believe that interventions with evidence of making parents happy are sufficient for commissioning them throughout a local area. Parents, too, are largely unaware of the differences between parenting programmes, so do not militate for things that work.

A third reason that good quality, proven parenting programmes are not used is that sometimes they have slightly upfront greater costs than ineffective ones, for example say costing a £1000 or sometimes more for the materials or DVDs. The fact that this is considered off-putting, when a team of say five staff with its overheads might be costing say £250,000 per year is extraordinary, since where their practice is ineffective, all that outlay is money wasted, and more importantly, children's lives deprived of enrichment. It is a matter of urgent need that services commissioned on their cost-effectiveness, rather than simply on cost alone.

A fourth reason effective approaches are not used is that a number of providers of parenting programmes have their own 'in-house' programmes and have a vested interest in promoting the approach in which they have already trained their staff. Understandably such providers may feel a sense of threat from evidence-based programmes, but surely if they are interested in helping families and children, it is incumbent upon them to use more effective practices?

A final reason is inertia – commissioners of parenting programmes may know there are more effective things out there, but there is little pressure on them to switch to more effective practices.

This situation is one that would be totally unacceptable say in the field of medicine – if parents discover that drugs or operations given to their children are out of date and ineffective, they are rightly very angry. However, the current standard of education of a wide range of the public and professionals concerned with childcare and parenting is low, and they do not know that what the standards of judging effectiveness are, and do not demand an evidence-based approach in this domain of their lives. In contrast, when buying a car or washing machine, many would go on to a magazine or website comparing different ones to get more information.

It might be thought that calling for this evidence-based approach is somehow painful and difficult. On the contrary, those that have gone down this path find that it is a rewarding experience for agencies and practitioners. Practitioners feel satisfied and empowered because they experience that what they are doing is effective, leading to positive change in the parents and children under their care. The practitioners own sense of effectiveness and satisfaction goes up, and typically the turnover within agencies goes down as they develop increasing skills. Taking such an approach is not in any sense mechanical, but leads to deeply rewarding personal experiences for all those concerned.

This book condenses findings that represent a revolution in the field of child development over the last thirty years. In three linked domains of enquiry major steps forward have been made: roughly thrity years ago, a whole raft of studies thoroughly demonstrated the causal influences of parenting on child outcomes. Then twenty years ago, there were many model trials of interventions showing that they could, under carefully controlled conditions, lead to great improvements in children's functioning in areas as diverse as their social behaviour, their aggressiveness, their ability to read and learn, and their happiness and wellbeing. Finally, in the last decade, a third and new domain of knowledge has emerged, implementation science. Findings here have shown that it is not good enough to simply transport the new ways of working into the community and expect them to be effective: great attention has to be given to the quality of the implementation. This book covers all three domains in depth and in a very accessible, readable way. It celebrates the good news that there is so much that can be done to improve the quality of parenting and make children happier and better adjusted.

Evidence-based support for children and families needs to be a policy agenda in its own right, and not co-opted into a workforce or values agenda. There needs to be government-wide commitment to implementing services that are proven to be effective, full stop. This book leads the way and will prove an invaluable guide to practitioners and commissioners alike. It comes out of the work of the National Academy for Parenting Research (www. parentingresearch.org.uk), which is dedicated to evaluating of practices that work best with parents and children. Kirsten Asmussen has been leading research teams that have evaluated the 130 or so parenting programmes in the UK, and also researched the implementation of ten of the best ones in England. The team has been at the forefront of developing constructive criteria to rate these, and offer helpful feedback to the programmes' authors where appropriate.

References

UNICEF (2007) An Overview of Child-wellbeing in Rich Countries. Downloadable from www.unicef. org.

Layard, Richard and Dunn, Judy (2009) *A Good Childhood*. London: Penguin

Scott S (2010) National dissemination of effective parenting programmes to improve child outcomes. *British Journal of Psychiatry* **196**, 1–3

1 Introduction

Why evidence-based parenting interventions?

Societies benefit when children thrive. Evidence suggests, however, that a significant number of children and young people living in industrial, English-speaking countries are not thriving. In the United Kingdom, one out of every ten children is assessed as having a mental health disorder annually (Green et al. 2005). In Australia, Canada, and the United States, this figure is higher, suggesting that between 12 and 14 per cent of all children have a diagnosable mental health problem in any given year (Costello et al. 2003, Green et al. 2005, McGorry et al. 2007, Waddell et al. 2005). Child mental health disorders include emotional problems, such as depression and anxiety, and behavioral problems, such as conduct disorders and hyperactivity (Kazdin 2003).

Between 35 and 40 per cent of all children will have been diagnosed with one, if not more, mental health problems by the age of 18 (Costello et al. 2003, Jaffee et al. 2005). When left untreated, mental health problems impair functioning well into adulthood, significantly interfering with the chances of finding a rewarding job or developing a positive romantic relationship (Patel et al. 2007). Between one-fourth and one-third of all adults suffer from a psychological disorder at any given point in time and slightly less than one-half will be diagnosed with a mental health problem during their lifetime (Kessler, Berglund et al. 2005, Kessler, Chiu et al. 2005). Approximately 50 per cent of all adult mental health problems are identified during childhood or adolescence (Belfer 2008, Costello et al. 2003).

Research suggests that child and adolescent mental health disorders are unfortunately on the rise. A British study comparing parental reports of children's behavior in the 1970s, 80s and 90s observed a 50 per cent increase in adolescent behavioral problems for each successive decade (Collishaw et al. 2004). Comparisons of young people's self-reports of their own wellbeing also suggest increases in child mental health problems, with twice as many adolescents reporting feelings of depression or anxiety today as young people reporting in the 1980s (Collishaw et al. 2010). Collectively, these findings suggest that childhood mental health problems may have more than doubled over the past forty years.

This trend is disturbing for a number of reasons. First, childhood mental health problems create multiple costs and hardships – including the personal costs incurred by those suffering from them and the financial costs involved in treating them. For example, a child with a diagnosed conduct disorder at age 10 can cost a community up to ten times as much as a child with no mental health problems, especially when crime- and school-related costs are taken into account (Cohen 2005, Scott 2001). Second, most childhood mental health problems are treatable and preventable (Fonagy et al. 2002, Kazdin 2003). Over the past 50 years, numerous effective interventions have been identified for preventing and/or treating childhood mental health disorders, as well as preventing the onset of further problems in adulthood (O'Connell et al. 2009, Patel et al. 2007, Scott 2010a).

Interestingly, many of the most effective treatments for childhood mental health problems are delivered to parents rather than children. This is because research evidence consistently suggests that parenting behaviors are highly associated with children's wellbeing. In particular, key parenting strategies, especially those that encourage and reward positive child behavior, reliably predict the development of pro-social skills and reduce the likelihood of child and adolescent conduct problems (Forgatch et al. 2009, Kazdin 2003, Martinez and Forgatch 2002). A positive parent–child relationship is also associated with children's ability to self-regulate and maintain a positive sense of self-worth (Baumrind 1991, Grolnick and Farkas 2002, Sroufe et al. 2005). These abilities, in turn, protect children from the negative emotions and thoughts typically associated with psychological difficulties in adulthood (Mrazek and Haggerty 1994).

Numerous parenting programs now exist to help parents learn appropriate strategies for supporting their children's development and managing their behavior (Sanders and Morawska 2006). Those with a particularly strong track record in improving parent and child outcomes are now referred to as **evidence-based** parenting interventions (Weisz and Kazdin 2010). Research suggests that programs which teach parents how to interact positively with their children and discourage negative child behaviors are particularly effective in reducing the likelihood of behavioral problems in adolescence and adulthood (Prinz and Jones 2003). Research also suggests that when these programs are available to entire communities, population-wide benefits can be achieved. These benefits typically include reductions in youth offending, reduced rates of substance misuse, reduced rates of child maltreatment and increased rates of school achievement (Aos et al. 2004, Brody et al. 2008, Bumbarger 2010, CPPRG 2007, Prinz et al. 2009). For these reasons, governments in a number of countries are now investing in policies and initiatives to improve the quality and availability of evidence-based parenting support, as well as expand the evidence base (O'Connell et al. 2009). The following sections provide an overview of how evidence-based initiatives and policies have improved the quality of parenting interventions in the United States, United Kingdom, Norway and Australia over the past twenty years.

Evidence-based parenting policy in the United States

Since the early 1990s, US policies aimed at children and parents have become increasingly informed by research evidence. This is due to a steady increase in scientific knowledge regarding the importance of the parent–child relationship and an improved understanding of the genetic and environmental factors that place this relationship at risk. US policies have also benefited from an increased consensus on what constitutes good evidence, informed by improved methodologies for testing hypotheses and analyzing research findings (O'Connell et al. 2009). The increased use of clinical trials to test the efficacy of family-based interventions has been particularly influential in informing US policy through the identification of programs that do and do not work (O'Connell et al. 2009). Information regarding the most effective interventions is now shared on numerous web directories which are increasingly used to inform federal- and state-wide funding decisions. The activity of consulting research evidence to inform government decision making is now referred to as 'evidence-based policy' and is considered by many to be a hallmark of modern democratic governments (Head 2008, Sanderson 2002).

Expanding the science: three influential reports

US policy makers have historically believed that unless parents abuse or neglect their children, parenting practices are personal matters that should not be subject to government policy or intervention (O'Connell et al. 2009). This perspective began to change, however, as findings from a number of government-funded research reports converged to suggest a strong link between parenting practices and child and adolescent mental health outcomes. Three reports were particularly influential in changing the US perspective in this respect: *Reducing Risks for Mental Disorders: Frontiers for Preventive Intervention Research* (Mrazek and Haggerty 1994), *From Neurons to Neighborhoods* (Shonkoff and Phillips 2000) and *Youth Violence: A Report of the Surgeon General* (US Surgeon General 2001).

Reducing Risks for Mental Disorders (Mzarek and Haggerty) was published by the Institute of Medicine in 1994 in response to a congressional request for a review on the status of research on the prevention of mental illness and problem behaviors. The report identified key risks known to be associated with the onset of mental health problems, with the aim of developing interventions that could reduce these risks. Maladaptive parenting behavior was identified as a primary risk for a variety of mental health problems, with child maltreatment, inappropriate disciplinary practices, problematic spousal relations and parental psychological dysfunction recognized as particular threats to children's wellbeing.

Reducing Risks also identified the need for mental health interventions to provide strong evidence of their effectiveness. In doing so, the report recommended that **randomized controlled trials**[1] (RCTs) be used whenever possible, since they provided the highest level of confidence of an intervention's efficacy. Since the report's publication in 1994, there has been a dramatic rise in the use of RCTs to test the impact of mental health treatments, with many government agencies now funding only programs underpinned by strong RCT evidence (O'Connell et al. 2009).

From Neurons to Neighborhoods (Shonkoff and Phillips) was published by the Institute of Medicine in 2000 to provide policy makers with an understanding of how scientific evidence could be used to support children's development through policy and practice. The report synthesized neurological evidence involving early brain development with findings from the behavioral sciences regarding emotional and cognitive development. A primary conclusion of the report was that nature and nurture are inextricably linked and that the quality of the parent–child relationship exerts a tremendous influence on children's emotional and intellectual development. A key recommendation of the report was to develop more interventions to support the parent–child relationship. In particular, *From Neurons to Neighborhoods* highlighted the need for programs that had clearly defined objectives and were underpinned by strong evaluation evidence:

> Model early childhood programs that deliver carefully designed interventions with well-defined objectives and that include well-designed evaluations have been shown to influence the developmental trajectories of children whose life course is threatened by socioeconomic disadvantage, family disruption, and diagnosed disabilities. Programs that combine child-focused educational activities with explicit attention to parent-child interaction patterns and relationship building appear to have the greatest impacts. In contrast, services that are based on generic family support, often without a clear delineation of intervention strategies matched directly to measurable objectives, and that are funded by more modest budgets, appear to be less effective.
>
> (Shonkoff and Phillips: 398)

Youth Violence: A Report of the Surgeon General (US Surgeon General 2001) was commissioned by President Clinton in 1999 in response to the Columbine shootings, with the aim of identifying evidence-based methods for keeping an event like Columbine from occurring again. In response to this request, the report developed a hierarchical model (informed, in part, on the *Maryland Scale of Scientific Methods* – see Box 2.4) to identify programs with evidence of effectiveness in reducing youth violence and delinquent behavior.

The report identified 27 programs, categorizing them as 'model' or 'promising' depending upon the quality of their evaluation evidence. 'Model' programs were interventions with rigorous evaluation evidence demonstrating 1) strong evidence of a deterrent effect against youth violence that was 2) sustainable over time and 3) replicated in multiple evaluations conducted in multiple, independent settings. A 'promising' program also had to demonstrate a strong deterrent effect through rigorous evaluation, although evidence of its sustainability or replicability might not yet have been established. Five of the seven model programs and ten out of the twenty promising programs included parents in their delivery models.

Youth Violence was also noteworthy through its introduction of the 'does not work' category that identified programs and practices with no evidence of reducing youth violence. Although none of the programs identified as not working included parents in their delivery model, many practices categorized as ineffective were popular and widespread. In fact, a number of common interventions such as peer counseling, boot camp and diversionary programs (e.g. Midnight Basketball) were identified as harmful, with some evaluation evidence suggesting that they actually increased the likelihood of youth offending. These findings led the Surgeon General to conclude that research and policy needed to 'build the science' so that more effective prevention and intervention programs could be made available to reduce the prevalence of youth violence.

Evidence of long-term benefits

As reports such as *Reducing Risks, From Neurons to Neighborhoods* and *Youth Violence* repeatedly stressed the need for evidence-based interventions, funding agencies increasingly began to favor programs that had undergone a randomized controlled trial and/or demonstrated sustainable, long-term effects. Numerous web-based directories were subsequently established to help local and national funding agencies identify programs with strong evaluation evidence. These directories included *Blueprints for Violence Prevention*, the Substance Abuse and Mental Health Services Administration (SAMHSA) *National Registry of Effective Prevention Programs* (NREPP) and the *What Works Clearinghouse* (sponsored by the US Department of Education). These directories were informed by a growing consensus of what constituted evidence of effectiveness,[2] as a well as promising long-term findings from several parenting programs developed in the 1960s and 70s.

Central to these findings were those from the longitudinal evaluations of the *Perry Preschool/HighScope* program and *Head Start* (see Boxes 1.1 and 2.1). Established in the 1960s, both programs combined enriching educational experiences with parental support to improve the school readiness of children aged 3 and 4 living in low-income households (Zigler and Styfco 1994). Participants in the original *Perry Preschool* randomized controlled trial were followed up until the age of 27, demonstrating significantly improved outcomes in comparison to those in the control group (Schweinhart et al. 1993). Specifically, *Perry Preschool* participants were significantly less likely to have undergone a police arrest, and receive public assistance and more likely to be employed (Schweinhart et al. 2005). Economists estimated that these benefits resulted in a tax saving of approximately $7 for

Box 1.1: The *Perry Preschool Program* longitudinal study

The *Perry Preschool* study began in 1962 to investigate the effects of the *High/Scope* preschool model. The *High/Scope* curriculum promotes children's early social and intellectual development through a hands-on educational environment which teaches children to plan, carry out, and review their own educational activities. Children attend preschool five days a week for two and a half hours a day for two years. During the initial roll-out of *Perry Preschool*, teachers conducted one and half hour home visits with the parents of the preschoolers on a weekly basis. Parents also attended small group meetings which were facilitated by program staff once a month.

The original study involved children from deprived communities with lower than average IQs. These children were randomly assigned to the program and comparison group and then assessed at regular intervals until their fortieth birthdays. Findings from the long-term evaluation have consistently suggested a variety of positive results for *Perry Preschool* participants, including a significantly lower rate of crime and delinquency, lower rates of teenage pregnancy and less dependency on welfare benefits. Program participants also demonstrate significantly higher levels of academic achievement, employment rates, annual income and pro-social behavior in comparison to those followed up in the comparison group. Although the original *Perry Preschool* is no longer running, the *High/Scope* curriculum continues in approximately one-fifth of all *Head Start* programs across the United States (Parks 2000, Schweinhart 2002).

every $1 invested in the program (Aos et al. 2004, Barnett 1996). Similar findings were observed in the evaluations of *Head Start*, with participants consistently demonstrating significantly lower rates of grade retention, higher rates of high school completion and higher rates of adult employment in comparison to those not enrolled in the program[3] (Currie and Thomas 1995). Like *Perry Preschool*, the benefit–cost ratio of *Head Start* was estimated to be $7 to $1 (Garces et al. 2002, Ludwig and Miller 2007, Nores et al. 2005).

At the same time that the long-term findings from *Head Start* and *Perry Preschool* were reported, similar positive findings were observed in a follow-up study of the *Nurse–Family Partnership* (NFP) home visiting program (see Box 1.2). Findings from three randomized controlled trials consistently demonstrated fewer child injuries, improved school readiness and increased rates of maternal employment among program participants (Kitzman et al. 1997). Longer-term benefits included significantly less child maltreatment, antisocial behavior and teen pregnancy among children fifteen years after their mothers completed the program (Eckenrode et al. 2010, Olds et al. 1997, 1998). Benefit–cost analyses indicated that these improved outcomes provided an economic return of $4 to $6 for every $1 invested in the program, depending on the risk level of the sample (Aos et al. 2004, Karoly et al. 2005).

Policy makers interpreted the combined findings from the *Perry Preschool*, *Head Start* and NFP programs to mean that large investments in early childhood programs could improve children's wellbeing and save taxpayers' money. On the basis of these findings, the US government expanded *Head Start* downwards to include mothers with infants through *Early Head Start* and increased funding for home visiting programs across the country (Astuto and Allen 2009, Gomby et al. 1999, Love et al. 2005).

Box 1.2: *The Nurse–Family Partnership Home Visiting Program*

Developed by David Olds in the 1970s, *Nurse–Family Partnership* (also referred to as NFP or the *Family–Nurse Partnership* in the UK) is an intensive home visiting program delivered by specially trained nurses to low-income, first-time, single mothers during the first two years of their child's life. Drawing from the theories of attachment, human ecology and self-efficacy (see Chapter 3 for a compete discussion) NFP aims to reduce the risks associated with child maltreatment and other undesirable child outcomes by addressing 1) the infant's health needs, 2) the mother's parenting skills and 3) the mother's access to community resources and opportunities for employment and education. Figure 1.1 (taken from Olds et al. 1997) provides a model of how various ecological elements (including NFP processes) work together to influence the mother's parenting behaviours.

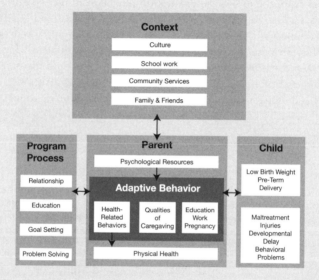

Figure 1.1   The *Nurse–Family Partnership* model of program influences (reprinted with permission from Olds et al. 1997)

NFP is underpinned by an extensive body of research, including three RCTs conducted with diverse populations in Elmira, New York (1977), Memphis, Tennessee (1988) and Denver, Colorado (1994). Follow-up studies continue to investigate the long-term outcomes for mothers and children participating in the three RCTs. Positive child and parent effects observed in at least two of the trials include:

* improved prenatal health
* fewer childhood injuries
* fewer subsequent pregnancies
* increased intervals between births
* increased maternal employment
* improved school readiness.

(More information about NFP can be found at: http://www.nursefamilypartnership.org.)

Evidence-based program implementation

The national expansion of home visiting in the mid 1990s meant that parenting support was more widely available than ever before. However, a special edition of the *Future of Children* published in the late 1990s (Gomby et al. 1999) observed that much more than strong evaluation evidence was necessary for programs to remain effective when implemented at scale. In a comparison of evaluation findings from six home visiting models (including NFP[4]), the *Future of Children* report found that only NFP achieved child and parent outcomes that were consistent across sites and sustainable over time. The authors attributed the overall lack of success of the other five programs to difficulties in recruiting parents and inconsistencies in their implementation (Gomby et al. 1999). Subsequent evaluations have since identified a lack of attention to important program details, including a clearly specified target population, a well-articulated **theory of change**, robust systems for ensuring program **fidelity** and sufficient practitioner training, as additional reasons why the other programs failed (Chaffin 2004, Duggan et al. 2004a and 2004b, Gomby 2007, Hebbeler and Gerlach-Downie 2002, Wagner and Clayton, 1999). By contrast, the NFP model specified many of these details through the use of research evidence (Olds et al. 2000). For example, the decision to target low-income, single mothers aged 19 or younger was based upon evidence suggesting that these women were more socially excluded and less likely than other women to access health services on their own, meaning that young mothers were more likely to benefit from home visiting support than other parents. The decision to target first-time mothers was also based on evidence suggesting that women would be more receptive to home visitation during their first pregnancy (Olds et al. 1997).

Another key feature of the NFP program was its clearly articulated theory of change. This theory of change included short- and long-term outcomes based on the scientifically supported theories which informed the development of the program. NFP's theory of change was also clearly evident in its home visiting activities, which were carefully taught to practitioners through intensive pre-program training and ongoing supervision. Practitioners nominated for NFP training were screened on the basis of their personal characteristics and qualifications in the nursing profession. The decision to use specially trained nurses was based upon experimental evidence suggesting that nurses were more effective than paraprofessionals in implementing the NFP model (Olds et al. 2004). Subsequent research has since observed that NFP's intended outcomes are supported by the high levels of 'technical assistance' it offers to host agencies (Mihalic and Irwin 2003). This assistance includes information about the infrastructures necessary to implement NFP, as well as ongoing coaching and consultation to practitioners and service managers.

Taking evidence-based parenting programs to scale

Collectively, the above findings illustrate the need for robust systems to facilitate the adoption and implementation of evidence-based parenting support. Research regarding evidence-based implementation is still in its infancy, however, and much still needs to be known about how program and agency factors jointly contribute to improved child and parent outcomes. For example, only a handful of studies have considered how a practitioner's knowledge and skill contribute to the efficacy of a parenting intervention (Eames et al. 2009, Scott et al. under review). Relatively few studies have also considered the extent to which coaching and practitioner supervision directly benefits parents and children. Information regarding the infrastructures necessary for agencies to implement programs is also lacking for many evidence-based programs. Answers to these questions are required, however, if policy makers hope to successfully implement evidence-based parenting support at scale within communities and countries. For this reason, scholars have called for an expansion of the evidence-based research agenda to include methods for improving program implementation (Kazak et al. 2010, O'Connell et al. 2009).

US policy makers have recently responded to these challenges through a series of federal, state and local initiatives aimed at expanding the availability of evidence-based interventions and translating research into practice (Kazak et al. 2010). For example, recommendations made by the Coalition for Evidence-Based Policy[5] have recently resulted in the Obama administration committing over $8 billion for the expansion of evidence-based home visitation programs over the next ten years. While the initial recommendation was to fund NFP only, funding has since been expanded to include other home visiting models underpinned by sound evaluation evidence. Programs with the strongest evidence are currently allocated the highest proportion of funds, with those with less evidence receiving less funding. Funded programs are also expected to provide evidence of effective implementation processes through rigorously collected monitoring data (Haskins et al. 2009a and 2009b).

Individual states are now also relying on evaluation evidence to inform the development of state-wide initiatives aimed at supporting children and parents. Washington State has been a particular leader in this area through the implementation of a 'portfolio'[6] of programs with strong evidence of deterring crime (Barnoski 2004). This work has been informed by the benefit–cost studies conducted by Steve Aos and his colleagues at the Washington State Institute for Public Policy (WSIPP). The WSIPP team identified a number of programs that were not only underpinned by strong evaluation evidence, but also showed evidence of reducing crime-related costs (Aos et al. 1998, Drake et al. 2009). Those identified with the highest benefit–cost ratios included programs that involved parents in their delivery models, such as NFP, *Functional Family Therapy* (FFT – see Chapter 4 for a complete discussion), and *Multi-dimensional Treatment Foster Care* (MTFC – see Box 7.1). Based upon Aos' analyses, Washington State has increased its investment in evidence-based programs (including parenting support) as part of a cost-saving strategy to lower crime and avert the need to build a new prison (Drake et al. 2009). Recent evaluation findings indicate 'encouraging early signs' of reductions in crime that are likely to offset crime-related costs in the predicted direction (Aos 2010).

Other states making investments in evidence-based parenting programs have similarly begun to observe measurable benefits at the state level. For example, the state of Pennsylvania has recently witnessed cost-saving decreases in juvenile delinquency and increases in school achievement in communities implementing evidence-based programs (including parenting programs) through the *Communities That Care* model (Feinberg et al. 2010, see Box 7.2). The state of South Carolina has also observed significant improvements in child and parent outcomes through the county-wide randomization of the *Triple P* program (see Box 1.3). Counties implementing a continuum of *Triple P* parenting services (from universally-based public awareness campaigns to highly targeted family therapy) demonstrated lower rates of child maltreatment in comparison to counties where the *Triple P* program was not implemented (Prinz et al. 2009).

Moving the research and policy agenda forward

In an effort to increase the state-wide dissemination of evidence-based practice, The National Research Council and Institute of Medicine recently commissioned the research review, *Preventing Mental, Emotional, and Behavioral Disorders among Young People* (O'Connell et al. 2009). This review observed that since the publication of *Reducing Risks* in 1994, considerable progress has been made in identifying what 'works' in the prevention of child mental health problems.

Box 1.3: *Triple P* – a multilevel parenting intervention

Triple P is a five-tier system of parental support designed for families with children between the ages of birth and 16 with mild to severe behavioral and emotional problems. The program draws from social learning theory, attachment theory and the ecological model (see Chapter 3 for a more complete discussion) to teach parents child behavior management skills, alongside methods for managing their moods and increasing their sense of self-efficacy. The five intervention tiers begin with a media-based public awareness campaign aimed at the entire population and end with individualized therapy targeting families who are confronting complex child problems:

- *Universal Triple P (Level 1)* uses media and informational strategies to make all parents aware of effective parenting strategies and facilitate parental help seeking.
- *Selected Triple P (Level 2)* involves brief and flexible consultation with individual parents or parenting seminars with large groups of parents.
- *Primary Care Triple P (Level 3)* manages discrete child behavior problems through four brief consultations that incorporate active skills training. These sessions involve the use of parenting tip sheets providing advice on common childhood problems.
- *Standard and Group Triple P (Level 4)* benefits children with identified problems by teaching parents specific child behavioral management strategies individually or within groups.
- *Enhanced Triple P (Level 5)* is directed at families with more complex problems and may include modules targeting coparenting behaviors addressing specific parent–child problems.

The individual *Triple P* intervention models have undergone multiple RCTs across multiple settings in a variety of countries, consistently demonstrating positive parent and child outcomes. Results consistently suggest clear improvements in parenting skills and mood, as well as reductions in children's attention and behavioral problems, with follow-up studies indicating that effects remain for up to three years (Bor et al. 2002, Markie-Dadds and Sanders 2006, Roberts et al. 2006, Sanders et al. 2000, Zubrick et al. 2005). A recent randomized trial involving counties in the state of South Carolina has additionally observed a significant drop in child maltreatment rates when all five *Triple P* interventions are implemented at scale within communities (Prinz et al. 2009).

However, the report also found that much more could be done to improve the implementation of evidence-based interventions within communities. In this respect, the report observed that there was a substantial gap between what was known through research and what was actually happening in practice. The report therefore recommended that the research agenda be expanded to include evidence-based methods for disseminating effective programs across diverse settings and agencies. To this end, the report asserted that dissemination efforts would be enhanced through the creation of a national, cross-departmental body that would direct research on the expansion of the evidence base and develop policies aimed at improving dissemination efforts. Additional recommendations from the report included the need for evidence-based and culturally sensitive methods to screen children for mental health problems, as well as methods for developing and evaluating effective mental health public awareness campaigns.

Box 1.4: Time-line of the development of evidence-based policy in the US

1991   The Society for Prevention Research (SPR) is established to advance the use of scientific knowledge to improve the efficacy of prevention and intervention programs.

1993   Findings from the longitudinal evaluation of the *High Scope/Perry Preschool* study are published, suggesting that children who participated in the program at age 3 are significantly more likely to be employed and significantly less likely to have committed a crime at age 27 (Schweinhart et al. 1993).

1994   The Institute of Medicine (IOM) publishes *Reducing Risks for Mental Disorders: Frontiers for Preventive Intervention Research*. This report identifies dysfunctional parenting as a risk factor for poor mental health outcomes and outlines a research agenda for testing the efficacy of mental health interventions.

Findings from the longitudinal evaluation of *Head Start* suggest significant long-term benefits for white children participating in the program at age 3 (Currie and Thomas 1995). The US government commits funds for the further development of the program so that it is effective with non-white program participants. The *Early Head Start* program is also launched to provide support for children aged 0–3.

1996   The US Department of Justice funds the Center for the Study and Prevention of Violence at the University of Colorado at Boulder to design and launch the *Blueprints for Violence Prevention* initiative to identify effective programs for reducing youth violence and associated risks.

Findings from a benefit-cost analysis of the *High Scope/Perry Preschool* Program are published, suggesting a $7 saving for every $1 invested in the program.

1997   The Center for Substance Abuse Prevention of the Substance Abuse and Mental Health Services Administration (SAMHSA) launches the *National Registry of Effective Prevention Programs* (NREPP) as a web-based directory of effective programs for reducing drug and alcohol misuse.

The *Maryland Scale of Scientific Methods* is published as a tool for evaluating interventions for deterring youth offending on the basis of the strength and quality of their research evidence (Sherman et al. 1998).

Findings from the longitudinal evaluation of the *Nurse–Family Partnership* (NFP) home visiting program suggest decreased rates of child maltreatment and antisocial behavior among adolescents whose mother participated in the program fifteen years earlier (Olds et al., 1997, 1998).

Washington State passes legislation to implement a portfolio of evidence-based programs as part of a state-wide strategy to reduce crime.

1999   The *Future of Children* publishes evaluation findings from six home visiting programs suggesting that only one (NFP) provides any consistent and long-lasting benefits for parents and children. The report observes that factors related to program implementation may have diminished the overall efficacy of the five other programs (Gomby et al. 1999).

2000   The Institute of Medicine publishes *From Neurons to Neighborhoods*, that describes the influence of the social and physical environment on early brain development. The report highlights the need for evidence-based programs that support the parent–child relationship.

The Society for Prevention Research publishes the first edition of its flagship journal, *Prevention Science*, which aims to share knowledge across disciplines in the theory, research and practice in the prevention of social problems.

2001 *Youth Violence: A Report of the Surgeon General* is published with the aim of identifying interventions for deterring youth violence in response to the Columbine shootings. The report identifies key risks in the perpetration of youth crime and identifies interventions that do and do not work in preventing it.

The *Coalition for Evidence-Based Policy* is established to promote the use of evidence-based research to inform funding decisions.

2002 The US Department of Education's Institute of Science establishes the *What Works Clearinghouse* to aid in the identification of evidence-based educational programs.

2004 The Society for Prevention Research publishes its *Standards of Evidence: Criteria for Efficacy, Effectiveness and Dissemination*.

2009 The Obama administration commits over $8 billion to assist states in the widespread dissemination of evidence-based home visitation programs.

The National Research Council and Institute of Medicine publish *Preventing Mental, Emotional and Behavioral Disorders among Young People* in an effort to track progress made since the publication of *Reducing Risks*, as well as outline a research and policy agenda for the future. The report recommends that a national entity be created to direct research into evidence-based practice and coordinate dissemination efforts.

Evidence-based parenting policy in the United Kingdom

In contrast to the United States, British policy makers have placed a relatively strong emphasis on expanding parenting support and a relatively weak emphasis on expanding the evidence base (Barrett 2007, James 2009). While a number of large-scale, community-based initiatives launched by the New Labour government have greatly increased the support available to parents, government policy has only actively encouraged the use of evidence-based parenting interventions since 2006 (James 2009). In addition, the use of RCTs for establishing the evidence base for family interventions is a relatively rare phenomenon in the UK, more often used in pilots of programs developed in other countries (such as *Incredible Years*, FFT and *Multisystemic Therapy*) than for British-based programs (Scott 2010a and Scott 2010b). Of the 135 parenting programs listed on the *Commissioning Toolkit*,[7] only 17 are underpinned by RCT evidence, and of those, only one has been developed in the UK.

Lessons from Sure Start

The need to expand parenting support was first recognized by the *Sure Start* initiative (Box 1.5). Now heralded as one of New Labour's 'greatest achievements' (Blair, *Guardian* 5 October 2006), *Sure Start* was the result of a 1998 Comprehensive Spending Review (CSR) that compared findings from an audit of children's services to findings from a review of research conducted in the US and UK (HM Treasury 1998). At the time, New Labour policy makers believed that complex, cross-cutting problems, such as social exclusion, were best addressed through 'joined-up' services delivered across governmental departments (Cabinet

Office 2000, Melhuish and Hall 2007). The CSR therefore placed an emphasis on identifying services which required departments to work together to meet the needs of children and families.

The CSR identified gaps in joined-up working across all children's services, but found that provision was especially sparse for children aged 4 and younger. At the time, midwifery and health visiting were the only universal services available to children under the age of 4 and the CSR observed that these health-based services were poorly accessed by families with young children living in poverty (Glass 1999, Welshman 2010). The evidence from the research review also highlighted the need for universally available support during the early years. Evidence for this included findings from the evaluations of *Head Start* and *Perry Preschool* that underscored the potential of early prevention programs for improving children's health and educational outcomes (Barnet 1995, Rutter 2006, Schweinhart et al. 1993, Welshman 2010, Zigler and Muenchow 1992, Zigler and Styfco 2004).

Sure Start was therefore launched with the aim of promoting 'the physical, intellectual and social development of babies and young children so that they [could] flourish at home and when they get to school' (*Sure Start* 2002). Like *Head Start* (and its younger sister, *Early Head Start*), *Sure Start* Local Programmes (SSLPs) aimed to meet the needs of families through an integrated package of health, education and community-based services, with support to parents and families as a key objective. This is where the similarities between *Sure Start* and *Head Start* ended, however. While *Head Start* services were available to only the most deprived families, *Sure Start* services were offered universally to all families living within deprived communities. In addition, SSLPs were encouraged to create and implement services as they saw fit, whereas *Head Start* provided a flexible yet clearly articulated model of intervention (Melhuish and Hall 2007). The New Labour government advocated this 'bottom-up' approach to encourage local authority ownership and promote service innovation. Although the national *Sure Start* unit provided guidance on evidence-based interventions, there was little incentive for SSLPs to consult or follow it (Barlow et al. 2007). The result was that *Sure Start* local programs 'let a thousand flowers bloom', with little consideration as to whether the services were evidence-based or achieved their intended outcomes (Lewis 2011: 7).

Another key difference between *Head Start* and *Sure Start* was the way in which the two initiatives were evaluated. Since its inception in the 1960s, *Head Start* has undergone multiple evaluations, with many studies including randomization and carefully matched control groups in their designs (Zigler and Muenchow 1992; see Chapter 2 for a more in-depth discussion). By contrast, the UK government refused the use of randomized controlled trials to evaluate the impact of *Sure Start*, despite the advice of the initiative's original research advisors (Rutter 2007). Reasons for rejecting the use of an RCT for *Sure Start*'s evaluation included the optimistic belief that *Sure Start* services would be effective and that denying individuals (or in this case, communities) access to them for the sake of a control group would be unethical (Rutter 2006). Barrett (2007) has additionally observed that the decision not to use an RCT reflected a general skepticism within the UK about the appropriateness of RCTs for investigating the efficacy of social interventions.

Whatever the reasons, *Sure Start*'s first impact evaluation ultimately involved a **cross-sectional**, **quasi-experimental** design (see Chapter 2 for a more in-depth discussion) that was considered to be the best option available, given the limitations imposed by the UK government (Rutter 2006). While the findings from this study observed some service innovation and community ownership, the overall conclusion was that *Sure Start* provided few measurable benefits for children and parents (Rutter 2006, 2007). In particular, the evaluation observed worse outcomes for highly vulnerable families living in *Sure Start* communities.

Box 1.5: *Sure Start*

Sure Start was first introduced by the *New Labour* government in 1998 to address child poverty and social exclusion through an improved package of support for families with children under the age of 4 living in the top 20 per cent of deprived communities in England and Wales. At the time it was announced, a budget of £540 million was allocated over a period of 3 years to fund 250 local programs. This was increased in 2000 by another £500 so that 500 local programs could be set up by 2004. *Sure Start*'s initial focus was to support children's physical, intellectual and emotional development through services that were coordinated through partnerships between agencies. In order to support partnership working, *Sure Start* local programmes (SSLPs) were governed by partnership boards whose membership consisted, in thirds, of representatives from voluntary agencies, statutory organizations and parents with young children living within the SSLP geographical areas.

In 2004, *Sure Start*'s aims shifted to reflect the goals of the newly announced *Every Child Matters* (ECM) policy agenda (DfES 2004). This meant that programs were to provide evidence of working towards the five ECM outcomes (be healthy, stay safe, enjoy and achieve, make a positive contribution and enjoy economic wellbeing) and that SSLPs would be operated through Children's Centres that would work as 'service hubs' to coordinate services for parents and children, including childcare. Programs would no longer be governed by partnership boards, but by Children's Trusts that were overseen by the local director of children's services. At the time, the UK government also expanded the program to less deprived communities, with a new target of 3,500 Children's Centres operating by 2010 (James 2009). In 2005, findings from *Sure Start*'s first national evaluation were announced, suggesting that families living in *Sure Start* communities were not much better off than those living in non-*Sure Start* areas. Moreover, highly vulnerable *Sure Start* families (e.g. those with single and/or teenage parents) were actually found to be doing worse than those not living in *Sure Start* communities (Belsky et al. 2006). These findings were disappointing, but did not deter the ongoing roll-out of the program. However, it did shift the initiative's initial focus on homegrown community-based interventions to more evidence-based family services. Findings from the second national evaluation subsequently observed some significant benefits for *Sure Start* families, including better access to family support services, improved home-learning environments and less negative parenting behaviors (Melhuish et al. 2008).

A report published by the Coalition government has recently recommended that Children's Centres target poor families in order to narrow the gap between poorer and richer children during the early years (Field 2010). Recommendations for the future development of Children's Centres include the increased availability of evidence-based parenting interventions for families who need them the most.

In *Sure Start* area households, where the mother was single or a teenager, or the parents were unemployed, the verbal ability of 3-year-olds was in fact significantly lower than in areas where there was no *Sure Start* local program (Belsky et al. 2006). While the specific reasons for these adverse effects continue to be debated to this day (Lewis 2010, Welshman 2010), program evaluators at the time theorized that more socially advantaged parents were better able to access *Sure Start* services, which in turn, decreased the resources available for those who were more vulnerable (Rutter 2006, 2007, Belsky et al. 2007). In other words, it is likely that the universal nature of *Sure Start* inadvertently interfered with the availability of services for the most deprived families.

Findings from subsequent *Sure Start* evaluations have additionally observed that the lack of consistency in services and the underuse of evidence-based interventions may have also reduced the efficacy of the initiative (Melhuish et al. 2008). In an evaluation of the impact of *Sure Start* parenting services, Barlow et al. (2007) found that a lack of attention to the evidence base frequently interfered with local programs' ability to achieve *Sure Start*'s objectives. In fact, the study noted that many local programs were openly prejudiced against the use of structured, evidence-based models, preferring the informal nature of their own home-grown interventions. This finding is not surprising, given the fact that the government actively encouraged programs to support locally developed programs. Barlow's study also found that parenting services were frequently delivered by individuals with no qualifications or experience in working with parents. When evidence-based interventions were offered, practitioners often made significant changes to the content, with only a third adhering to the program's original model.

Collectively, the above findings suggested that *Sure Start* suffered from many of the same deficiencies as the US home visitation programs did in the 1990s. In a comparison between *Sure Start* and NFP, Sir Michael Rutter (2006) observed that the lack of a specific target group (e.g. families living in deprived communities rather than low-income families), poor grounding in empirically tested theories, no consistency in program goals, a lack of adherence to a manual or protocol and no specifications for practitioner training all likely contributed to *Sure Start*'s inability to achieve its intended outcomes. In effect, UK policy makers ignored key details in the planning and operation of services that would have increased the quality, and most likely the efficacy, of *Sure Start* services. Rutter (2006, 2007) recommended that going forward, *Sure Start* should combine its universal focus with interventions targeting more vulnerable families. Rutter also recommended that in the future, *Sure Start* interventions be based upon explicit, evidence-based curriculums, delivered by appropriately trained practitioners.

The extent to which Rutter's recommendations were taken on board remains unclear, although there is some evidence to suggest that *Sure Start* services became more focused through the introduction of the *Every Child Matters* agenda in 2003 and the *Respect* agenda in 2006 (Lewis 2011 – see following sections). Findings from the second national evaluation of *Sure Start* suggested that these changes may have improved outcomes for families, with *Sure Start* parents accessing more family support services, providing better home-learning environments and exhibiting less negative parenting behavior than a **historic control** sample of families living in *Sure Start* communities prior to the launch of the initiative (Melhuish et al. 2008). *Sure Start* evaluators have since attributed these improvements to the more widespread use of clearly focused family interventions, citing the implementation of the evidence-based *Incredible Years* (Box 1.7) parenting program in *Sure Start* programs in Wales as a positive example (Hutchings et al. 2007). The extent to which these benefits will be sustained or replicated over time, however, has yet to be determined.

Parenting Orders

Parenting Orders were introduced as part of the Crime and Disorder Act in 1998. In keeping with New Labour's electioneering slogan 'tough on crime, tough on the causes of crime' the Act introduced a range of punitive measures to prevent and discourage youth offending.

These measures included Anti-Social Behaviour Orders (ASBOs) issued to individuals, aged 10 or older, who were engaging in behavior that 'was likely to cause alarm, harassment, or distress to one or more persons not of the same household as him or herself' (Crime and Disorder Act 1998: s.1(i)(a)). The Act recognized that many of those engaging in these behaviors or 'nuisance crimes' were children and young people (Campbell and Markesinis 2002). Parenting Orders were thus created alongside ASBOs as a way of reinforcing the responsibilities of parents for managing their children's behavior (Koffman 2008).

Parenting Orders may be issued in response to criminal or antisocial behavior by a young person (i.e. a criminal order), or to school refusal or persistent truancy (i.e. an education order). They carry with them a requirement that parents engage with a parenting support and/or education service in a form directed by the court or their local Youth Offending Team[8] for a period of time which is generally around three months. Categorized as a supportive intervention, Parenting Orders are not considered a punishment, but rather as 'a positive way of bolstering parental responsibility and helping parents develop their skills' (Respect Task Force 2006). However, failure to comply with the terms of the Order can result in criminal breach proceedings, necessitating a return to court that may lead to a fine or to the issuance of a further Order. For this reason, some have criticized Parenting Orders as a means for penalizing parents for the crimes of their children (Coleman and Roker 2007).

The kind of support offered through Parenting Orders largely depends upon the reasons underpinning the order and the range of parenting services available through the YOT and local community. An early evaluation of the Youth Justice Board's Parenting Programme[9] observed that Parenting Order-related services typically included group-based parent management training, home visiting, telephone support and family therapy (Ghate and Ramella 2002). Although some YOTs delivered 'off the shelf' or evidence-based models of parenting support, they frequently adapted them to the needs of their team or their target population.

The evaluation also observed some positive benefits from parenting services offered in conjunction with Parenting Orders, including reductions in reoffending rates and improvements in parents' self-reported attitudes and behaviors. However, these findings should be interpreted with much caution, since the study design did not use a comparison group and involved only those parents who completed all questionnaires. Thus, parents who dropped out of the study or were dissatisfied with the Parenting Order were not represented, suggesting that the study's findings may have been biased towards better functioning families. In addition, the authors acknowledge that there was no way of determining whether the observed reduced recidivism rates were due to parents' participation in the program or to other interventions delivered in conjunction with the Order.

On Track / Children's Fund

On Track was launched in 1999 by the Home Office as part the of New Labour's Crime Reduction Programme. The initiative was the result of findings from the research review, *Reducing Offending*, commissioned by the Home Office in 1998 to identify cost-effective strategies for reversing the 5 per cent annual increase in crime occurring in the UK since the 1920s (Nuttall et al. 1998). *Reducing Offending* examined the characteristics of 15 American programs with strong evidence of preventing antisocial behavior in an effort to identify delivery models (as opposed to specific programs) that were likely to reduce crime. Delivery models identified as effective included family-based models (e.g. home visiting, group-based parent training and family preservation programs) and school-based models (e.g. anti-bullying programs and school–family partnerships).

Although *Reducing Offending* emphasized delivery methods over specific programs, several preventive interventions (including *Perry Preschool*, *Head Start* and NFP) were used as examples of how the risks associated with antisocial behavior could be reduced through family and school-based support. One of these was the *Fast Track* program developed by the Conduct Problems Prevention Research Group (CPRG) in the early 1990s (CPPRG 1992 – see Box 1.6). *Fast Track* combined an evidence-based school curriculum (PATHS) with targeted support for 5-year-olds identified as at-risk for antisocial behavior. This 'multi-component' approach was particularly attractive to UK policy makers who were keen to introduce methods that encouraged partnership working at the local authority level (Ghate et al. 2008).

On Track was thus launched as a crime-reduction demonstration project in 24 disadvantaged communities across England and Wales. *On Track* was delivered through five core interventions targeting children aged 4–12 that included home visiting, preschool education, family therapy, parent management training and home–school partnerships. Although the government encouraged *On Track* programs to adopt evidence-based models, the guidance was very general and the exact form of service delivery was ultimately left to the discretion of each *On Track* local program. This meant that local programs were essentially free to develop and deliver their own content within each of the five core intervention categories. In addition, *On Track* local programs were allowed to offer services within a sixth, specialist category that could include service models that did not fit within the five core categories. In the end, the majority of support offered through the *On Track* initiative fell within this sixth, specialist category, resulting in a hodgepodge of school- and family-based services, some of which were evidence-based, but most of which were not (Ghate et al. 2008).

In 2001, the responsibility for *On Track* was passed from the Home Office to the Department for Education and Skills (DfES), where it became integrated into the *Children's Fund* initiative. Introduced in 2001, *Children's Fund* activities were more focused towards reducing the risks of social exclusion as opposed to those associated with youth crime. This had the effect of shifting *On Track*'s focus from parents and families to schools and peer groups.

The evaluation findings from both *On Track* and the *Children's Fund* suggested few positive gains from either initiative. Once again, the UK government decided against the use of RCTs for investigating the impact of either initiative, so both evaluations adopted a mixed-methods approach which synthesized qualitative and quasi-experimental methods. The balance of these investigations provided little evidence of *On Track*'s effectiveness, often suggesting conflicting results. For example, while the school cohort study observed decreases in children's self-reports of antisocial behavior over time, the community impact study found that antisocial behavior actually increased in *On Track* areas (Ghate et al. 2008). Although the *Children's Fund* evaluation did not directly consider the impact of the initiative on child and parent outcomes, it found that *Children's Fund* services were not particularly successful in reaching socially excluded children and parents. The authors attributed this to the fact that many *Children's Fund* partnerships had difficulty knowing how to identify and target the at-risk populations living within their communities through the use of population data. The report also observed that the initiative would have been more successful if more services had targeted parents as part of their delivery models (Edwards et al. 2006).

Every Child Matters

In 2000, 8-year-old Victoria Climbié died in the north London Borough of Haringey as a result of the abuse and neglect inflicted upon her by her guardians. Revelations made in the aftermath of her death suggested that the many professionals involved in her case

Box 1.6: *Fast Track*

Fast Track is described as a 'multicomponent' approach providing a mixture of universal and targeted support tailored to a child's individual needs. The universal component involves the PATHS curriculum (Promoting Alternative Thinking Strategies) that is provided to all children during their first three years of primary school. PATHS promotes child mastery in four domains known to foster resilience in children: 1) friendship skills and pro-social behavior, 2) emotional understanding and self-control, 3) effective communication and conflict resolution skills and 4) problem-solving strategies. Multiple evaluations have demonstrated that the PATHS curriculum reduces aggressive and hyperactive behavior in classroom settings (CPPRG 1999, Greenberg et al. 1995).

In addition to participating in PATHS, 5-year-old children identified as 'high risk' by their teachers through the use of a standardized screening tool receive a package of support which includes the following components:

- **Parent training groups** parent training is provided via a 22-session curriculum emphasizing the use of praise and the careful monitoring of child activities. Parent training also reinforces the self-control and problem-solving strategies taught in the PATHS curriculum. Parent-and-child sharing activities take place for one half hour after each parent training session in order to facilitate positive parent–child interactions under the guidance of a trained professional.
- **Home visiting** parents also receive bi-weekly home visits or telephone contacts aimed at helping them apply the skills that are covered during the parent training groups.
- **Social skills training** children participate in 22 group sessions of social skills training that focus on pro-social behavior and play skills.
- **Academic tutoring** children also receive academic tutoring to increase their reading skills via a phonics-based reading program. This is done to promote a sense of mastery and reduce the risk of academic failure. Tutoring sessions take place three times a week and a parent attends at least one of these sessions to ensure that the child's reading skills are reinforced at home.

Numerous evaluations of *Fast Track* suggest that program participation reduces the risk of antisocial behavior and improves children's achievement. Findings from a ten year follow-up study suggest that children assigned to *Fast Track* interventions are significantly more likely to demonstrate improved social and academic skills in the short term and significantly less likely be diagnosed with a conduct disorder or receive a police arrest in the long term. In addition, high-risk children's parents are significantly less likely to report using harsh discipline in their homes (CPPRG 2007).

missed important opportunities to protect her. The government subsequently set up a public inquiry, headed by Lord Laming, to investigate the extent to which her death could have been prevented. The resulting report observed that on at least 12 occasions, workers from health, police and social services failed to intervene when they should have. Lord Laming observed that 'a lack of good practice', 'a gross failure of the system' and 'widespread organizational malaise' (Laming 2003: 3–4) were all to blame for Victoria's death. The report concluded with 108 recommendations to reform the social work system.

In September 2003, the *Every Child Matters* (ECM) Green Paper[10] was published in response to Lord Laming's recommendations (HM Treasury 2003). In addressing the failures of the child protection system identified in Laming's report, *Every Child Matters* placed a strong emphasis on the importance of early intervention and recommended that agencies work together to improve children's lives through five key outcomes: be healthy, stay safe, enjoy and achieve, make a positive contribution and achieve economic wellbeing. In this respect, *Every Child Matters* proposed much more than an overhaul of the child protection system, by suggesting a complete reform of all of children's services (Parton 2006). Child maltreatment was thus just one of a number of negative child outcomes which could be prevented through improved coordination between health, education and social work services. By targeting key risks, *Every Child Matters* proposed that agencies could work together to prevent the occurrence of a wide range of adverse child outcomes, including school failure, teen pregnancy, child substance misuse, antisocial behavior and youth offending.

Every Child Matters also recognized the importance of the parent–child relationship in supporting children's development and emphasized the need for local authorities to provide good-quality support to parents as well as children. *Every Child Matters* guidance suggested that this could be accomplished through local authorities relocating their parenting support (once provided through adult social services) within their children's services departments. In ECM terms, this realignment put parenting support at the 'heart' of children's services and introduced a range of universal and targeted parenting interventions that supported the agenda's five key outcomes. The green paper also announced that parents would receive further support through the *Parenting Fund*,[11] which would allocate £25 million over three years to small grant holders (primarily within the voluntary sector) to develop services for parents who were traditionally not well served through statutory provision.

The *Every Child Matters* green paper was subsequently brought into legislation through the Children Act 2004 (HM Government 2004). This Act imposed a duty on local authorities to promote cooperation between statutory agencies and other appropriate bodies in implementing children's services that worked towards the five *Every Child Matters* outcomes. Cooperation between agencies was to be coordinated through Children's Trusts and overseen by the director of children's services. Although Children's Trusts could include representatives from a wide range of agencies, in practice they typically involved partners from education, social work and health (James 2009).

The Respect Action Plan

Up until the end of 2005, the central government put strong pressure on local authorities to increase the services offered to parents, but paid relatively little attention to the extent to which these services improved outcomes for children or communities. The need for parenting support that measurably improved child outcomes became increasingly recognized, however, in the policies and initiatives introduced by the *Respect Action Plan* in 2006 (Scott 2010a, Welshman 2010). Launched at the beginning of Prime Minister Tony Blair's third term, the *Plan* set forth measures for correcting negative parenting behaviors as part of a wider strategy targeting antisocial behavior. These measures included an expanded use of Parenting Orders, increased support for parents with a child undergoing sentencing and the introduction of *Family Intervention Projects* (FIPs). The FIPs initiative was based on the *Dundee Families Project* scheme in Scotland, which aimed to reduce the offending of highly disruptive families by sentencing them to live in residential units where they received ongoing support and surveillance. FIPs adopt a similar approach by combining intensive family support with legal sanctions to motivate families to change their disruptive behavior (White et al. 2008).

The *Respect Action Plan* additionally introduced measures to help local authorities identify and implement effective parenting interventions. These measures included:

- Advice on how directors of children's services and Children's Trusts could commission parenting support in response to local needs
- A toolkit to help commissioners identify effective parenting programs
- A requirement that every local authority appoint a senior 'parents' champion' to coordinate parenting services that would support the objectives identified in its Children and Young People's Plan.[12]

The *Respect Action Plan* also announced plans to set up a national parenting academy that would improve the size and quality of the children's and parents' workforce. This decision was informed, in part, by findings from the evaluations of *Sure Start* and the youth offending program which identified significant shortages in the availability of practitioners with the skills and qualifications necessary to deliver effective parenting support (Ball 2002, Ghate and Ramella 2002, Tunstill et al. 2005). It was envisioned that the academy would provide training and supervision to a wide variety of qualified professionals, including social workers, psychologists, community safety officers and youth justice workers. In the months that followed the launch of the *Respect* agenda, the government provided local authorities with funding for practitioners to work in the following roles:

- ***Respect* Parenting Practitioners** who would be hired and trained to deliver evidence-based parenting interventions to families with children at risk for or engaged in antisocial behavior
- **Parenting Experts** who were similar to *Respect* parenting practitioners, but instead worked with vulnerable families experiencing difficulties with substance misuse, mental health and/or domestic violence
- **FIPs workers** who were to assess the needs of families and coordinate services accordingly for families receiving support through *Family Intervention Projects*
- **Parent Support Advisors**, who were originally introduced in 2005 to provide preventive support to parents in schools (HM Treasury 2005).

Evidence-based parenting interventions

In July 2006, evidence-based parenting support was 'officially' introduced to the UK through the launch of the *Parenting Early Intervention Pathfinders* (PEIPs) pilot. The aim of this scheme was to make effective parenting interventions available to families with children aged 8 to 13 who were considered at risk for antisocial behavior. During the PEIPs pilot stage (2006/2007), 18 local authorities were offered funding to implement one of three evidence-based parenting programs: *Incredible Years*, *Triple P* and *Strengthening Families, Strengthening Communities* (SFSC). All three of these programs teach parents appropriate discipline and boundary-setting strategies within the theoretical context of social learning theory (see Chapter 3 for a more in-depth discussion). Two of the programs (*Incredible Years*, see Box 1.7 and *Triple P*, see Box 1.3) are also underpinned by strong RCT evidence suggesting that they significantly reduce antisocial behavior. Although the use of evidence-based parenting programs had been recommended to local authorities in the past,[13] this was the first time that specific models had been nationally coordinated as part of a crime reduction strategy.

Findings from the first evaluation of the PEIPs pilot suggested that all three parenting interventions significantly improved parents' attitudes and behaviors, as well as their self-reported perceptions of their children's behavior (Lindsay et al. 2008). These findings should be interpreted with caution, however, since the study did not make use of a control group, nor did it follow up parents who dropped out of the program, suggesting a strong bias towards positive program effects. The UK government nevertheless interpreted them to mean that all three interventions had the potential to be effective within the UK and expanded the program to run in 24 additional local authorities in 2008 and 2009 and all local authorities by 2011.

In 2007, the UK government made a further investment in evidence-based parenting support through the introduction of NFP (called *Family–Nurse Partnership* in the UK) in ten pilot sites across England. Positive findings from its first evaluation[14] (Barnes et al. 2008) prompted the government to expand the pilot to twenty additional sites in 2009. The program is now operating in over fifty local authorities and has recently been endorsed for further expansion by the Coalition government.

Parenting Commissioners

In the autumn of 2006, the UK government required English local authorities to appoint a local parenting champion in the form of a parenting commissioner, whose role was to develop a local parenting strategy (DfES 2006). The *Every Parent Matters* guidelines (DfES 2007) subsequently advised local authorities to develop a parenting strategy within their Children and Young People's Plan and to appoint a parenting commissioner to carry it out. Ideally, parenting strategies were to be developed in consultation with parents, children and young people and were to include a range of universal and targeted interventions based upon local need. In addition, these services were to be evidence-based and delivered by individuals with the appropriate skills and qualifications. Coincident with the publication of *Every Parent Matters*, £7.5 million was made available to local authorities to hire a parenting commissioner and develop a parenting strategy.

The National Academy for Parenting Practitioners

The National Academy for Parenting Practitioners (NAPP) was launched in April 2007 as a collaborative effort between two leading national charities (Parenting UK and the Family and Parenting Institute) and King's College London. It was intended as a center of excellence that would provide training in evidence-based parenting program models and conduct research to expand the evidence base. Although criticized by some as 'the nanny state school for good parenting' (Womack, *Telegraph* 14 November 2006), NAPP reflected a government commitment to improved services for parents and children. As Beverley Hughes, former Minister of State for Children, Young People and Families, emphasized at the Academy's launch, 'we are not taking any risks with the advice that we offer parents'.

A key feature of NAPP was the emphasis on research to inform practice. The research team, led by Professor Stephen Scott at King's College London, had an established reputation of conducting rigorous evaluations of parenting interventions and was one of the

Box 1.7: The *Incredible Years* program

Incredible Years is a parent training intervention designed to promote social competence and prevent conduct problems in children aged 0 to 12 years. The range of programs on offer includes *Incredible Years* BASIC, *Babies*, *Toddlers* and *School Age*. *Incredible Years* may be offered universally to all parents living within a community or targeted at families whose children are at risk for behavioral problems. The *Incredible Years* program model is based on social learning theory, teaching parents skills known to promote children's competence and reduce negative behavior including: 1) how to play with children, 2) the effective use of praise to promote positive behavior, 3) the effective use of limit setting and of disciplinary strategies, to discourage misbehavior and 4) how to support child learning. *Incredible Years* ADVANCE can be offered as a supplement to the other three programs, teaching parents improved communication, anger management and problem-solving strategies.

A series of RCTs have observed that participation in the *Incredible Years* program consistently results in the following:

- Increases in parents' use of praise
- Reductions in parents' use of criticism and negative commands
- Increases in parents' use of effective limit setting
- Reductions in parental depression and increases in parental self-confidence
- Increases in positive family communication and problem solving
- Reduced conduct problems in children's interactions with parents and increases in their positive affect and compliance with parental commands.

A long-term follow up of the program has also observed that positive program effects are likely sustained for over 12 years (Webster-Stratton et al. 2010). A recent UK cost study has additionally found that effective implementation of the program could result in a 13.3 per cent internal rate of return (O'Neill et al. 2010).

few teams in the UK to use randomized controlled trials in its study designs. The NAPP research arm included an RCT of the SPOKES intervention (Box 1.8) and the first UK RCT of *Functional Family Therapy* (see Chapter 4). Additional research included three **case series trials** involving interventions targeting high-needs families, foster parents and parents with 'callous-unemotional' children. NAPP-sponsored research also included the standardization of instruments to assess parenting, as well as a cost study of parenting programs.

The NAPP research team was also assigned responsibility for the *Commissioning Toolkit*, a web-based system announced in the *Respect Action Plan* to help commissioners identify effective parenting interventions. In addition to providing information about the nature and quality of parenting programs, the *Toolkit* sets standards for parenting practice at the national level. This is done through the use of the *Parenting Programme Evaluation Tool* (PPET), which is similar to other internationally recognized evaluation systems (e.g. *Blueprints for Violence Prevention*) in that it rates parenting programs in terms of the quality of their evaluation evidence. However, the PPET also rates parenting interventions in terms of the specificity of the target population, their content and their training systems. The aim of adding these extra categories was

Box 1.8: Supporting Parents on Kids' Education in Schools (SPOKES)

The SPOKES (Supporting Parents on Kids' Education in Schools) Literacy Program aims to provide parents with skills they can use at home to support their children's reading at the time their children begin school. An essential element of the program is the 'Pause Prompt Praise' approach to reading, where the parent is taught to pause for five seconds if a child has difficulty reading an unknown word. If, after five seconds, the child does not succeed on his or her own, the parent gives a specific prompt and then praises the child for complying (after McNaughton et al. 1987). Parents learn this strategy through activities involving role play, homework and a home visit.

Two RCTs of the intervention used in combination with the *Incredible Years* program demonstrate significant improvements in parents' sensitivity to their children when reading to them (Scott et al. 2010a, Scott et al. 2010b, Sylva et al. 2008). The first SPOKES trial additionally showed significantly improved reading outcomes and reduced behavioral problems one year following program completion (Scott et al. 2010a, Sylva et al. 2008). The National Academy of Parenting Research (NAPR) is currently conducting a third trial of SPOKES (called the *Helping Children Achieve* trial) to test the efficacy of the SPOKES intervention on its own in comparison to the *Incredible Years* intervention on its own, as well as the combined use of SPOKES and *Incredible Years* interventions. Preliminary findings suggest that SPOKES on its own may be as effective as the *Incredible Years* program in improving children's behavioral outcomes (Beckett et al. 2010).

to improve program standards across a variety of dimensions, as well as highlight promising programs that had not yet undergone an RCT (Scott 2010a).

NAPP research also included the ongoing evaluation of its core training offer, involving 6,000 training places in one of three strands of training:

- 4,000 training places in one of ten evidence-based parenting program models
- 600 training places in a Level 3 qualification course teaching practitioners the skills and principles underpinning parenting work
- 1,400 training places in one of six workshops covering special themes in working with parents, including working with young parents, fathers and parents who misuse drugs and alcohol.

A primary aim of training evaluation was to provide 'real-time' information on the progress of the training offer so that improvements could be made on an ongoing basis. Preliminary findings from the ongoing evaluation suggest that of the 3,162 practitioners attending the evidence-based parent training, approximately 42 per cent went on to deliver a parenting group within six months of their training. While this percentage is somewhat lower than what NAPP had originally anticipated, it suggests that evidence-based parenting support is now widely available to parents living across England, potentially having reached at least 5,000 children[15] within 6 months of the start of NAPP's training offer.

The extent to which the NAPP training will improve outcomes for parents has yet to be determined, however. Although many of the evidence-based parenting programs specified a bachelor's qualification (or higher) in a helping profession (e.g. social work, psychology or nursing) for program delivery, less than one-third of those participating in the NAPP offer met this specification. As the research discussed in Chapter 5 suggests, practitioner characteristics, including their skills and qualifications, stand to significantly impact on the efficacy of parenting interventions.

In March 2010, the National Academy for Parenting Practitioners was closed by the UK government. The training activities were transferred to the Children's Workforce Development Council and the research activities continue through the work of the National Academy for Parenting Research at King's College London.

Investing to save: Birmingham's Brighter Futures

Birmingham City Council is the first British local authority to develop a city-wide strategy to improve child and parent outcomes. Like the US state of Washington, Birmingham aims to do this by making a portfolio of evidence-based programs (including *Family–Nurse Partnership*, *Incredible Years*, PATHS and *Triple P*) available to its 260,000 child residents. What is unique about Birmingham's approach is that it plans to invest £42 million in these prevention programs with the aim of earning a £102 million return on this investment over a ten year period. It is anticipated that this return will be achieved through savings earned in high-end services (e.g. prison and foster care) in the later phases of the strategy. The scheme is underpinned by a monitoring and evaluation system that will provide ongoing information about how and where the money should be spent as the initiative unfolds (Birmingham City Council 2007). The details of this scheme and the processes which informed it are described in greater detail in Chapter 7 and Box 7.5.

The Coalition government: taking the evidence-based practice agenda forward

In May 2010, the New Labour government was voted out of office and replaced by a coalition of the Conservative and Liberal Democrat parties. A key priority of this new government has been to reduce the UK's large budget deficit through the introduction of 'austerity' measures. These measures include dramatic reductions in local authority funding and a substantial downsizing of central government bodies.

Despite these cuts, the Coalition government has renewed the UK's commitment to evidence-based family interventions. Two ministerial reports have particularly identified the need for evidence-based interventions to maximize children's potential and reduce the imbalances created by poverty. The first of these, written by Frank Field (2010), suggests that the gap between the rich and poor is most likely rectified through improved 'Foundation Years' (ages 0–5) provision. Should this proposal be taken forward, local authorities will be expected to show progress towards a national set of 'Life Chance Indicators' (measures of children's cognitive, social and emotional development) through the commissioning of evidence-based interventions for young children and their parents.

The second report, written by Graham Allen (2011), takes Field's proposals one step further by identifying specific evidence-based interventions (many of which are described in this book) that are the most likely to improve children's life chances. Allen's report goes on to suggest that these interventions be piloted in 'Early Intervention Places', involving 26 local authorities that will offer a menu of evidence-based interventions to the parents and children living in their communities. This effort will be supported through an 'Early Intervention Foundation', which will encourage the dissemination of the evidence-based interventions and provide support for workforce and evaluation issues. It is intended that the foundation will be independent of central government and supported through funding provided by private and philanthropic organizations.

International dissemination of evidence-based parenting support

The US and the UK are not the only countries to have implemented national strategies to increase the availability of evidence-based parenting support. Over the past ten years Norway has implemented a 'suite' of parenting programs (including the Oregon Social Learning Center's parent management training model (see Box 3.2), *Incredible Years* (Box 1.7) and FFT (see Chapter 4)) through health services and schools across the country as part of a wider strategy to improve school achievement and reduce behavioral problems (Ogden et al. 2005). This effort is overseen by the Norwegian Center for Studies of Conduct Problems and Innovative Practice, which plays a role similar to that of NAPP in the coordination of training and research (Ogden et al. 2005). Dissemination processes have been underway since 1997 and RCT evidence suggests significant improvements in parent and child behaviors (Ogden and Hagen 2008).

Australia has had similar success with the population-wide dissemination of *Triple P* in ten communities. This effort is coordinated by the *National Mental Health Promotion, Prevention and Early Intervention Action Plan* as part of a national initiative to reduce depression in children and adults. Findings from a quasi-experimental study observed significant reductions in the number of children with behavioral and emotional problems, as well as fewer parents reporting depression, stress and coercive parenting behaviors in communities where *Triple P* services were available (Sanders et al. 2008).

Summary and conclusion

Over the past fifty years, thousands of interventions have been developed to improve children's life circumstances. These interventions range from universally available school-based prevention programs, to individually delivered interventions targeting families with serious problems. All of these programs have good intentions and many of them are well liked. Only a few of them actually work, however. Despite their best intentions, most prevention and intervention programs do not have any evidence of improving children's circumstances and some even result in harm. Even when not harmful, ineffective parenting programs waste the money of taxpayers and the time of families who are in desperate need of effective treatments. For these reasons it is essential that services delivered to children and parents have some evidence of being effective.

Fortunately, there are now a growing number of prevention and intervention programs that reliably result in long-term benefits for children. Research now suggests that when these programs are implemented properly, community-wide benefits can be achieved. The lessons summarized in this chapter suggest, however, that developing and implementing effective interventions is hard to do. Policies that try to do too much, too soon are particularly unlikely to be effective, as the examples of *Sure Start* in the UK and the 1990s home visitation initiative in the US suggest. In order to be effective, interventions require careful planning and development so that important program details are fully understood. These details include a well-specified target population, an evidence-based theory of change and robust systems for training and implementation. Robust research designs are also necessary to understand how and when programs are effective.

Box 1.9: Time-line of events in UK parenting policy

1998 The national *Sure Start* initiative is launched in an effort to improve outcomes for children aged 4 and younger. This is to be achieved through services developed and coordinated at the community level. Funding is made available for 250 *Sure Start* local programs.

Parenting Orders are established as part of the Crime and Disorder Act 1998. Parenting Orders require that parents attend family therapy or parent education services in conjunction with their child receiving a criminal or educational order.

The *Supporting Families* green paper announces the *Family and Parenting Institute* to 'provide helpful guidance and develop more and better parenting support' (Home Office 1998: 6).

1999 The *On Track* initiative is launched as part of a government strategy to reduce the risks associated with youth offending through prevention services targeting families with children aged 4 to 12. The initiative is introduced in 24 deprived communities in England and Wales.

2000 An additional £5 million is allocated to increase the number of *Sure Start* local programs to 500.

Victoria Climbié is murdered by her guardians in north London. Her death sparks a public inquiry that results in an overhaul of the child protection system.

2001 The *Children's Fund* is launched to improve outcomes for children at risk for social exclusion. *On Track* programs are merged into the *Children's Fund* initiative.

2002 Plans to establish *Sure Start* Children's Centres are announced, whereby *Sure Start* local programs are be converted into centers offering 'good quality childcare, early years education, health services, family support, parental outreach and a base for childminders' (HM Treasury 2002: 33).

2003 Findings from the investigation into Victoria Climbié's death are announced. The *Every Child Matters* (ECM) Green Paper is published as a result and children's services are required to work toward the five ECM outcomes: be healthy, stay safe, enjoy and achieve, make a positive contribution and achieve economic wellbeing.

2004 Plans to increase funding for Children's Centres are announced with a target of 3,500 being set up by 2010. This announcement changes the focus of the initiative from disadvantaged communities to all communities.

The *Every Child Matters* green paper is put into legislation through the Children Act 2004. Children's Trusts are established to coordinate activities from education, health, social work and other agencies to provide a seamless system of children's services.

The Department of Health announces a national services framework for the delivery of children's, young people's and maternity services (DoH/DfES 2004a, DoH/DfES 2004b).

2005 Findings from the first national evaluation of *Sure Start* suggest that there is little evidence that the initiative has resulted in improved outcomes for families living in *Sure Start* communities. Outcomes were, in fact, worse for vulnerable families, including those headed by a lone parent or a teen mother living in *Sure Start* communities (Belsky et al. 2006).

2006 The *Respect Action Plan* is published, announcing plans for *Family Intervention Projects* and a national parenting academy that will train practitioners to work with parents.

The *Parenting Early Intervention Pathfinders* pilot is launched, providing evidence-based parenting support in 18 communities across the country.

Local authorities are provided with guidance on the hiring of parenting commissioners.

2007 Findings from the second national evaluation of *Sure Start* indicate that the initiative is linked to improved outcomes for families living in *Sure Start* communities, including improved home-learning environments, increased access to family support services and decreased negative parenting behaviors (Melhuish and Hall 2007).

The National Academy for Parenting Practitioners (NAPP) is established to train 4,000 practitioners in the delivery of evidence-based parenting programs.

The *Family–Nurse Partnership* program is piloted in ten local authorities.

2008 The *Think Family* approach is introduced through the *Family Pathfinder* program. This initiative encourages professionals to adopt a family focus when working with complex cases.

2009 A public *Think Fathers* campaign is launched to encourage services to become more 'dad friendly'.

2010 NAPP closes and the training of parenting practitioners is transferred to the Children's Workforce Development Council. The research of NAPP is carried forward by the National Academy for Parenting Research (NAPR) at King's College London.

The Coalition government is elected. The new government introduces 'austerity' measures, including reductions in local authority funding and in numbers of central government employees, in an effort to reduce the budget deficit.

An independent review on poverty and life chances (the Field report) emphasizes the need for improved services for families with children aged 5 and younger. The report also introduces a new framework for measuring reductions in poverty and effects through the use of cognitive, emotional and home environment 'Life Chance Indicators'.

2011 The Allen report is published, introducing a menu of evidence-based early interventions that will be disseminated through an independent Early Intervention Foundation.

The success of evidence-based parenting interventions also depends upon strong government policies and infrastructures to coordinate training, conduct research and disseminate knowledge. The lessons described in this chapter suggest that local, home-grown interventions are unlikely to be effective unless substantial investments are made in their development and evaluation. For this reason, a number of countries are now applying substantial funds to the implementation of parenting interventions which are underpinned by strong research evidence. These strides are most often facilitated through a central body that assumes responsibility for coordinating training, directing research and disseminating practice knowledge. Improvements in the availability of effective parenting interventions are also only possible through the hard work and dedication of individuals who understand the principles underpinning parenting work and appreciate the need for strong evidence. The chapters that follow describe the knowledge necessary to deliver evidence-based parenting support and the processes required to make it happen.

Box 1.10: Key points

- The prevalence of childhood mental health disorders is high. Ten per cent of children within the UK are estimated to have a mental health disorder. Within the US, Canada and Australia, the prevalence of childhood mental health problems is estimated at between 14 and 20 per cent.
- 35 to 40 per cent of all children will be diagnosed with a mental health problem by the age of 18.
- Approximately one-half of all adults will be diagnosed with a mental health disorder during their lifetime. Fifty per cent of all adult mental health disorders are diagnosed during childhood.
- Childhood mental health problems are expensive. A child diagnosed with a conduct disorder at age 10 can cost a community up to ten times as much as a child with no mental health problems.
- Mental health problems, including conduct disorders, are curable and preventable.
- Parenting behaviors significantly contribute to children's wellbeing. High levels of warmth and sensitivity and effective disciplinary strategies are particularly associated with children's behavioral and emotional outcomes.
- A number of parenting interventions with a consistent track record of improving child behavioral and emotional outcomes now exist.
- Research evidence now suggests that many parenting interventions are cost-effective.
- Since the early 1990s, the US government has made significant investments in obtaining RCT evidence on social interventions.
- The US government now advises local authorities to invest only in social programs underpinned by RCT evidence.
- Since the late 1990s, the UK government has rigorously promoted parenting interventions.
- Since 2006, the UK government has encouraged local authorities to implement evidence-based parenting interventions.
- A number of communities within the US, UK, Australia and Norway have started to achieve community-wide benefits through the wide-scale implementation of parenting interventions at multiple levels of need.
- Effective implementation of parenting interventions is difficult and requires high levels of program, agency and government support.

Notes

1 RCTs are considered to be the most rigorous way of attributing positive outcomes to an interven-tion and not other known or unknown biases. As the name implies, participants are randomly assigned to one or more treatment groups and a control group to ensure that any confounding factors are evenly distributed across all groups. An overview of the rationale and use of RCTs is provided in full in Chapter 2.
2 Although discrepancies exist between the criteria used to evaluate the quality of research evidence, many systems recognize the elements similar to those identified in the *Maryland Scale*. See, for example, Borkovec and Castonguay 1998, Chambless and Hollon 1998, Flay et al. 2005.
3 Findings from the evaluation of *Head Start* to date have not been as consistent or as strong as those observed in the *Perry Preschool Program* and other early education programs, such as *Early Head Start* (Sawhill and Baron 2010).
4 The programs discussed in the report included NFP, Hawaii's *Healthy Start*, *Parents as Teachers* (PAT), *Home Instruction Program for Preschool Youngsters* (HIPPY), the *Comprehensive Child Development Program* and *Healthy Families America* (HFA).
5 Established in 2001 to support the dissemination of evidence-based social interventions.
6 The term portfolio refers to a continuum of universal and targeted evidence-based services avail-able at the community level.
7 The *Commissioning Toolkit* is a UK-based directory of evidence-based parenting programs available in the UK. See Chapter 2 for a complete overview.
8 Youth Offending Teams (YOTs) were also established by the Crime and Disorder Act 1998 as multi-disciplinary teams operating within existing local authority structures to develop and imple-ment prevention and intervention services for youth offenders. The activities of YOTs are overseen by the Youth Justice Board (YJB) also established in 1998 and recently brought within the functions of the Ministry of Justice.
9 An initiative aimed at supporting the development of parenting projects developed in conjunction with Parenting Orders.
10 A Green Paper is a government report containing a tentative proposal without any commitment to action, although it is often a first step in changing the law.
11 The decision to create the *Parenting Fund* was the result of the 2002 CSR, thus predating the *Every Child Matters* green paper.
12 Children's and Young People's Plans were also introduced through the *Every Child Matters* agenda, requiring local authorities to develop strategies for their children's services that were underpinned by specific actions and outputs linked to the five *Every Child Matters* outcomes.
13 It should be noted that a number of local authorities had already implemented evidence-based parenting programs with funding from the *Sure Start* and *On Track* initiatives.
14 The initial evaluation of the *Family–Nurse Partnership* program was a feasibility study using qualitative methods and did not assess impact.
15 This figure is based on the following assumptions: of the 3,162 attending, 42 per cent deliver training within the first six months. If, on average, two practitioners deliver a parenting group to an average of eight parents, each with two children, the following calculation can be made = 5,312.

2 Understanding the evidence base

What is evidence-based practice?

David Sackett, a pioneer in the field of evidence-based medicine, is accredited with providing the most widely used definition of evidence-based practice:

> Evidence-based practice is the integration of the best research evidence with clinical expertise and patient values.
>
> (Sackett et al. 2000 as quoted in IOM 2001: 147)

This definition suggests that three intersecting components are necessary to provide parents and children with evidence-based support: 1) knowledge of the best research evidence, 2) an understanding and respect for client values and 3) practitioner expertise. Haynes et al. (2002) have recently added a fourth component to this definition to include a consideration of the client's circumstances and the constraints of the clinical setting (Figure 2.1). The point at which the four components intersect is where evidence-based practice begins.

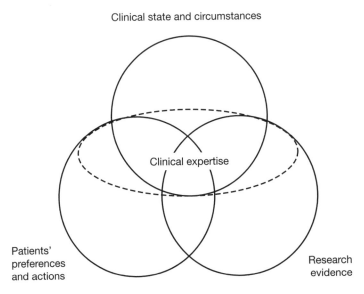

Figure 2.1 Model of the key elements of evidence-based practice (reprinted with permission from Haynes et al. 2002)

A practitioner must understand each of these four components in order to successfully deliver evidence-based support to parents and children. This chapter describes the processes involved in the first component – how to understand and find the best research evidence. It begins with the example of *Head Start* to illustrate how research evidence can be used to understand an intervention's efficacy. It then discusses the methods used to measure impact and establish an evidence base. The chapter concludes with an overview of how practitioners can find evidence-based information to support their day-to-day work with parents and children.

The need for a strong evidence base: lessons from *Head Start*

As described in Chapter 1, the US *Head Start* initiative (Box 2.1) has been historically influential in the development of US and UK policies aimed at young children and their parents (Glass 1999; Welshman, 2010). It is highly unlikely that this would have been the case, however, if there had not been convincing evidence of *Head Start*'s effectiveness in the early phases of its development (Zigler and Muenchow 1992, Zigler and Styfco 2004).

The idea for *Head Start* began in the early 1960s at a time when US policy makers sincerely believed that social inequalities could be corrected through large-scale government initiatives. As part of Democratic President Johnson's 'war on poverty', *Head Start* aimed to reverse the negative effects of growing up poor by providing a range of services which supported the 'whole child'. To this end, *Head Start* was initially developed as an eight-week summer program offering disadvantaged preschool children and their parents a comprehensive package of education, health and community support (Zigler and Styfco 1994: 272).

Given *Head Start*'s holistic approach, it is surprising that its first evaluations considered children's cognitive development only. *Head Start*'s first evaluations involved **standardized measures** in the form of IQ tests which were given to children at the beginning of the first summer pilot and then again at the end. These studies typically observed an astonishingly high increase of eight to ten IQ points upon program completion, which was much higher than what would happen by chance. Those evaluating the program considered these to be extraordinary gains and policy makers quickly embraced them as strong evidence of *Head Start*'s success. On the basis of these early evaluation findings, *Head Start* was quickly transformed from an eight-week summer 'camp' to a fully fledged preschool program reaching over a half a million children, with an annual budget of $96.4 million (Zigler and Muenchow 1992).

Head Start's promising evaluation findings were not sufficient for the Republican administration that followed, however. By the time Richard Nixon was elected in 1968, the national evaluation of *Head Start* was underway. This study found that the gains in IQ originally observed were completely lost within three years of program completion (Cicirelli 1969, Lee et al. 1988, Zigler and Muenchow 1992). This 'fade-out' was enough for many Republican leaders to call for *Head Start* to be abolished and it is highly likely that this would have occurred, had it not been for the program's initial positive evaluation findings (Zigler and Muenchow 1992). Within its first three years, parents and politicians were so convinced of *Head Start*'s 'success' that its critics were forced to commission additional research before scrapping the program on the basis that its impact was short lived (Vinovskis 2005).

This was bad and good news for *Head Start*. It was bad in the sense that the findings from the national evaluation suddenly put the program on the defensive, but good because it provided program developers with the opportunity to better articulate *Head Start*'s program goals and identify more appropriate measures (Zigler and Muenchow 1992, Zigler and

Box 2.1: *Head Start*

Head Start is a federally funded US preschool program aiming to promote the school readiness of economically disadvantaged 3- and 4-year-olds. *Head Start* was established in the mid 1960s and its budget was voted into law by Congress through the Head Start Act in 1981. The program has since been reauthorized multiple times and was significantly expanded in 1994 to include the *Early Head Start* program for low-income families with children under the age of 3. *Head Start* local programs are collectively allocated a budget of over $7 billion per year and now reach over 900,000 children (Office of Head Start 2010).

   Head Start is administered through federal grants provided to local and private profit and non-profit agencies which provide a range of services to children and parents, based on local resources and community need. *Head Start* local programs are encouraged to coordinate these services through collaborative community partnerships. However, all programs must provide a daily preschool curriculum that supports children's early literacy and math skills as part of *Head Start*'s core offer.

   Local programs must also provide support to the parents of *Head Start* participants. Many programs do this through monthly home visits, where parents' personal strengths and weaknesses are discussed within a solution-focused framework. Parents are also actively encouraged to involve themselves in the governance of their child's *Head Start* program. To this end, *Head Start* performance standards require that at least 51 per cent of the members of its governing body are parents with children enrolled in the program (Schumacher 2003).

   The development of *Head Start* has been informed through a rigorous evaluation program since its first pilot study in the mid 1960s. These studies repeatedly suggest that program participants consistently demonstrate significant short-term cognitive gains which rapidly fade out once they enter primary school. The reasons for this fade-out remain unclear, although many assume that *Head Start*'s initial benefits are difficult to maintain when children attend low-quality primary schools after leaving the program (Lee and Loeb 1995, Zigler and Muenchow 1992). Longer-term studies suggest, however, that *Head Start* benefits re-emerge once participants enter the job market. Specifically, *Head Start* children are significantly less likely to be held back a grade, are more likely to graduate from high school and are more likely to get a job (Currie and Thomas 1995, McKey et al. 1985).

   It should also be noted that the positive findings involving *Head Start*'s long-term outcomes have not been observed through a rigorously designed evaluation involving randomization and a comparison group. Instead, the majority of *Head Start*'s longitudinal research has involved **cross-sectional studies** which are likely to contain a number of unknown biases. To date, only one RCT has been conducted with *Head Start* participants. Findings from this study have reconfirmed *Head Start*'s significant short-term benefits followed by a rapid fade-out (Puma et al. 2005, 2010). The extent to which **sleeper effects** will re-emerge when these children become older has yet to be determined (O'Connell et al. 2009, Sawhill and Baron 2010).

Styfco 2004). To this end, researchers determined that measures of IQ were not sufficient for evaluating *Head Start*'s efficacy and more varied and rigorous evaluation methods were required (Schrag et al. 2004).

Hence, a series of evaluations followed which measured the long-term impact of the program, as well as its efficacy in comparison to other preschool models. These investigations confirmed the findings from the first national evaluation, observing an initial gain in IQ followed by a rapid fade-out during the elementary school years (Bronfenbrenner 1974). However, many of these studies also found that *Head Start* participants gained important skills that did not fade out over time (Lee et al. 1988 – see Box 2.1 for a more complete discussion). As noted in Chapter 1, these positive outcomes, now referred to as *Head Start*'s 'sleeper' effects, have since been used to understand the program's cost-effectiveness, suggesting a potential tax saving of $7 for every $1 spent (Garces et al. 2002, Ludwig and Miller 2007, Nores et al. 2005). Collectively, *Head Start*'s evaluations helped the program to survive dramatic budget cuts in the 1970s and 80s and contributed to the program's expansion in the 1990s. Although the implications of the evaluation findings are often debated, *Head Start*'s program of research is considered an integral part of its ongoing development (Henrich 2004, Puma et al. 2010). In the words of *Head Start*'s founder, Ed Zigler, 'research, which almost killed *Head Start*, would finally help save it' (Zigler and Muenchow 1992: 170).

Understanding impact

Experimental and observational research

A wide variety of research designs have been used throughout *Head Start*'s history to understand the impact of the program. Its initial evaluations used standardized measures administered before and after program participation to gain a preliminary understanding of the program's impact. Subsequent studies involved the use of **randomized controlled trials**, **cohort studies** and **cross-sectional** studies to understand the extent to which *Head Start* was effective. Some of these studies suggested that *Head Start* provided few benefits for children, whereas others indicated that program participation was associated with a variety of positive child outcomes. Given these conflicting findings, it can be difficult to determine which studies were correct. In order to do this, one must be able to **critically appraise** the *strength* of the evaluation evidence and this requires an understanding of the advantages and weaknesses of various research designs.

Grimes and Schulz (2002) have developed a useful framework for understanding the different kinds of designs employed to investigate whether or not a treatment is effective. As Figure 2.2 suggests, **empirical** research designs can be classified as either **experimental** or **observational**. Experimental studies are literally set up as experiments which involve a treatment and a comparison group so that comparisons between the two groups can be made. Participants' exposure to a treatment is controlled through assignment to the treatment or comparison group.

Experimental studies fall into one of two categories, depending on whether participants are randomly assigned to the treatment or control group. As the name implies, randomized controlled designs randomly assign participants to a treatment and non-treatment group or groups. Non-randomized trials make use of a control group, but assignment to this group is determined by non-random factors. Strictly speaking, the term **experimental** should be reserved for RCTs only and **quasi-experimental** should be used to describe controlled trials that do not use randomization, as well as observational studies, which are described below (Cook and Campbell 1979).

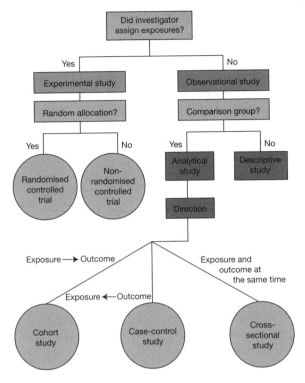

Figure 2.2 A taxonomy of research designs (reprinted with permission from Grimes and Schulz 2002)

Observational studies involve the use of research methods to systematically observe activities that happen naturally, independently of the study. This means that allocation to the treatment is not fully under the control of the researcher. If the observational study involves a comparison group, it is considered an **analytic study**. If it does not involve a comparison group, it is considered a **descriptive study**. Analytic studies are used to test hypotheses by comparing observations between two groups. Examples of analytic studies include cohort studies, cross-sectional studies and case-control studies. Descriptive studies can use either statistical or **qualitative methods** to describe observations and relationships, but they cannot verify whether a treatment is effective.

Experimental research

Randomized controlled trials

Randomized controlled trials (Figure 2.3) are widely considered to be the most rigorous way of measuring impact and comparing the relative effectiveness of alternative interventions. As the term 'randomized' implies, participants from a sufficiently large **sample** are randomly assigned[1] to one or more **treatment groups** and a **control group**. This is done to ensure that any known or unknown biases are evenly distributed across all groups. A control group may involve a **placebo** or no treatment at all. Once the intervention is completed, the outcomes for the treatment group are compared with the

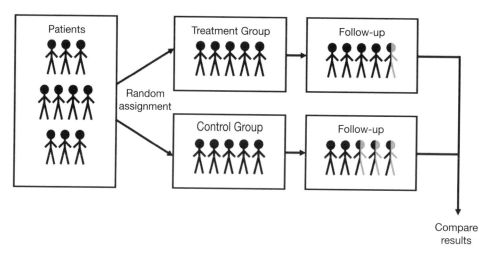

Figure 2.3 Example of an RCT design with a treatment and control group

control group to determine the extent to which any observed change can be attributed to the treatment.

Blinding is another method used to reduce bias in RCTs. Blinding refers to a participant's or researcher's lack of knowledge regarding treatment assignment. In studies involving a comparison treatment, it is possible to blind the participants from knowing whether they have been assigned to the treatment or comparison group. Researchers measuring the treatment's effects can also be blinded from knowing what group a subject participated in. The term **double-blind** is used to refer to studies where both the participants and the researchers are blind to who belongs in the treatment and control groups.

Tests of statistical significance and effect sizes

A **statistically significant** difference between treatment and control group outcomes provides tentative evidence that an intervention is effective. **Significance tests** involve statistical calculations to determine whether to accept or reject the **null hypothesis** – i.e. to confirm that the observed difference is greater than what might happen by chance. Rejecting the null hypothesis when it is true (i.e. concluding a treatment is effective when it is not) is a **type I error**. Accepting the null hypothesis when it is false (i.e. concluding that the treatment is not effective when it is) is a **type II error**.

The significance of an observed difference is usually reported in terms of a **p value** that reports the probability of the difference being greater than what would occur by chance. Most studies require a p value of less than or equal to 0.05 to avoid making a type I error by concluding that the observed result is not related to chance. This means that the observed relationship could only happen by chance 5 per cent of the time – i.e. one out of 20 times.

Type II errors involve the conclusion that the treatment is not effective when it is. Statisticians refer to the need for **statistical power** to avoid making a type II error. Factors that determine the power of a statistical test include the probability of making a type I error (rejecting the null hypothesis when it is true), the probability of making a type II error (accepting the null hypothesis when it is false), the sample size and the particular statistical test being used. While it is beyond the scope of this book to describe the various ways of increasing statistical power, it is generally fair to say that a large sample size greatly increases a study's statistical power and greatly reduces the likelihood of a type II error. However, this principle should not be interpreted to mean that bigger is always better. Although big samples will improve the likelihood of finding a statistically significant difference, a statistically significant difference may not be particularly large or meaningful. For this reason, calculating an **effect size** is the preferred method for determining the extent to which a treatment is effective. An effect size estimates the magnitude of the difference between the treatment and control groups. As Figure 2.4 illustrates, an effect size is the standardized mean difference between two populations.

An effect size is calculated by taking the difference between two means and dividing it by the standard deviation of either one or both populations. Cohen's *d* is a common method used for calculating effect sizes.[2]

$$d = \frac{\overline{x}_1 - \overline{x}_2}{S}$$

In this equation, $\overline{x}_1$ = the mean change for the treatment group, $\overline{x}_2$ = the mean change for the control group and S = the standard deviation.

In evaluation studies, effect sizes are typically reported in terms of standard units derived from **means** and **standard deviations**. For example, an effect size of 0.5 suggests a one-half standard deviation increase in treatment outcomes. The use of a standard unit allows comparisons to be made across treatments to assess each treatment's relative impact. As a rule of thumb, an effect size of 0.2 involving Cohen's *d* is considered to be a small effect, 0.5 a moderate effect and 0.8 a large effect. Typically, large effect sizes suggest a strong impact on child outcomes and small effect sizes suggest a more modest effect, although the meaning of

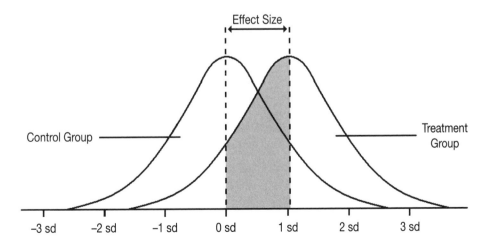

Figure 2.4   The effect size between two group outcomes

the effect size should always be considered within the context of the research hypothesis and the aims of the study (McCartney and Rosenthal 2000). It is also important to remember that a small effect size does not necessarily mean that a program is ineffective. While many interventions achieve large effect sizes of 0.7 or higher, they are also often expensive to deliver – thus reducing the overall benefits of the program. By comparison, prevention programs are typically less expensive to deliver, so a modest effect size of 0.2 or 0.3 may still be of value if its benefits offset the program's costs (Dodge 2009, Foster et al. 2003, McCartney and Rosenthal 2000).

Arguments for and against the use of RCTs

As discussed in Chapter 1, some policy makers resist the use of RCTs on ethical and practical grounds (see Box 2.2 for an overview). The most commonly used ethical argument operates under the assumption that the treatment being tested is highly likely to work and therefore denying participants access to the treatment for the sake of an experiment is unethical. The counter-argument to this assumption is that some of the best-intended programs do not always work, as the example in Box 2.3 suggests.

Box 2.2: Arguments against the use of RCTs and their counter-arguments (Rosen et al. 2006)

Argument	Counter-argument
Withholding an intervention from individuals is unfair or unethical.	Unless the program has been proved to work, it cannot be known if withholding a treatment is unethical. Many popular ideas have been proven to be ineffective and sometimes even harmful. There are ways of improving clients' access to an intervention, however, through the use of a wait-list control group. In these cases, study participants are randomly assigned to the treatment or a wait list. If the treatment appears to be effective, it can be offered to the wait list.
Social interventions often have many complex outcomes. RCTs tend to focus on only one or two outcomes and their measures are often overly simplistic.	Good interventions include a theory of change that specifies short- and long-term behavioral outcomes. Short behavioral outcomes can often be measured through standardized instruments or observational coding. Well-designed RCTs also aim to measure multiple outcomes.
Social interventions cannot be expected to achieve change in a short period of time.	Good social interventions are able to identify short- and long-term goals. RCTs should also include a follow-up as part of their design.

Social interventions often address issues that are hard to evaluate.	It is true that some interventions are difficult to investigate through the use of an RCT. This includes changes in public policy or public awareness campaigns. However, evaluators should first explore the feasibility of an RCT before ruling out its use.
Findings from RCTs cannot be generalized, as they are conducted with a narrowly defined group of people under artificial conditions. In other words, they have low **external validity**.	This is a valid criticism of some RCTs if steps are not taken to make sure that the sample is representative of the target population or if the clinical setting is too artificial. These limitations can be overcome by evaluators making sure that study participants are representative of the intervention's target population and that study conditions reflect normal practice. In many instances, it is also recommended that interventions undergo multiple RCTs in diverse settings with diverse populations.
Findings from RCTs apply only to individuals and not to communities.	This can be overcome by randomizing communities (sometimes referred to as **cluster randomization**) rather than individuals, as was done in the *Triple P* trial in South Carolina (see Box 1.3).
RCTs cannot be tailored to local need and do not take the views of participants into account.	This problem can be overcome if individuals representative of program participants are consulted in the design of the intervention. This step is also likely to improve the efficacy of the intervention. See Chapter 6 for further discussion.
RCTs are too expensive.	In truth, RCT designs are not any more expensive than other evaluation designs. The reason why they are perceived as expensive is because of the need for large sample sizes, which sometimes can take a long time to recruit and randomize into the study. However, other research designs also require the use of large samples. The expense of an RCT should be considered within the context of expenses incurred by inaccurate conclusions informed by poorly designed studies.

An additional argument against the use of RCTs involves the fact that social programs often aim to improve multiple outcomes and that RCTs may narrowly focus on the wrong outcomes. This was certainly the case with the first *Head Start* evaluations, where fade-out was attributed to the use of IQ to evaluate the effectiveness of the program instead of other measures that might have been more relevant. This limitation can be overcome, however, by carefully considering the program's key outcomes and selecting the measures accordingly during the planning stages of the evaluation.

Box 2.3: Negative effects of the *Cambridge-Somerville* program

The *Cambridge-Somerville* program was developed in the 1930s in eastern Massachusetts to prevent juvenile delinquency. Boys between the age of 5 and 13 were randomly assigned to a control and a treatment group. Boys in the treatment group received bi-monthly visits from a youth counselor, who provided support to the family and coordinated additional services for the boys as needed. This support often included academic tutoring, attendance at a summer camp and participation in extra-curricular groups such as scouting, the YMCA and other community programs. Boys assigned to the control group received no additional support, but completed the evaluation measures throughout the course of the study.

A 30-year follow-up study observed that the Cambridge-Somerville program had no positive impact on delinquency, the participants' opportunities for employment or their overall health. In fact, boys who participated in the program were significantly more likely to have been re-arrested for a criminal offence, to have developed a substance misuse problem, to have a low paying job, to have poor physical or psychological health or to have died, in comparison to boys not participating in the program. Joan McCord, the program's evaluator, interpreted these findings to mean that there were features of the program (also referred to as **iatrogenic effects**) that actually increased the participants' level of risk. While McCord did not identify any specific program feature that may have increased the boys' level of risk, she did speculate that the program may have inadvertently encouraged the boys and their parents to become dependent on the counselors, which in turn reduced their ability to function independently after the program was over (McCord 1978).

A re-analysis of the findings, comparing the program experiences of the participants with the worst outcomes to those exhibiting fewer problems, observed that the boys who attended a summer camp (approximately one-quarter) were the most likely to have recommitted a crime and to have serious physical and mental health problems. This suggested that the camp experience inadvertently provided the boys with the opportunity to exchange deviant ideas and reinforce each other's antisocial attitudes, ultimately increasing their risks of worse developmental outcomes (Dishion et al. 1999).

RCTs are also frequently rejected because they are perceived as expensive and they lack generalizability (also referred to as external validity – see following sections). As Box 2.2 suggests, these problems, too, can be overcome if care is taken in the planning stages of the evaluation. However, it is true that a single RCT is often not sufficient for verifying whether an intervention is effective. As the example of *Head Start* demonstrates, good interventions are evaluated on an ongoing basis and the best ones include multiple RCTs to repeatedly test their effectiveness and inform their ongoing development (Flay 1986).

Non-randomized controlled trials

Randomized controlled trials are considered to be the 'gold standard' of research designs because all biases are evenly distributed between the control and treatment groups. Random assignment thus improves the **internal validity** of the study by making it easier to attribute observed effects to the treatment rather than to other, confounding factors. However, as noted in the previous section, RCTs are commonly rejected for a variety of reasons, with a common issue being difficulty in recruiting participants. Even when the evaluator believes in the merits of randomization, individuals often refuse participation because they do not have the time, or they do not want their access to the treatment to be determined by a computer algorithm or coin-toss (Jenkins 2007). While some clients may feel entitled to a new intervention, others might reject it because it has not yet been proven. The evaluator then has the difficult choice of waiting a long time to recruit participants or considering alternative methods to random assignment.

Non-randomized controlled trials can involve concurrent or historic samples. In a **concurrent controlled trial**, the participant or practitioner determines allocation to the control or treatment group. For example, participants may be offered the choice to try a new treatment, or a practitioner may offer a new parenting intervention to one group of parents, while providing an older one to another group. Under both circumstances, high levels of bias related to both practitioner and parent characteristics may enter the study, ultimately threatening the internal validity of the study's findings (see following section).

Another example of a non-randomized design involves the use of a **historic control**, where the outcomes of individuals participating in a treatment are then compared to outcomes from comparable individuals in the past who did not receive the treatment. A simple example of this would be to introduce a new curriculum to a school and compare the achievement rates of pupils who received the curriculum to those of pupils who did not receive it the year previously. While historic controls provide a practical way to compare treatment outcomes, they also introduce biases to the study that may occur through the passage of time. Changes in school personnel, school policies, demographics of the student population and historical events can all create biases which are highly likely to impact the treatment outcome.

Carefully matching the treatment and control groups is another way of reducing bias in non-randomized controlled studies. Design biases can also sometimes be controlled for through statistical methods. However, these methods are limited in their ability to control for all the factors that could potentially confound a non-randomized experiment. Evaluators must therefore consider all the ways that bias may contribute to a non-randomized study before concluding that a treatment is effective (Shadish et al. 2002).

Observational research

Descriptive studies

As mentioned previously, observational studies are distinguished by the fact that relatively little is under the control of the researcher. For this reason, observational studies are sometimes referred to as natural experiments (Shadish et al. 2002). Although observational designs lack the internal validity associated with experimental design, they have increased **external validity** because they systematically observe associations between interventions and treatments in everyday settings. When observational studies do not have access to a comparison group they are considered **descriptive**. Descriptive studies should never be used to determine whether a treatment is effective. They can, however, be very useful for understanding the characteristics of various target populations and can sometimes be used to establish a baseline. Examples of descriptive studies include **case series trials**, involving observations on a series of individuals, before and after an intervention, **correlational studies**, which consider the interaction between a number of variables and **longitudinal studies** (not involving a treatment and control group), which track changes in participant outcomes over time.

Cross-sectional studies

Analytic studies facilitate hypothesis testing by comparing outcomes from separate groups. A 'quick and dirty' way of comparing groups is through a cross-sectional study. Cross-sectional studies do not make use of pre- and post-treatment measures, but instead compare data for groups of participants collected at one point in time.

A cross-sectional design was used for the first *Sure Start* impact evaluation, where children and parents living in *Sure Start* and non-*Sure Start* communities were compared through observational measures collected at one point in time. This design was chosen over an RCT on the basis that *Sure Start* targeted communities rather than individuals. Although arguments have been made that an area-based randomized design could (and should) have been used to assign communities to the *Sure Start* program (as was done with the *Triple P* trial in South Carolina, see Chapter 1), this ultimately was not practical, due to the rapid roll-out of the program (Belsky et al. 2007, Rutter 2006, 2007).

While a cross-sectional design is a good way to get quick information about differences between groups, it limits the conclusions that can be made about the effect of a treatment, since it does not measure change over time. Cross-sectional studies also rely on the assumption that the comparison and treatment groups are similarly matched. In the case of the first *Sure Start* evaluation, efforts were made to match communities, but the *Sure Start* areas were nevertheless more deprived. Some have argued that this may have contributed to the disappointing findings observed in this study (Meadows 2007, Rutter 2007).

Case-control studies

Case-control studies are used in instances where researchers are interested in exploring the origins of a fairly rare phenomenon, such as extreme forms of youth violence, child maltreatment and unusual mental health disorders. This is done by retrospectively comparing a group of individuals with the outcome of interest (e.g. youths who commit murder) to those who do not have that outcome. Case-control methods were used in the retrospective analysis of the Cambridge-Somerville study (Box 2.3), which observed that summer camp participation increased the risk of poor adult outcomes.

Cohort studies

Cohort studies prospectively follow separate groups of participants (cohorts) over a long period of time. Cohort studies investigating the potential effects of an intervention recruit a control and a treatment group prior to the intervention and then follow them for months, years or even decades. Cohort studies can also be RCTs if randomization is used to assign participants to the treatment and control groups. This was the case with the Cambridge-Somerville study, where boys were randomly assigned to the program or control group and then prospectively followed for a 30-year period. Cohort studies using randomization and non-randomization have also been used to investigate the effectiveness of *Head Start* (Lee et al. 1990, Puma et al. 2005).

Understanding and reducing threats to internal validity

In order to verify whether an intervention is effective, one must be able to attribute the cause of the outcome to the treatment. In order to assume this causality, three conditions must be met (from Shadish et al. 2002):

- **Temporal precedence**: the cause precedes effect
- **Covariation of the cause and effect**: there must be a change that could possibly cause the effect
- **No plausible alternative explanations**: this means that it is not likely that something other than the treatment caused the effect.

Internal validity refers to an evaluation design's ability to infer cause and effect. Factors that confound this ability (e.g. other plausible explanations) are referred to as **threats to internal validity** (Campbell 1957).

A good evaluation design minimizes or eliminates threats to internal validity. As noted previously, RCTs are considered the gold standard of evaluation design because the use of a comparison group and randomization substantially reduces the threats to internal validity. However, even the best-designed RCTs are subject to a variety of threats that can confound the results and reduce the ability to attribute causality to the treatment. A variety of authors have developed systems for classifying the different kinds of confounds, including Campbell (1957), Sackett (1979) and Feinstein (1985). While it is beyond the scope of this book to describe all the factors that could potentially confound an evaluation's results, several are discussed below.

Selection bias

Selection bias occurs when there is a difference between the treatment and the comparison groups. As mentioned previously, randomization should minimize selection biases. When randomization is not possible, researchers should take measures to ensure that the treatment and comparison groups are as similar as possible. However, as the example of *Sure Start* suggests, this is more easily said than done. Despite efforts to carefully match *Sure Start* communities to non-*Sure Start* communities on a number of demographic dimensions, *Sure Start* communities were nevertheless more deprived. When the evaluation findings from the first impact study suggested worse outcomes for *Sure Start* communities, it became difficult to attribute these findings to the presence of *Sure Start* or to the fact that *Sure Start* communities were more disadvantaged to begin with (Belsky et al. 2007). Similar issues have plagued the cohort evaluations of *Head Start* (see Lee et al. 1990). Although it is possible to statistically control for group differences, selection bias is always a potential threat to studies that lack randomization.

Information bias

Information bias (also referred to as measurement bias, observation bias, or instrument decay) occurs on account of inconsistencies or inaccuracies in the data collection methods. For example, it is not uncommon for differences to occur in the way in which data is collected. Take the case of a school intervention where post-treatment measures were administered in the morning for the treatment group and in the afternoon for the comparison group. This creates the potential confound of those completing the measures in the morning being more alert and therefore doing better. Other examples of information bias include changes in the wording or ordering of questionnaires and coding 'drift' occurring on account of researchers' understanding of the outcomes they are rating or coding (Grimes and Schulz 2002b).

Information bias can be reduced if evaluators ensure that procedures and instruments remain the same for all participants and all conditions through the use of protocols that standardize the administration of measures across evaluation sites. Information bias is also greatly reduced by the use of standardized measures that have both **construct validity** and **test/retest reliability**. Construct validity means that the measures actually test what they claim they test. For example, when developing a measure of ADHD, data collected from the new measure should be compared to data collected from similar measures to look for consistency. Test/retest reliability means that the measure will produce the same findings when repeated with the same subjects. Standardized measures will be discussed in greater depth in the section describing methods for collecting and analyzing data.

Differential attrition

Differential attrition biases occur when post-treatment change is assessed with data collected only from those who complete the treatment, since there are often differences between participants who complete the program and those who drop out. For example, research suggests that parents experiencing high levels of stress are more likely to drop out of parenting programs than those who are experiencing less stress (Kazdin 1990, Kazdin and Mazurick 1994, Kazdin et al. 1993). Measuring the outcomes of program completers is therefore likely to overestimate the treatment's efficacy, since the findings will be biased towards the higher-functioning parents.

A method for avoiding differential attrition bias is to adopt an **intention-to-treat** evaluation design. Intention-to-treat means that all participants complete the post-treatment measures, regardless of whether they complete the treatment. Thus, the post-treatment scores of program drop-outs are included in the analysis of the study even if they attended only one session. Although some argue that this could artificially deflate a treatment's effect, it is considered a necessary step to reduce the likelihood of grossly overestimating the treatment's effects.

Increasing external validity: from efficacy to effectiveness

Although a randomized controlled trial is widely considered to be the most rigorous method for understanding the impact of a program, a single trial is generally not sufficient. This is because most trials are implemented within clinical or university settings, where it is possible to control multiple factors, including the **target population**, the intensity with which the treatment is provided (also known as **dosage**), practitioner skill and **fidelity**. Once an intervention is transported into community settings, however, most of these factors are no longer under the program developer's control. In this respect, RCTs conducted in clinical or university settings are likely to have low **external validity**.

Take, for example, a new program developed for the parents of children with ADHD. The first trial of the program is delivered by the same individuals who developed the program's content. This virtually ensures that the program is delivered with **fidelity** – i.e. there is an exact fit between the program's model and the way it is implemented. It also ensures that the program is delivered by individuals who understand the content and know how to work with parents with difficult children. In addition, the program developers have access to the appropriate treatment group, as they get referrals for children with ADHD on a weekly basis and have reliable methods for assessing them. Thus, the **eligibility criteria** of the intervention (e.g. only children with ADHD) are also met. A clinical trial may also use methods to incentivize attendance (e.g. monetary rewards, gift vouchers) to ensure that attendance is high so that participants all have the same 'dosage'. (See Chapter 5 for a more in-depth discussion of how eligibility criteria, dosage and fidelity affect program outcomes.) Such high levels of program-developer control are likely to have a favorable influence on the treatment's overall efficacy (Weisz et al. 2005).

Once the program model is delivered in a community setting, program developers often lose control over many key program elements. For example, it is not uncommon for agencies to decrease the specificity of a program's eligibility requirements to improve program participation. However, it is likely that the impact of the program will be less for a parent with a child who does not have ADHD. Similarly, program effects are likely to be weaker if key elements of the intervention model are changed (i.e. loss of fidelity) or parents do not attend all the meetings (i.e. did not receive the proper dosage).

Flay (1986) recommends that a series of trials, falling within the categories listed below, are necessary to fully understand an intervention's effectiveness in real-world settings:

- **Efficacy trials**, which determine the extent to which an intervention is effective under ideal circumstances.
- **Effectiveness trials**, which consider the extent to which a program with demonstrated efficacy under optimal conditions remains effective in real-world settings.
- **Implementation effectiveness**, which considers the conditions under which the intervention is acceptable to the target population and remains effective under these conditions.
- **Program evaluation**, which applies to interventions with unknown efficacy that are already implemented at scale. This kind of evaluation is different than an efficacy trial, because the extent to which the intervention is effective under optimal conditions has not yet been determined.

Flay recommends that the use of efficacy, effectiveness and implementation effectiveness trials should reflect the phase of the intervention's development. Thus, an efficacy trial should be considered required **basic research** before an effectiveness trial, and most certainly before an intervention is implemented at scale. This is likely one of the reasons why the majority of the US home visiting programs described in Chapter 1 failed to achieve their intended outcomes. Developers had not yet fully determined their efficacy under optimal conditions, so it was difficult for them to identify the factors necessary to effectively implement the interventions in new settings.

Hierarchies of evidence

The previous sections make clear that much research is required before an intervention can be considered effective. Interventions and programs vary greatly, however, in terms of the amount and quality of their research evidence. A number of organizations have therefore developed hierarchical systems to judge the quality of an intervention's evidence. Most of these systems place treatments underpinned by multiple RCTs at the top of the hierarchies and studies that do not include a comparison group at the bottom (APA 2002, Chambless and Hollon 1998, Evans 2003, Flay et al. 2005, Sackett et al. 1996, Sherman et al. 1998).

A number of organizations also provide thresholds for determining whether or not an intervention is effective. For example, the *Maryland Scale of Scientific Methods* was developed in the mid 1990s to identify programs that 'work', 'do not work', are 'promising' or have 'unknown' effects in reducing youth offending (see Box 2.4).

Box 2.4: The *Maryland Scale of Scientific Methods*

The *Maryland Scale of Scientific Methods* can be used to understand the strength and quality of an intervention's evaluation evidence. The scale rates evaluation designs on a continuum of 1 to 5 (1 being the lowest and 5 being the highest). The scale's criteria consider both the quality of the evaluation design and the extent to which confounding factors have been adequately taken into account.

The scale has been used by a number of organizations to identify the extent to which a program 'works', 'does not work', is 'promising' or has 'unknown' effects. Criteria used to identify whether a program works include the quality of the program's evaluation design (i.e. was a randomized controlled trial used?), the strength of a program's effect (measured in terms of its effect size), the sustainability of this effect (i.e. does it last over time?) and the extent to which the effect has been replicated through multiple evaluations conducted in multiple settings. Programs that **work** have undergone at least two evaluations involving a comparison group demonstrating a positive significant effect. Programs that are **promising** have undergone at least one evaluation involving a comparison group.

The Society for Prevention Research has more recently issued criteria for determining whether a program is efficacious, effective or ready for wide-scale dissemination (Flay et al. 2005; see Box 2.5).

Hierarchies of evidence have also been developed to understand the efficacy of various methods of clinical practice. These hierarchies recognize the importance of RCTs, but also identify **systematic reviews** as a best source of evidence. Hierarchical frameworks, such as the example provided in Figure 2.5, also recognize the use of expert opinion when no other evidence is available (Evans 2003).

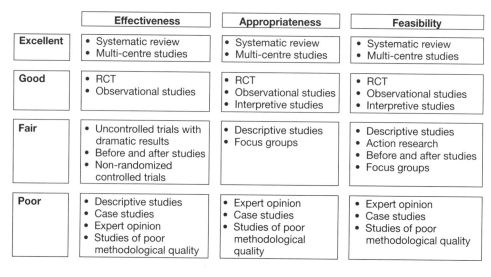

	Effectiveness	Appropriateness	Feasibility
Excellent	• Systematic review • Multi-centre studies	• Systematic review • Multi-centre studies	• Systematic review • Multi-centre studies
Good	• RCT • Observational studies	• RCT • Observational studies • Interpretive studies	• RCT • Observational studies • Interpretive studies
Fair	• Uncontrolled trials with dramatic results • Before and after studies • Non-randomized controlled trials	• Descriptive studies • Focus groups	• Descriptive studies • Action research • Before and after studies • Focus groups
Poor	• Descriptive studies • Case studies • Expert opinion • Studies of poor methodological quality	• Expert opinion • Case studies • Studies of poor methodological quality	• Expert opinion • Case studies • Studies of poor methodological quality

Figure 2.5   Hierarchy of evidence: ranking of research evidence evaluating health care interventions (reprinted with permission from Evans 2003)

Box 2.5: The Society for Prevention Research's Standards of Evidence (Flay et al. 2005)

The Society for Prevention Research (SPR) developed the Standards of Evidence to help policy makers, commissioners and practitioners identify the extent to which a program is effective and ready for wide-scale dissemination.

Programs judged as **efficacious** have undergone at least two trials under ideal conditions that have:

- Used a sufficiently large sample that is representative of the program's target population
- Used standardized measures and data collection procedures
- Analyzed the findings with the appropriate statistical methods
- Observed at least one significant positive long-term outcome.

Programs judged as effective must have met all of the requirements of an efficacious program, but must also have:

- Manuals, training and implementation support so that an external agency can implement the program and achieve positive outcomes
- Undergone a sufficiently rigorous evaluation in real-world settings involving the target population
- Outcomes that are significant and are of practical value
- A clear understanding of who the outcomes do and do not apply to.

Programs judged as ready for wide-scale dissemination must meet all of the standards for efficacious and effective programs, but must also:

- Have the capacity to go to scale through the availability of training materials, training personnel, etc.
- Have accurate information regarding costs and cost-benefits
- Include monitoring and evaluation tools that will enable host agencies to monitor the effectiveness of the program in their own settings.

Systematic reviews are used to understand the overall efficacy of a treatment method. Systematic reviews involve the systematic searching of scientific databases to identify appraise, select and synthesize all the research evidence relevant to a specific research question. Typically, these questions involve the efficacy of a treatment approach rather than a specific treatment model. For example, Dretzke et al. (2009) comprehensively searched 20 scientific databases to identify randomized controlled trials that considered whether parenting programs, in general, were an effective method for reducing the risks associated with child conduct problems. The review identified 57 RCTs which collectively showed favorable effects across the treatment groups, suggesting that parenting programs generally reduced the risks associated with child conduct disorders. The review did not, however, confirm the efficacy of individual parenting interventions.

At the bottom of most hierarchies are qualitative findings, expert opinion and anecdotal opinion. Although these methods cannot be used to determine whether a treatment is effective, they can provide insight as to why, when or how a treatment is effective. In addition, there are many times when there are an insufficient number of good-quality RCTs to determine if an intervention is effective. In these instances, practitioners need to weigh the balance of other forms of evidence, depending upon the needs of their clients and the constraints of their organization (Evans 2003, Sackett et al. 1996).

Data collection and measurement

Validity and reliability

Good-quality data is critical to the success of every research study. Even the best-designed RCT will fail if the data underpinning it is inconsistent or inaccurate. For this reason, a good evaluation design must also include accurate, reliable and objective methods for collecting information and measuring an intervention's efficacy. While it is beyond the scope of this book to describe all of the different ways data can be collected, categorized and analyzed, it is useful to consider a few of the most common methods to provide an understanding of how good-quality data contributes to the understanding of an intervention's efficacy.

Simply put, measurement involves the assignment of numerical values to observations or events according to a set of rules (Stevens 1946). In order to accurately measure a treatment's efficacy, it is crucial that the methods used are valid. Validity, when applied to measurement, means that *a measure measures what it intends to measure*. Good research measures should be valid in four different ways:

- **Face validity** suggests that the measure accurately reflects what it intends to measure in a common-sense way. Thus, a measure of aggression might measure the frequency of aggressive acts – such as shouting, snarling, hitting, etc. – not of other behaviors – such as smiling, laughing or crying.
- **Content validity** refers to the extent to which a measure adequately captures all aspects of the concept being measured. For example, a measure of self-esteem should obtain sufficient information related to the concept – i.e. the feelings, attitudes and behaviors associated with self-esteem – without measuring other similar concepts, such as narcissism, prejudice, etc.
- **Criterion validity** applies to the extent to which a measure is a good predictor of the trait it is measuring, either now or in the future. For example, intelligence tests are said to have high criterion validity because they correlate well with other measures of intelligence (such as school achievement and aptitude tests, etc.) and are good predictors of future intellectual performance.
- **Construct validity** refers to the extent to which a measure is an accurate reflection of the concept being measured. For example, the initial evaluations of *Head Start* used IQ tests to measure the efficacy of the program because it was assumed that IQ would be associated with the main goals of the program, including school readiness and social competence. While the initial increase in IQ observed in the first *Head Start* evaluations appeared to confirm this conclusion, the longer-term follow-ups suggested otherwise, indicating that IQ had poor construct validity when it came to measuring school readiness and social competence. The rapid gain in IQ typically observed over the duration of the program has since been linked to motivational factors related to the administration of the IQ test, rather than the test itself (Schrag et al. 2004, Zigler and Butterfield 1968, Zigler and Trickett 1978).

Reliability refers to a measure's ability to consistently measure concepts, attitudes and behaviors. Good research measures should demonstrate three kinds of reliability:

- **Test/retest reliability** refers to a measure's ability to obtain the same results every time it is administered. IQ tests typically have high test/retest reliability, with individuals consistently obtaining the same score each time they take it.

- **Inter-item reliability** refers to the extent to which measurement items (e.g. questions) included to measure the same concept are, in fact, related to each other. For example, in measures of self-esteem, all items measuring self-esteem should correlate with one another.
- **Inter-observer reliability** refers to the extent to which different researchers (interviewers, observers, etc.) achieve the same results with the same measure. For example, the evaluation of *Sure Start* used video-tapes of parents and children interacting with each other to assess the quality of the parent–child relationship. These tapes were then coded with an observational tool to score the interactions between the parent and child. This tool had high inter-observer reliability, meaning that the scores of two separate observers consistently matched.

Objective vs. subjective data

By definition, objective measures are systems for assigning the same values to the same objects or concepts over and over again. In this respect, a weighing scale is an objective measure, as is a ruler or a yard-stick. Psychometrically valid measures can similarly objectively measure behavior, personality, perceptions, attitudes, beliefs, intelligence and feelings. Objective measures should be used whenever possible to gather information about a treatment's efficacy. Examples of commonly used measures include standardized instruments and observational rating scales, which are both described in the sections below.

Subjective measures, on the other hand, are methods used to capture participants' subjective experience of a treatment or program. Examples of subjective methods include satisfaction surveys and qualitative investigations which explore opinions and attitudes. While these methods may provide insight as to *why* a treatment is effective, subjective measures should not be used to verify whether an intervention *is* effective.

The use of standardized validated measures

A key way to understand a program's efficacy is to test whether change has occurred between the beginning and end of the treatment. In order to do this accurately, the same measure must be administered once before the treatment takes place and then again afterwards. A **t-test** can then be used to measure whether the pre- and post-treatment change is significant. Although it is not possible to attribute this change to the treatment without a comparison group, a significant change in the predicted direction is a positive sign that an intervention may work. For this reason, it is considered good practice to measure pre- and post-treatment change before investing in a randomized controlled trial. Pre- and post-treatment measures are also a good way for organizations to monitor the efficacy of their services.

It is considered good practice to use **standardized valid measures** to assess pre and post change whenever possible. Standardized measures are questionnaires and assessment tools that have been psychometrically tested as valid and reliable. In other words, they have demonstrated face, content, criterion and construct validity and they reliably produce the same findings when they are repeated. Just as scales need to be calibrated, measures need to go through a fair number of revisions before they can be considered valid and reliable. It is near impossible for a researcher to establish the validity of a measure at the same time that he or she is trying to investigate whether or not a treatment is effective.

The initial evaluations of *Head Start* involving IQ testing illustrate how standardized measures can be used in a preliminary way to investigate the efficacy of an intervention.

IQ tests are **norm-referenced** standardized measures of cognitive functioning. 'Norm-referenced' means that individual performance is compared to a population-based average. 'Standardized' means that measures are administered in the same, standardized way every time. IQ tests are also recognized for having high levels of test/retest reliability. In the *Head Start* studies, the participants' IQ was assessed pre and post program. Changes in IQ that may have occurred over the duration of the *Head Start* program were then assessed against those observed amongst the norm-referenced IQ scores. The 8- to 10-point improvement observed within the *Head Start* group was significantly higher than the changes observed within the norm-referenced sample, suggesting that the program was likely to be effective, since such changes are rarely observed within normal preschool populations.

Other examples of standardized measures include the *Strengths and Difficulties Questionnaire* (SDQ), the *Child Behavioral Checklist* (CBCL) and the *Eyberg Child Behavior Inventory*. All three of these instruments have undergone extensive psychometric validation and are considered to be good measures of children's behavior and emotional functioning. Comprehensive lists of standardized parent and child measures are provided in Tables 2.1 and 2.2.

Table 2.1 Standardized measures for assessing parenting behaviors

Name of measure	Description of measure	Administration	How to obtain
Measures of parental competency and sense of efficacy			
Parenting Daily Hassles	A 20-item scale used to assess the frequency and intensity of 20 experiences that can be a 'hassle' to parents. The totals for the frequency and intensity items can be obtained. Two dimensions can also be calculated. Dimensions include: challenging behavior (e.g. 'being nagged, whined at, or complained to') and parenting tasks ('difficulties getting kids ready for outings on time').	Parent questionnaire. It is particularly suited for parents or caregivers of young children.	Free Available at: http://www.dh.gov. uk/en/Publications andstatistics/ Publications/ PublicationsPolicy AndGuidance/DH_ 4008144
Parenting Sense of Competence Scale (PSOC) – 'Being a Parent'	This 17-item scale measures satisfaction with the parenting role (reflecting the extent of parental frustration, anxiety and motivation) and feelings of efficacy as a parent (reflecting competence, problem-solving ability and capability in the parenting role).	Parent questionnaire	Free, but permission must be received, to use scale contact: JPWanders@aol. com. Scale available at: http://www. fasttrackproject.org/ allmeasures.htm Gibaud-Wallston and Wandersman (1978)

Name of measure	Description of measure	Administration	How to obtain
Parenting Stress Index (PSI)	A measure of child characteristics, parent characteristics and parent–child relationship associated with the presence of parenting stress and troubled relationships. The full version contains 101 items, but a 36-item short version is available. Child subscales include: Distractibility/ Hyperactivity, Adaptability, Reinforces Parents, Demandingness, Mood and Acceptability. Parental subscales include: Competence, Social Isolation, Attachment, Health, Role Restriction, Depression and Relationship with Spouse. The total score and the subscale, Sense of Competence in Parenting Role, is of particular interest for this expected outcome.	Parent questionnaire. PSI can be used with parents whose children are 12 years of age or younger (main focus on preschool children)	$62.00 – Manual; $175.00 – Manual and re-usable forms. Scale and manual available from: www.mhs.com www.parinc.com Scale developed by Abidin (1995)

Parent's use of discipline and behavior management

Name of measure	Description of measure	Administration	How to obtain
Alabama Parenting Questionnaire	A questionnaire measuring parenting practices shown to be associated with behavioral problems in children. The longer version of the questionnaire has 42 items and measures five factors: Positive Parenting, Poor Monitoring/Supervision, Inconsistent Parenting, Parental Involvement and Corporal Punishment. A shortened version has nine items and measures the first three factors.	Parent questionnaire & Child questionnaire	Free measure, but not manual. Manual available from Consulting Psychologists Press. Form available at: http://fs.uno.edu/pfrick/ APQ.html Scale developed by Frick (1991)
Conflict Tactics Scale: Parent–Child interaction (CTS–PC)	A measure of psychological and physical maltreatment and neglect of children by parents, as well as nonviolent modes of discipline. The scales include items that describe constructive conflict tactics and verbal aggression; the measure's primary focus is on physically aggressive acts of intimidation and coercion. Dimensions include: Aggression, Violence, Nonviolent Discipline, Psychological Aggression, Physical Assault, Neglect, Weekly Discipline and Sexual Abuse.	Parent questionnaire; Child self-report questionnaire also available. CTS–PC can be used with parents of children aged 10 to 18	$54.50 – Handbook only; $82.50 – Handbook and forms. Permission required from M.A. Straus. Available at: www.wpspublish.com/ Scale developed by Straus (1979)
Parenting Scale	A measure of three styles of dysfunctional parenting: over-reactivity (authoritarian discipline, anger and irritability), verbosity (overly long reprimands or reliance on talking) and laxness (permissive discipline). The measure contains 30 items and is intended to be independent of child misbehavior. It can therefore be used to identify parents of children at risk of developing severe behavior problems before problems develop.	Parent questionnaire	Free Forms available at: http://www.health.vic. gov.au/communityhealth/ downloads/p_scale.pdf Scale developed by Arnold et al. (1993)

Continued overleaf

Name of measure	Description of measure	Administration	How to obtain
Family relationships			
Dyadic Adjustment Scale (DAS)	A measure consisting of 32 items measuring relationship satisfaction and couple's adjustment in a relationship. Dimensions include: Consensus, Satisfaction, Cohesion and Affectional Expression. The measure is worded such that it is applicable to married or cohabiting dyads.	Parent questionnaire	$45.00 – Forms (×20); $70.00 – Manual and forms. Available at: www.mhs.com Scale developed by Spanier (1976)
Conflict Tactics Scale: Parent–Child interaction (CTS–PC)	A measure of psychological and physical maltreatment and neglect of children by parents, as well as nonviolent modes of discipline. The scales include items that describe constructive conflict tactics and verbal aggression; the measure's primary focus is on physically aggressive acts of intimidation and coercion. Dimensions include: Aggression, Violence, Nonviolent Discipline, Psychological Aggression, Physical Assault, Neglect, Weekly Discipline and Sexual Abuse.	Parent questionnaire; Child self-report questionnaire also available. CTS–PC can be used with parents of children aged 10 to 18	$54.50 – Handbook only; $82.50 – Handbook and forms. Permission required from M.A. Straus. Available at: www.wpspublish.com/ Scale developed by Straus (1979)
McMasters Family Assessment Device	A measure consisting of 53 items which assesses dimensions of family functioning and overall health and pathology of the family. Dimensions include: Problem Solving, Communication, Roles, Affective Responsiveness, Affective Involvement and Behavior Control.	Parent questionnaire & Child questionnaire	Copyrighted instrument with scoring available in: Ryan et al. (2005) Can also be purchased by contacting Dr Christine Ryan at: Ryan@Brown.edu Scale developed by Epstein et al. (1983)
Parenting Stress Index (PSI)	A measure of child characteristics, parent characteristics and parent–child relationship associated with the presence of parenting stress and troubled relationships. The full version contains 101 items, but a 36-item short version is available. Child subscales include: Distractibility/ Hyperactivity, Adaptability, Reinforces Parents, Demandingness, Mood and Acceptability. Parental subscales include: Competence, Social Isolation, Attachment, Health, Role Restriction, Depression and Relationship with Spouse. The total score and the subscale, Relationship with Spouse/Parenting Partner, is of particular interest for this expected outcome.	Parent questionnaire. PSI can be used with parents whose children are 12 years of age or younger (main focus on preschool children)	$62.00 – Manual; $175.00 – Manual and re-usable forms. Scale and manual available from: www.mhs.com www.parinc.com Scale developed by Abidin (1995)

Name of measure	Description of measure	Administration	How to obtain
Parental mental health			
Beck Anxiety Inventory (BAI)	A measure of the severity of anxiety which contains 21 items. Each item refers to a symptom of anxiety and contains a list of four statements arranged in increasing severity from not at all to severe.	Parent questionnaire	$49.00 – forms (×25); $109.00 – manual and forms (×25). Available at: http://harcourtassessment.com Scale developed by Beck et al. (1988)
Beck Depression Inventory (BDI-II)	A measure of the severity of depressive symptoms containing 21 items. Each item refers to a symptom of depression and contains a list of four statements arranged in increasing severity. Subscales include: somatic-affective factor and a cognitive factor.	Parent questionnaire	$49.00 – forms (×25); $109.00 – manual and forms (×25). Available at: http://harcourtassessment.com Scale developed by Beck et al. (1996)
Depression Anxiety Stress Scale (DASS)	A measure of three dimensions: Depression, Anxiety and Stress. Each dimension contains 14 items, each with a four-point scale relating to the extent to which the parent has experienced each item over the past week.	Parent questionnaire	Free forms and scoring sheets but not manual; $55.00 – manual. Available at: http://www2.psy.unsw.edu.au/groups/dass/ Scale developed by Lovibond and Lovibond (1995)
Drinker Inventory of Consequences (DrInC)	A measure of the overall consequences to document changes in consequences over time and with treatment interventions. Contains 50 items evaluating five alcohol-related areas: Physical, Intrapersonal, Social Responsibility, Interpersonal and Impulse Control over lifetime (DrInC-2L) and since last interview (DrInC-2R).	Parent questionnaire	Free Available at: http://casaa.unm.edu/inst.html Scale developed by Miller et al. (1995)
Inventory of Drug Use Consequences (InDUC)	A measure of the overall consequences of substance misuse as a way to document changes in consequences over time and with treatment interventions. Contains 50 items evaluating substance misuse-related areas: Physical, Intrapersonal, Social Responsibility, Interpersonal and Impulse Control over lifetime (InDUC-2L) and since last interview (InDUC-2R).	Parent questionnaire	Free Available at: http://casaa.unm.edu/inst.html Scale developed by Tonigan and Miller (2002)
Timeline Followback (TLFB)	A measure of the frequency and quantity of substance use on a daily basis. The measure uses a calendar as a guide, along with other memory aids to help the parent provide a retrospective estimate of daily drinking or drug use over a specified time period (up to one year).	Parent questionnaire	Free forms but not manual; $39.95 – manual and $99.50 – training video can also be purchased. Available at: http://www.nova.edu/gsc/ Scale developed by Sobell and Sobell (1992)

Table 2.2 Standardized measures for assessing child behaviors, emotional wellbeing and achievement

Name of measure	Description of measure	Outcomes measured	Administration	How to obtain
Beck Youth Inventories (Anger Inventory)	The *Beck Youth Inventory* consists of five 20-item scales that can be used separately or in combination. Designed for children and adolescents aged 7 to 18, the instruments measure emotional and social impairment in five specific areas: Depression, Anxiety, Anger, Disruptive Behavior and Self-concept. The Anger Inventory includes items about perceptions of mistreatment, negative thoughts about others, feelings of anger, and physiological arousal. Beck's Anxiety Inventory (BAI) is a questionnaire intended to assess general anxiety symptoms in children and adolescents aged 7–14 years. It contains 21 items and takes 5–10 minutes to complete. This scale can be used for measuring improvements with treatments on anxiety symptoms. The Beck Depression Inventory (BDI, BDI-II), is a 21-question multiple-choice self-report inventory, one of the most widely used instruments for measuring the severity of depression. It is designed for individuals aged 13 and over, and contains items relating to symptoms of depression such as hopelessness and irritability, cognitions such as guilt or feelings of being punished, as well as physical symptoms such as fatigue and weight loss. The Disruptive Behavior Inventory taps into behaviors and attitudes associated with Conduct Disorder and Oppositional Defiant Disorder.	Behavior, Emotions	Children and adolescents; suitable for group or individual administration	£40.50 for scoring forms; £57.50 for manual. Contact: Pearson Assessment http://www. psychcorp.co.uk/ Tel: 0845 630 88 88 Email: info@ psychcorp.co.uk
Child Behavior Checklist (CBCL)	A questionnaire used to measure a child's problem behaviors and competencies. The first section consists of 20 competence items and the second section consists of 120 items on behavior or emotional problems during the past 6 months. Two versions of this instrument exist: one for children aged 1½–5 and another for ages 6–18. Dimensions measured include: Aggressive Behavior, Anxious/Depressed Behavior, Attention Problems, Delinquent Rule-Breaking Behavior, Social Problems, Somatic Complaints, Thought Problems, Withdrawn Symptoms, Externalizing and Internalizing Behaviors.	Behavior, Emotions	Parent/teacher questionnaire. A youth and direct observation version also available. Can be self-administered or part of an interview.	£8 – Reusable form; £22 – standard forms; £34 for manual. Contact: Achenbach System of Empirically Based Assessment http://www1.aston. ac.uk/lhs/aseba/ Email: lhs_aseba@ aston.ac.uk

Name of measure	Description of measure	Outcomes measured	Administration	How to obtain
Child Health Questionnaire	The *Child Health Questionnaire* (CHQ) was developed for children and adolescents 5 years of age and older. The CHQ assesses a child's physical, emotional, and social wellbeing from the perspective of a parent or guardian (CHQ-PF50 and PF-28 (short form)) or, in some instances, the child directly (CHQ-CF87, for children 10 years of age and older). Areas measured include: physical functioning, bodily pain or discomfort, general health, change in health, limitations in schoolwork, limitations in activities with friends, mental health, behavior, self-esteem, family cohesion, limitations in family activities, emotional or time impact on the parent. Example item: 'How much of the time do you think your child: felt lonely; acted nervous; bothered or upset?'	Health, Emotions, Self-esteem, Achievement	Parent or child (10 yrs+) report	Landgraf and Ware (Landgraf et al. 1996) www.healthact.com/chq.html
Child Health and Illness Profile	The *Child Health and Illness Profile* (CHIP) describes the health and wellbeing of youths aged 6–17. There is a child/parent version (ages 6–11) which takes 15 minutes to complete, and an adolescent version (ages 11–17) which takes 25 minutes to complete. The child version taps into 4 domains of health: Satisfaction, Comfort, Resilience and Risk Avoidance. Child version reports symptoms of illness and wellbeing, health-related behaviors, problem behavior, school performance, and involvement with family and peers are reported. The majority of items assess frequency of events, typically over the past 4 weeks, using a 5-point response format (never to always), e.g. 'Over the past 4 weeks how often did you feel really worried?' Items on the Child Report Form (CRF) are illustrated with cartoon-type characters. The adolescent version taps into 5 health-related domains: Satisfaction, Comfort, Risk Avoidance, Resilience, and Achievement. The adolescent version reports symptoms of illness and of health-protective behaviors, satisfaction with health and with themselves, problem behavior, school performance, and involvement with family.	Achievement, Health, Wellbeing	Child, adolescent and parent versions	http://www.childhealthprofile.org/ chipinfo@jhsph.edu Free for academic and school researchers and evaluators. Developed by Starfield & Riley (1998)
Eyberg's Child Behavior Inventory	Designed to assess the current frequency and severity of disruptive behaviors in the home and school settings, as well as the extent to which parents and/or teachers find the behavior troublesome. This 38-item measure distinguishes normal behavior problems from conduct-disordered behavior in children and adolescents aged 2 to 16.	Behavior, Achievement	Parent/teacher questionnaire; suitable for group administration or via telephone	£33 – forms only; £45 for manual. Contact: Ann Arbor Publishers http://www.annarbor.co.uk/ Created by Sheila Eyberg, PhD

Continued overleaf

Name of measure	Description of measure	Outcomes measured	Administration	How to obtain
Moods and Feelings Questionnaire	Child and/or parent is asked to rate on a 3-point scale (true, sometimes, not true) statements in relation to how they/their child have felt over the past two weeks e.g. I (she/he) felt awful or unhappy. There is a full-length (33 item) or shortened version (13 items) for both child and parent	Emotions	Child and parent reports	Developed by Angold et al. (1995)
Multidimensional Anxiety Scale for Children (MASC)	Assess anxiety symptoms across clinically significant symptom domains with this empirically derived instrument. The MASC consists of the following scales and indexes: Physical Symptoms Scale, Social Anxiety Scale, Harm Avoidance Scale, Separation/Panic Scale, Anxiety Disorders Index, Total Anxiety Index, Inconsistency Index. The MASC has a 4th-grade reading level and can be used in a number of settings such as schools, outpatient clinics, and child protective services. The MASC-10, a 10-item version, is designed for repeated testing. The MASC-10 takes approximately 5 minutes to administer and score and is particularly suited for group-testing situations.	Emotions	Child report	www. pearsonassessments. com Complete MASC kit: $86 Complete MASC and MASC-10 kit: $113 Developed by March (1997)
Strengths & Difficulties Questionnaire (SDQ)	A behavioral screening questionnaire for children aged 4 to 16, a preschool-age version is available for children aged 3 to 4. The measure has been translated into over 60 languages. Five scores are generated: emotional symptoms, conduct problems, hyperactivity/inattention, peer relationship problems and pro-social behaviour.	Behavior, Emotions, Peer relations	Parent/teacher questionnaire. A youth (ages 11–16) version also available	Free Measures and Scoring guidance. Download forms at: http://www.sdqinfo. com Scale is available without permission or charge for non-commercial purposes. Developed by Goodman (1997)

It is important to note that standardized measures may not yet exist for some treatments (Decker 2008). This was the case for the early *Head Start* evaluations, where IQ tests were used to evaluate the program because measures of school readiness and social competence were not readily available. Another limitation to standardized measures is that they are not always validated with the appropriate population. This was another criticism made against the use of IQ tests with the *Head Start* participants, as they were validated with a predominately white, middle-class sample, but were nevertheless used to assess change amongst disadvantaged minority-ethnic children. Additional drawbacks of validated measures include the fact that they often require appropriately trained professionals to administer them and they frequently require permission for use that may involve some form of payment.

Observational methods

Observational methods refer to the use of standardized observational systems to rate children's and parents' behaviors on a variety of dimensions. Observational measures are frequently referred to as the 'gold standard' of measurement because they assess actual behaviors rather than children's and parents' self-reports. Observational methods impose structure over the observational process through the use of rating scales that quantify human behaviors. Researchers are trained to use these scales by establishing **inter-observer reliability** between themselves and a head rater. If it is difficult to establish inter-observer reliability between observers, it can mean that the rating scale is not accurately assessing behavior, or the observers have not been properly trained.

Observations are often made of video-taped interactions between parents and children. Video-taping makes it easy to watch certain behaviors repeatedly and also ensures that raters are 'blind' to other factors that may be affecting the family. Observational studies can take place in controlled laboratory settings or in more natural surroundings, such as a home or classroom.

Observational methods may be used in randomized controlled trials or cross-sectional studies. Observational methods were used in both *Sure Start* impact evaluations, where trained researchers went into participants' homes and rated mother-and-child interactions. These ratings were then converted into scores that were used for comparisons between the *Sure Start* and non-*Sure Start* samples. Observational methods have also been used in many of the studies informing the development of evidence-based parenting programs, which will be described in greater detail in Chapter 3.

Understanding process: the various uses of qualitative research

The use of standardized measures and statistical tests provides **quantitative** evidence of an intervention's efficacy. **Quantitative methods** are widely considered to be the most robust way of measuring impact because they can be used efficiently with large samples and their objective nature reduces the potential of evaluator or practitioner bias. However, quantitative methods have their drawbacks. While they are the best way of determining *whether* an intervention works, they cannot necessarily clarify *why* or *how* an intervention works. Nor can they fully explain why an intervention *does not* work. When this information is required, **qualitative methods** are useful, as they can contextualize quantitative findings and may provide answers to important questions the evaluator may not have originally thought to ask. Qualitative research is particularly useful for exploring the relevance of an intervention as it is being developed. Qualitative studies can also be used to follow up quantitative studies to understand why an intervention may or may not have worked.

Take, for example, a service manager who is concerned about a school-based agency offering an evidence-based parenting group in the evenings at a school during term time. The program has been running for over a year and quantitative assessments involving standardized pre and post measures of previous groups suggest that parents are generally satisfied with the intervention and that their parenting skills measurably improve. However, one of the training programs suddenly has a high attrition rate, with over half of the participants dropping out between half and two-thirds of the way through the program. The service manager is not sure if this drop-out is related to the characteristics of the practitioner facilitating the group, the parents who attend the group or some other issue that she has not identified.

The service manager is concerned that the program is not meeting the needs of the parents who dropped out. She compares the characteristics (e.g. **demographics**) of the parents who completed the course against those who dropped out and cannot see any obvious differences between the groups. The service manager wonders whether the parents did not like the practitioner, but knows that this individual has successfully run parenting groups in the past. She considers contacting the parents herself, but does not really have the time, and also wonders whether the parents will give her an honest answer. It is important that she finds out why half of the parents left the intervention, since it is expensive to run and its overall impact will be reduced if attendance is not sufficiently high.

The service manager therefore decides to hire an independent evaluator to conduct **semi-structured interviews** with the parents to find out why some dropped out. The use of an independent evaluator will improve the likelihood that the respondents are honest and that the interpretation of the findings is objective. The use of open-ended questions will allow the evaluator to consider issues that the service manager and practitioner may not have already thought of. Once the evaluator contacts the parents, he learns that while all of them liked the group facilitator and the content of the course, the next series of *Strictly Come Dancing* started midway during the group. Those who dropped out did so because the show's time conflicted with the group, but were reluctant to tell the practitioner because they were afraid they would be perceived as bad parents by putting a television show before improving their parenting skills. Once the service manager discovered that this was the problem, she was able to explore ways of proactively addressing this issue at the beginning of the next parenting intervention.

Focus groups are another method for finding out why and how an intervention works. For example, Miller and Sambell (2003) wanted to understand how parents' perceptions of parenting groups influenced their willingness to attend. They did not have the resources to do lengthy interviews with many parents, so they conducted a series of seven focus groups consisting of 4–6 parents each. The focus groups involved researchers asking participants a number of open-ended questions about the reasons why they might and might not attend a parenting group. The focus group sessions were tape-recorded and then transcribed. The researchers then carefully read the transcriptions and analyzed them for themes arising from the data.

The researchers observed that when parents seek help, they usually do so for reasons falling into one of three categories: dispensing, relating or reflecting. *Dispensing* support generally comes in the form of specific information or advice that enables the parent to 'fix' their child. An example of dispensing support might include advice on how to set limits. Parents are likely to pay greater attention to dispensing advice if they know that it is coming from an expert. *Relating* support, on the other hand, does not involve advice, but instead addresses parents' emotional needs. Parenting seeking *relating* support often want validation and reassurance that their feelings and experiences as a parent are normal. Examples of relating support include opportunities for parents to share their frustrations with other parents. The third category, *reflecting* support, includes any form of information or training that enhances parents' understanding of their children. This goes beyond wanting to know *what* one should do as a parent (the dispensing model), but *why* one should do it. Miller and Sambell found that all parents seek support for a variety of reasons, but primarily come for dispensing support. In fact, parents are likely to be disappointed with parenting interventions if they do not provide them with specific advice that will help them manage their children.

Finding evidence-based interventions and programs

Systematic literature searches

By definition, evidence-based practice means keeping up to date with the current best evidence. This is becoming an increasingly difficult task, however. It is estimated that at least one scientific journal article is published every minute of every day. At the time of this writing, it is estimated that the online database PubMed holds over 19 million citations and Scopus has indexed over 40 million (Hull 2010). In addition, the knowledge 'turnover' is occurring at an increasingly rapid pace. Within the field of medicine, it is estimated that a student graduating in the 1950s knew about 80 per cent of what there was to know about medicine and most of this knowledge would have remained up-to-date for about 25 years. It is estimated that these days a graduating medical student will know only 40 per cent of what there is to know and half of this knowledge will be out of date within 10 years (Dawes et al. 2005). As discussed in Chapter 1, the field of family and parenting support has witnessed a similar rapid expansion. Literally hundreds of interventions have been developed and a growing number have been tested in real-world settings. We now know much more about interventions that work for children and parents, as well as those that do not work, than we did 20 years ago (O'Connell et al. 2009).

Given the size of the evidence base, it is difficult for practitioners to continually stay current with the research evidence. Fortunately, a number of strategies now exist to help practitioners systematically search for the information they need, when they need it. These strategies include thorough and objective methods for systematically searching scientific databases to identify evidence-based interventions for parents and children. The Cochrane Collaboration (Higgins and Green 2008) recommends that a systematic search of the research literature include the following steps:

1   Formulate the problem or search question
2   Locate and select the studies
3   Critically appraise the studies
4   Collect the data
5   Analyze the results
6   Interpret the results
7   Apply the findings.

Good questions get good answers

Systematic literature searches are particularly useful when decisions must be made regarding service provision (Mulrow 1994). The most productive searches begin with a clear and structured question that is specific to a practitioner's or service agency's needs. Melnyk and

Fineout-Overholt (2010) recommend using the acronym PICOT to formulate clear literature search questions:

- **Population** refers to the people the question is investigating – e.g. their age, gender, needs, location, role, etc.
- **Intervention** refers to the method for addressing the population's needs
- **Comparison** can involve another intervention or no intervention
- **Outcome** refers to what the intervention may wish to achieve
- **Time** refers to the time period when the intervention may be relevant.

Take the example of a maternity service team that is concerned that it is not adequately detecting and providing support for mothers with postnatal depression (PND). It wants to conduct a systematic review to find out whether any specific interventions could be implemented through its practice. It formulates the following PICOT question:

> Does additional therapeutic support (intervention) during the first six months postpartum (time) reduce the symptoms of postnatal depression (outcome) in mothers (population) in comparison to standard postnatal care (comparison)?

Searching the literature

Once the research question is formulated, the team must then determine where to look for information. While it is beyond the scope of this book to provide the specific details of search methods (good overviews are provided in Aveyard and Sharp 2009, Dawes et al. 2005, Gibbs 2003 and Melnyk and Fineout-Overholt 2010), literature reviews typically involve the following three steps:

1   **Identify the sources of data**. Many search engines and databases are available for a variety of different subject areas. Ovid, Medline, PsychoInfo, Social Care Online, Science Direct, the BMJ Index and Cochrane Database of Systematic Reviews are examples of comprehensive databases covering research from the fields of psychiatry, psychology, education and social work. Google can be a good place to explore a search topic, but is not specific enough to effectively search literature within restricted subject areas.
2   **Identify appropriate search terms**. Identifying key terms is not an exact science and often involves a bit of trial and error. A good place to start is to explore the topic on Google, identify one or two good articles and identify their key words.
3   **Establish the selection criteria**. Selection criteria involve both inclusion and exclusion criteria. Examples of **inclusion criteria** include specific dates (e.g. 1995 onwards), published literature only[3] (as opposed to dissertations and unpublished studies), specific settings and language(s). Exclusion criteria might include non-English languages, unpublished research, dates, specific populations, etc.

Literature searches typically result in thousands of hits, even when the search terms are clear and specific. Returning to the example of the primary care team, its initial search returned over 15,000 hits. It was able to reduce its hits to 945 after it refined its search terms several times. After sorting out the duplications, the team identified 340 articles which the members each reviewed independently with respect to the selection criteria. There was 90 per cent agreement between the team members regarding the studies, resulting in 83 studies that required further review.

Critical appraisal

Once all studies meeting the selection criteria are identified, it is time to assess the quality of the research through critical appraisal. There are three key questions to consider when critically appraising a piece of research:

- What are the results of the study?
- Are the results valid?
- Are the results relevant?

In order to answer these questions, one must have knowledge of how research is conducted and what constitutes valid research findings. The first half of this chapter provided an overview of the issues involved in determining the extent to which an intervention is effective. This same knowledge forms the starting point for critically appraising a research study. Box 2.6 provides an overview of questions[4] to consider when critically appraising an **experimental study**.

Answering the questions outlined in Box 2.6 will provide a good understanding of the results of the study and the extent to which they are valid. However, they cannot determine whether the findings are relevant for an individual practitioner or agency. The extent to which the findings are relevant can be determined only by the specific needs of the individuals appraising the research.

Returning to the example of the maternity services team, its literature search returned five systematic reviews, three of which included a meta-review. A **meta-review** (also called a meta-analysis) considers the findings of multiple studies investigating similar interventions

---

Box 2.6: Questions for appraising an experimental study

- What were the characteristics of the participants?
- Were the groups similar at the start of the study?
- Were the participants representative of the target population?
- What was the treatment?
- What was (were) the comparison(s)?
- Aside from the treatment, were both groups treated equally?
- Were all the participants properly accounted for at the conclusion of the study? In other words, did the study include an intention-to-treat analysis?
- Did the study use randomization?
- Were the participants and researchers blind to the treatment and comparison group assignments?
- Was the length of the study appropriate?
- Did the study appropriately consider all potential threats to internal validity?
- What was the effect?
- How generalizable are the findings?

and statistically combines their effect sizes to calculate a **meta-effect size**. A meta-effect size is believed to be a more powerful estimate of the true effect size of a treatment than a single effect size.

Two meta reviews suggested that home visiting PND services resulted in a high meta-effect. Moreover, one review identified a specific treatment for PND demonstrating substantial effect sizes in community settings that could be delivered by appropriately trained nurses. After reading these articles, the maternity nurse team was pleased to have identified a specific treatment for PND that was practical for its agency to deliver. This allowed the team to investigate opportunities for additional training so that it could learn how to deliver the treatment.

Systems that summarize and synthesize research

As the maternity nurse team's example suggests, literature searches can be time consuming and not necessarily practical when time and resources are scarce. For this reason, a number of organizations provide systems and services which summarize and synthesize research findings. Haynes (2006) has observed that these systems can be organized into what he calls the '5S' hierarchical model, provided in Figure 2.6, that places individual research studies on the bottom and computerized decision-support systems on the top.

When the maternity nurse team began its search, it identified both individual studies and **systematic reviews**. Systematic reviews are defined as 'concise studies of the best available evidence that address sharply defined clinical questions' (Mulrow et al. 1997: 389). Systematic reviews examine the evidence by systematically searching databases for research studies in a given topic area. Once the search is complete, the reviews synthesize the findings in a way that is meaningful for practice. As mentioned previously, the maternity nurse's

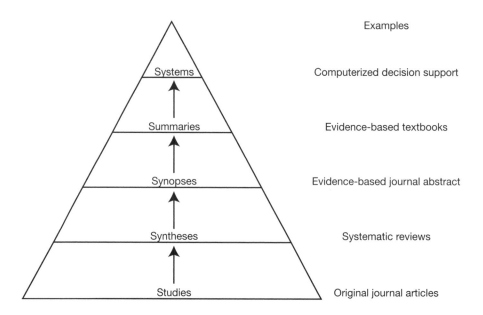

Figure 2.6 The '5S' levels of organization of evidence from health care research (reprinted with permission from Haynes 2006)

search identified several meta-reviews which aggregated the findings from similar studies to report a meta-effect.

Systematic reviews conducted by the Cochrane Collaboration are widely considered to be the most rigorous. Each review begins with a protocol that outlines the review question, the assessment criteria and the ways in which the researchers will manage the review process. The Cochrane Collaboration also manages the Cochrane Library, which houses a collection of seven electronic databases, one of which is the Cochrane Database of Systematic Reviews (CDSR). The Cochrane Library 2010, Issue 9 included 4,372 published reviews and 1,950 protocols.

The Campbell Collaboration was formed in 2000 as the sister organization to the Cochrane Collaboration in the US. While the Cochrane Collaboration primarily focuses on research pertaining to human health, the Campbell Collaboration reviews research in the areas of education, criminal justice, social policy and social care. Information about the Cochrane Collaboration can be found at http://www.cochrane.org. Information about the Campbell Collaboration can be found at http://www.campbellcollaboration.org/.

Moving up the '5S' hierarchy, **synopses** refer to academic journals which provide information on important advances in evidence-based practice on a regular basis. These journals use strict criteria to identify top-quality studies which are then appraised by clinicians for their validity and relevance. Examples of these journals in the field of medicine include *Evidence-Based Medicine* and *ACP Journal Club*.

Summaries aim to integrate the best available evidence (from studies, systematic reviews, etc.) to inform practice decisions about a specific health problem. In this sense, summaries make explicit recommendations, whereas studies, syntheses and synopses leave the decision making to the practitioner or service manager. Examples of summaries include evidence-based textbooks and information publicized on websites such as *Social Care Online* (managed by the Social Care Institute for Excellence (SCIE) available at http://www.scie-socialcare-online.org.uk and *Research into Practice* at http://www.rip.org.uk. The National Institute for Health and Clinical Excellence (NICE) also provides up-to-date information and guidance on promoting good physical and mental health. More information about NICE can be found at http://www.nice.org.uk.

Computerized decision-support systems (CDSS) are at the very top of the '5S' hierarchy. Ideally, CDSS allow practitioners to identify the most up-to-date research evidence that matches a specific client's individual circumstances. However, Haynes cautions that these systems are still relatively limited in their scope and are rarely up-to-date. Within the field of medicine *Clinical Evidence* aims to provide up-to-date research evidence applying to a wide variety of child mental health issues within the UK. The *Physician's Information and Education Resource* (PIER) plays a similar role in the US.

Web-based rating systems

The systems described through the '5S' hierarchy are particularly good for identifying interventions which aim to improve children's mental health outcomes through the use of clinical treatments. However, these websites contain relatively little information about prevention or intervention programs which can be implemented through schools and communities. Information about these kinds of interventions is better accessed via a number of US and UK websites sponsored by agencies which review and rate the quality of specific evidence-based programs. Within the US, these agencies include *Blueprints for Violence Prevention* and SAMHSA (the Substance Abuse and Mental Health Services Administration). *Blueprints for*

Violence Prevention rates programs via a rigorous system that considers the extent to which there is 1) strong evidence of improved outcomes (measured via rigorously conducted RCTs), that is 2) observable over a sustained period of time and is 3) replicable across multiple settings. Programs receiving a *model* rating must meet all three criteria via multiple research trials (e.g. effectiveness trials). Programs identified *promising* need only to have provided strong evidence of a short-term outcome. The *Blueprints for Violence* website can be accessed at http://www.colorado.edu/cspv/blueprints/.

The National Registry of Evidence-based Programs and Practices (NREPP, managed by SAMHSA) rates programs in terms of the quality of their evidence in terms of specific outcomes (e.g. juvenile delinquency, school achievement, etc.) and their 'readiness for dissemination' on a scale from 1 to 4. Both *Blueprints* and NREPP also provide information regarding programs' cost-effectiveness, staffing requirements (including qualifications and training needs), the settings in which programs work and the administration costs.

Within the UK, the Children's Workforce Development Council and the National Academy for Parenting Research co-sponsor the *Commissioning Toolkit*. The *Toolkit* provides commissioners of family-based services with an understanding of what constitutes an effective parenting intervention by rating programs on a scale from 0 to 4 in terms of four elements:

- **Element 1: The quality of the specification of the target population** considers the extent to which the program specifies who it is designed for (e.g. eligibility requirements, including age of participants, ethnicity, or mental health needs) and processes for assessing families for treatment.
- **Element 2: The quality of the program content and processes** assesses the program's theoretical framework, its learning outcomes, the format of learning and the resources available to practitioners for delivering the program.
- **Element 3: How practitioners are trained and supported to deliver the program in a consistent and effective manner** considers information regarding the experience and qualifications required of practitioners to deliver the program, the quality of practitioner training, supervisory arrangements and systems for implementing the program and monitoring fidelity.
- **Element 4: The quality of the evaluations used to prove the effectiveness of the program in achieving its targeted outcomes** considers the quality of the research underpinning the program's effectiveness, including the degree to which the program achieved its intended outcomes and the extent to which multiple RCTs were used to establish its evidence base.

Summary and conclusion

By definition, evidence-based practice requires a solid understanding of research evidence. This means being able to understand the strengths and limitations of various research designs and the factors that may threaten their validity. Evidence-based practice also involves knowing how to stay current with the most recent research findings and make use of them in everyday practice. This chapter provided an overview of the ways in which an evidence base is established and methods for identifying and critically appraising research studies. The following chapter will consider the ways in which research has improved our knowledge of the parent–child relationship and has informed the development of evidence-based parenting programs.

Box 2.7: Key points

- Evidence-based practice involves four intersecting components: 1) knowledge of the best research evidence, 2) an understanding and respect for client values, 3) practitioner expertise and 4) consideration of the client's circumstances and the constraints of the intervention setting.
- Well-designed and -conducted evaluation is necessary to understand the efficacy of a parenting intervention.
- Evaluation designs broadly fall into one of two categories: experimental and observational.
- Experimental studies involve the random assignment of participants to a treatment and a control group. This is referred to as a randomized controlled trial (RCT).
- Quasi-experimental studies are similar to experimental studies because they involve a comparison group, but lack randomization.
- Observational studies involve the use of research methods to systematically observe activities as they naturally happen.
- RCTs are widely considered to be the most rigorous way of assessing the effectiveness of an intervention. This is because all known and unknown biases are randomly distributed across the treatment and comparison groups.
- Findings from RCTs are often reported in terms of effect sizes. An effect size is the magnitude of the difference between the experimental outcome of the treatment and controls group(s).
- The use of RCTs is often rejected on practical and ethical grounds. These objections can be overcome, however, through the use of good designs that include wait lists.
- Less rigorous methods to test the efficacy of an intervention include cross-sectional designs, case-control studies and cohort studies.
- Internal validity refers to the extent to which cause and effect can be inferred from an evaluation's design.
- A threat to internal validity is a factor that confounds the extent to which cause and effect can be inferred from an evaluation's design.
- Intention-to-treat refers to evaluation designs that collect evaluation evidence on study subjects even if they have dropped out of the treatment.
- External validity refers to the extent to which findings from a study can be generalized to real-world settings.
- The term 'efficacy trial' refers to RCTs conducted within optimal research settings. Efficacy trials often have high internal validity but low external validity.
- Effectiveness trials refer to RCTs conducted in real-world settings.
- The quality of an intervention's evidence can be considered in terms of a hierarchical scale. Multiple effectiveness trials are at the high end of the scale, with cross-sectional designs at the bottom.
- Systematic review evidence can also be used to understand the overall efficacy of a treatment method. Systematic reviews involve the systematic searching of scientific databases to select and synthesize the available research evidence with respect to a particular intervention.
- Qualitative methods cannot be used to understand an intervention's efficacy, but they can shed light on how or why an intervention works.

Notes

1   Random assignment is usually determined through the use of a computer algorithm.
2   Effect sizes can also be calculated to assess the difference between correlations (McCartney and Rosenthal 2000).
3   Limiting searches to published literature only has the advantage of identifying the best-quality studies, as most of these appear in peer-reviewed journals. However, there is an inherent bias in this practice because most research is submitted to peer-review only if it contains positive results. Thus, information about negative findings or ineffective treatments may not be identified.
4   Multiple resources exist for critically appraising research studies. See Dawe et al. (2005), Gibbs (2003) and Melnyk and Fineout-Overholt (2010) for further reading.

3 Evidence-based theories of parenting

Introduction

Evidence-based parenting support involves understanding the research literature and putting it into practice. The previous chapter provided an overview of what constitutes good research. This chapter considers more specifically the ways in which research has informed the development of evidence-based parenting interventions.

Evidence-based parenting programs are not only supported by experimental research confirming their efficacy, they are also underpinned by sound theoretical frameworks that are informed by research in the fields of child development and parenting. Findings from this research consistently suggest the following:

1   Certain parenting behaviors, particularly warm and loving support combined with high supervision, protect children in ways that allow them to mature into happy and healthy adults.
2   Disruptive and unpredictable parenting behaviors, especially inconsistent or harsh discipline and poor supervision, place children at risk for a variety of negative outcomes, including low achievement, poor mental health and antisocial behavior.
3   Children differ with respect to the benefits they receive from warm and enriching parenting support and the extent to which disruptive and inconsistent parenting behaviors place them at risk.

Most evidence-based parenting interventions make use of these findings by teaching parents effective strategies for supporting their children's development in a way that is sensitive to parents' culture and personal needs. This section provides an overview of the key theoretical frameworks that form the basis of most evidence-based parenting interventions.

Evidence from the neurosciences

Early brain development

Developmental psychologists have long been interested in understanding the relative contribution of nature versus nurture in children's development. While it is now obvious that this is no longer an 'either or' debate, there is still much to learn about how genetic and environmental factors work together to produce a happy and healthy child. Up until recently, researchers could only speculate about how the environment influences children's neurological development. However, new advances in **magnetic resonance imaging** and animal experimentation have made it possible for researchers to directly consider how environmental and genetic factors interact. While much of this research is still in its 'infancy', scientists are now in a better position to consider whether conclusions once based upon observational findings are supported by neuroscientific 'facts'.

In order to understand brain development, early neuroscientific research traditionally focused on comparisons between the number of cells present at birth and in adulthood (Shonkoff and Phillips 2000). These studies suggested a relatively small difference, leading many scientists to erroneously conclude that much of the child's brain is developed at birth and that brain cell production and organization are genetically determined. More recent research suggests that this is not the case, however. While a healthy child is indeed born into the world with an astonishingly high number of brain cells (approximately 100 billion!), most of these are in an immature state. At birth, many cells have not been activated and the connections between them have yet to be established. While we know that some of these processes are genetically determined, we now also know that the environment makes a substantial contribution to how the brain matures (Perry 2002, Stiles 2008).

Figure 3.1 provides an example of a brain cell (also called a **neuron**). Brain cells are designed to connect with other brain cells. On the upper left-hand side is the cell body, surrounded by an outgrowth of **dendrites**. Stemming from the cell body is the **axon**. The length of an axon depends upon its purpose – with some axons extending over a metre in length. Most axons are surrounded by a fatty, **myelin** sheath, which provides insulation and

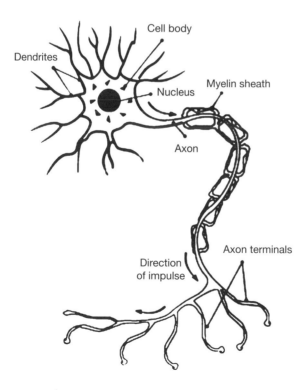

Figure 3.1 Drawing of a neuron.

improves the axon's conductivity. At the end of the neuron are its **terminal buttons** or branches. These buttons contain **neurotransmitters** that fire signals to electro-chemical receptors located on the dendritic ends of other neurons.

The brain is made up of concentrations of grey and white matter. **Grey matter** refers to the pink/grey concentrations of neural cell bodies, dendrites and non-myelinated axons that form on the brain's surface. **White matter** refers to the myelinated axon tracts (revealed as white when preserved in formaldehyde) that extend from the cell bodies to connect the nerve cells to each other. The point at which a neuron connects to another neuron is called a **synapse** (Figure 3.2). Brain activity is determined by trillions of synapses that fire continuously. A terminal branch of an axon may form as many as 1,000 synapses with other neurons. Dendrites, on the receiving end of the cell body, may accept signals from hundreds, if not thousands, of other neurons (Stiles 2008).

The formation of brain cells (also referred to as **neurogenesis**) predominantly occurs at between 6 and 18 weeks of gestation (Rakic 1995, Rakic and Sidman 1968). During this period, approximately 225,000 cortical neurons are generated per minute (Uylings 2001). As they are formed, the neurons migrate to their respective regions within the brain, where they differentiate to perform separate functions (Fox et al. 2010, Rakic 1988). By the twenty-sixth week, the majority of neurons will have reached their final destination and their dendritic branches will have started to grow (Uylings 2006). The prenatal formation and migration of neurons are believed to be **activity-independent**, meaning that they are driven by genetic processes and do not require environmental input. Despite their independent nature, their success is nevertheless determined by the quality of the fetal environment. For example, there is clear evidence that a wide range of substances (including drugs and alcohol) have a

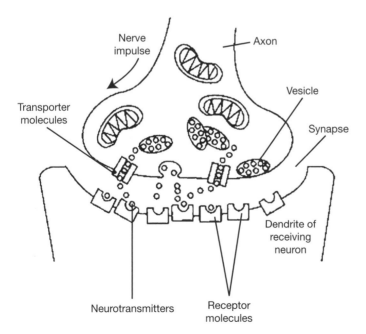

Figure 3.2   A synaptic connection between neurons

neurotoxic effect on prenatal brain development (Fox et al. 2010, Uylings 2006). A growing body of evidence now also suggests that high levels of stress-related maternal **cortisol** in early pregnancy can interfere with the organization and programming of developing neurons as the brain begins to form trillions of synapses and pathways between the neurons (Davis et al. 2007, Davis and Sandman 2010, Gutteling et al. 2005). These connections are vital because they enable the infant to process important environmental information through all five senses – sight, sound, smell, taste and touch.

Activity-dependent synaptic processes are typically classified as either **experience-expectant** or **experience-dependent**. Experience-expectant processes are triggered by stimuli that naturally occur in most infant environments. The word 'expectant' is used because the brain is genetically wired to expect and rely on a particular kind of environmental stimulus. For example, when patterned light hits a newborn's retina for the first time, it activates a chain of genetic events that determine the development of important neural pathways, including those that process light and other visual information. Experience-expectant responses (such as exposure to light and sound) are ubiquitous and necessary for normal development in all human infants (Shonkoff and Phillips 2000).

Experience-dependent (or adaptive) processes, on the other hand, are not reliant upon species-specific environmental stimuli (including light, sound, etc.). While environmental inputs actively contribute to the development of the brain's structure, experiences are not predetermined or anticipated by the synapses at any particular stage. Experience-dependent processes are instead reliant on an individual's unique interaction with his or her environment (Greenough and Black 1992). For instance, there is evidence to suggest that the neural areas that govern finger movements in the hand are more highly developed in individuals who play stringed instruments (Elbert et al. 1995). In this respect, experience-dependent processes constitute what we define as 'learning' and play a significant role in determining how information is stored and processed by the brain.

Experience-expectant and experience-dependent processes take place during separate but overlapping time periods. During the prenatal stage and at birth, genetically based, experience-expectant processes trigger an overproduction of synaptic connections that continues throughout the first two years of life. By the age of 2, the infant will have over 1,000 trillion connections, which is twice as many as his or her parents have. Although the brain will continue to make connections throughout the child's lifetime, they will have reached their highest density by the age of 3, with 15,000 synapses per neuron. Figure 3.3 provides a comparison of the brain's dendritic growth and connectivity at birth and then again at 3 years.

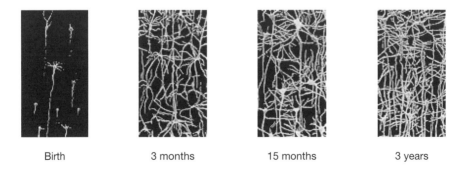

| Birth | 3 months | 15 months | 3 years |

Figure 3.3   Dendritic growth from birth to three years

This process, also known as **synaptic overproduction** (or synaptic 'blooming'), takes place predominantly during the first three years of life. From an evolutionary standpoint, synaptic overproduction is considered to be highly adaptive, as it enables young children to learn a wide variety of things. Synaptic connectivity is also influenced by the extent to which synapses are used. Neural pathways that are frequently used (through learning and experience) become stronger and more efficient. This process is further reinforced through neural **myelination**, whereby a protective layer of fatty myelin grows around the axon to insulate it (Deoni et al. 2011). Myelination further improves the efficiency of synaptic connections, as it serves a purpose similar to the plastic coating surrounding an electrical wire by increasing the axon's conductivity.

While synaptic overproduction increases the brain's potential for learning, it also reduces its efficiency. Redundant and unnecessary synaptic connections frequently interfere with the young brain's ability to effectively process information. For this reason, connections that are not used eventually wither and die through a **synaptic pruning** process that takes place throughout the remainder of childhood until the adult number is reached. The end result is an adult brain that has far fewer, but more efficient, synaptic connections.

Synaptic overproduction and pruning cycles differ within each region of the developing brain. For example, the density of synapses per neuron in the visual cortex reaches its peak at 150 percent of the adult level at the age of 4 months and then gradually decreases to the adult level by the age of 4 years (Huttenlocher 1990). In the regions governing language and speech development, synaptic pruning occurs more gradually – reaching adult levels in late adolescence. In regions governing higher-order cognitive reasoning, the synaptic pruning process is not complete until early adulthood (Huttenlocher and Dabholkar 1997, Shonkoff and Phillips 2000).

It is worth noting that synaptic pruning is a characteristic of experience-expectant processes that predominantly occur in childhood. By contrast, experience-dependent processes, involving the formation and strengthening of new neural connections (as opposed to synaptic pruning), appear to continue throughout the life span (Davis 2004, Shonkoff and Phillips 2000). In fact, evidence now suggests that some regions of the brain (the hippocampus and olfactory bulb in particular) continue to generate new neurons and integrate them into mature synaptic systems well into adulthood. It is assumed that this ability provides the brain with ongoing flexibility to process and respond to the new demands within an ever-changing adult environment (Kelsh et al. 2010, Song et al. 2005).

Critical periods

Although it is clear that experience-dependent processes continue throughout the life span, evidence suggests that the brain's basic architecture is more or less established by the age of 3. This has led some to view the first three years of life as a sensitive or **critical period** for determining the course of a child's future cognitive and emotional development (National Scientific Council on the Developing Child 2007). Indeed, animal research suggests that there are sensitive time frames during which animal babies imprint or bond with their parents. The outcomes of these periods frequently determine whether the animal survives into adulthood. Research with humans similarly suggests that there are critical periods during which experience-expectant outcomes must be established (Knudson 2004). A clear example of this is the case of infants who are born with cataracts. If the cataracts are not removed by the age of 2, vision will not develop because the experience-expectant synapses will not have been fully activated and some connections will have been 'pruned' away (Shonkoff and Phillips 2000).

The implications of the above findings suggest that parents play an extremely important role in supporting their children's brain development. They do this first by providing their children with a proper diet that supports cell growth and myelination. Parents also contribute to their children's neurological development by providing appropriate stimulation within critical periods. For example, there is some evidence to suggest that parental stimulation, in the form of 'serve and return' face play, helps infants to learn how to regulate their arousal states at critical points during their development. Optimal levels of infant arousal are linked to children's improved cognitive and emotional development (Kertes et al. 2009, National Scientific Council in the Developing Child 2004).

'Serve and return' face play often begins with the baby cooing at its mother. The mother responds by smiling and gently vocalizing the baby's emotional state by saying something like *Look at you! Aren't we happy today?* The baby might then smile and gurgle and the mother may then respond by gently poking her baby. At this point the baby might laugh and squeal, which is then reinforced by another gentle poke by the mother and another vocalization, such as *You're such a little character.*

Through this gentle interaction, the parent and infant work together to create optimal arousal states in the infant, where the infant remains alert and content. A parent's role in this process is to 'scaffold' the infant's emotion regulation by providing repetitive vocal, facial and tactile stimulation that is appropriately matched to the infant's level of arousal. When a parent responds in a way that is frightening or otherwise poorly attuned to the infant's state, the infant often experiences stress (Beebe 2000, Kochanska 2002, Stern et al. 1977, Tronick et al. 1982).

Research with animals suggests that optimal arousal states during infancy lay the foundation for optimal brain development as children mature. Specifically, too much or too little stimulation is stressful for animal young and can result in too much or too little production of cortisol. For example, high levels of cortisol during critical periods can inhibit myelin production and damage the hippocampus. Such damage has been linked to deficits in learning, memory and emotion regulation in young animals (Loman and Gunnar 2010, Gunnar and Quevedo 2007, National Scientific Council in the Developing Child 2005).

Research with humans has similarly linked high levels of stress to brain abnormalities. The research of Bruce Perry provides an especially dramatic example of the damage that can occur when children are raised in conditions of extreme neglect and sensory deprivation. In a study comparing MRI and CT scans of the brains of 'globally' neglected 3-year-olds (i.e. children who received minimal exposure to language, touch and social interactions), neglected children's brains were observed to be significantly smaller than the brains of children reared in normal environments. In particular, the neglected children's brains exhibited substantially enlarged **lateral ventricles** and significantly less grey and white matter (Perry 2002).

Similar damage has been observed in the brains of maltreated children suffering from post-traumatic stress disorder (PTSD). In a series of carefully controlled studies, De Bellis and his colleagues found that PTSD children had significantly smaller **corpora callosa** (a region of white matter responsible for communication between the hemispheres), as well as enlarged ventricles and smaller volumes of grey and white matter (De Bellis et al. 1999a, 1999b, 2002). De Bellis et al. further observed that the extent of the brain's damage was positively correlated with the duration of the maltreatment. In other words, the longer and more intense the maltreatment, the more significant the structural damage to the brain. Interestingly, the brain's structural damage was more pronounced for boys than for girls (De Bellis and Keshavan 2003). These findings have since been replicated by Teicher and his colleagues, who have also observed substantial reductions in the corpora callosa of maltreated and neglected children, as well as increased damage amongst boys (Teicher et al. 1997, 2004, 2006).

Research involving children who have spent significant periods of time in institutionalized environments has also documented abnormalities in brain structure, although the pattern of damage is somewhat different than that observed with maltreated children. For example, Mehta et al. (2009) have noted enlarged **amygdalas** (an abnormality linked to increases in aggression) in the brains of children who spent a significant portion of their early childhood in Romanian orphanages. These children also displayed reduced volumes of grey and white matter, although they did not exhibit reductions in the size of their corpora callosa.

The structural abnormalities observed in the above studies (e.g. reduced corpus callosum and reduced brain volume) have all been linked to a wide variety of childhood and adult psychiatric disorders, including schizophrenia, bipolar disorder and major depression. Such damage has also been linked to impairments in cognitive functioning. For example, Pollack et al. (2010) have documented deficits in the visual memories and attention regulation of 8- and 9-year-olds who spent a significant portion of their infancy in deprived institutionalized care. Impairments in cognitive and emotional development have been similarly noted in children raised by depressed mothers (Murray and Cooper 1997, National Scientific Council on the Developing Child 2009, Schore 2001).

Thus it is clear that early deprivation (in the form neglect, abuse and long periods in non-stimulating institutionalized settings) can result in pronounced and lasting deficits in brain functioning. The extent to which such deprivation permanently damages the brain remains unclear, however. For example, there is some evidence to suggest that structural brain damage can be reversed if children are removed from adverse circumstances and placed in enriching environments. To this end, Perry (2002) observed that when severely neglected children were removed from their homes and placed in warm and nurturing foster homes, some (not all) of their brain's function and volume were recovered. Perry further noted that the degree of recovery was inversely proportional to the age at which children were removed from their deprived environments. The earlier in life this happened and the less time they spent in a neglectful home, the more significant the recovery.

Perry's observations are echoed in studies of children raised in deprived institutional environments. For example, Nelson et al. (2007) observed significant cognitive recoveries amongst Romanian orphans randomly removed from institutions and placed in foster care. Full cognitive recoveries have also been noted among Romanian orphans placed in supportive adoptive homes within six months of their birth. Marked cognitive deficits are typically observed, however, in the majority of children who remain in deprived institutional care for substantial periods of time after the age of 6 months (e.g. see Pollak et al. 2010 noted above, Rutter et al. 2010). Even amongst these children, however, significant recoveries have been observed (Beckett et al. 2006, Kreppner et al. 2007).

Collectively, the above findings suggest that while the effects of severe early deprivation are indeed negative, they are by no means universal, nor irreversible (Kreppner et al. 2007, O'Connor et al. 2003, Rutter et al. 2004, Rutter et al. 2010). Moreover, they attest to the highly malleable and self-righting nature of the young brain, indicating that harmful and aberrant experiences early in life do not necessarily determine a child's fate and that genetic and neurobiological processes can and do facilitate resilience and flexible adaptation (Cicchetti 2002, Cicchetti and Tucker 1994, Cicchetti 2003). While efforts are indeed necessary to support children's early development and protect them from harm, the balance of the evidence also suggests that interventions remain necessary to support children's resilience and recovery in the aftermath of adversity.

Adolescent brain development

There is now a fair amount of evidence to suggest that pre-adolescence and the early teen years constitute a second period of synaptic overproduction. Hormones released during the onset of puberty (typically at around the age of 9) trigger a rapid increase in the connections between brain cells in the prefrontal cortex that continues until the child is between the ages of 12 and 13 (Blakemore and Choudhury 2006, Giedd 2004). This is then followed by a second period of synaptic pruning that carries on until early adulthood, with some adult brains not reaching full maturity until the mid 20s (Dahl and Hariri 2005, Giedd 2004).

Evidence suggests that this increased synaptic activity interferes with the adolescent's ability to process information, much as it did in infancy. Moreover, synaptic overproduction in the prefrontal cortex appears to reduce teenagers' ability to manage strong emotions brought on by the swelling of the amygdala, which is also due to increased hormonal activity during puberty (Baird et al. 1999, Giedd 2004, Kelley et al. 2004). This suggests that neurobiological processes contribute to the moodiness and irritability exhibited by many teenagers. These findings also suggest that adolescents are far less mature than was once assumed and this has implications for how they are educated and parented. In particular, it is likely that the quality of the parenting environment is just as important during the teenage years as it is in early childhood. Indeed, Whittle et al. (2008, 2009) have observed a significant link between punitive parenting behaviors and an enlarged amygdala in teenage boys, which has, in turn, been linked to increases in the boys' aggressive behavior.

Implications for parenting support

While findings from neuroscientific research have not yet made their way into any specific evidence-based parenting program, they have strongly influenced the development of recent US and UK government policies aimed at young children and their parents. As mentioned in the first chapter, the *Sure Start* initiative was launched in direct response to neuroscientific evidence involving children's early brain development. The Allen review (see Chapter 1) also draws heavily on neuroscientific evidence in its recommendations for early years interventions. While this emphasis on the early years is well founded, it is important that it does not pre-empt the support to parents available during other stages of children's development. Indeed, one of the conclusions of the *From Neurons to Neighborhoods* report (see Chapter 1) was that a disproportionate amount of attention is paid to the period between birth to 3, stating that support 'begins too late and ends too soon' (Shonkoff and Phillips 2000: 7). Although evidence suggests that the brain's architecture is established in the first few years of life, it is also clear that the brain remains extremely malleable as children mature. Evidence now also suggests that experience-dependent learning occurs at all stages of development, including the adult years.

It should also be noted that many of the findings reported in the previous sections consider children's developmental outcomes within the context of extreme deprivation and may not apply to normal parenting environments (Belsky and de Haan 2010). From this perspective, we still do not know what kinds of parental stimulation are required for optimal brain development and how much is 'good enough'. For example, we have yet to understand what constitutes a 'normal' vs. 'enhanced' external environment and the extent to which extremely enhanced circumstances (i.e. those found in affluent homes) continue to improve neurological outcomes over and above what is provided in the average Western household (Fox et al. 2010).

Researchers and practitioners should also keep in mind that while it is likely that parenting and environmental factors make a strong contribution to children's development, genetic factors also continue to influence child outcomes at all stages of development. This is especially true when it comes to genetically determined learning disorders, such as ADHD, dyslexia and autism. In these instances, parents are likely to require support that addresses the unique impacts of their child's disorder. For example, Sonuga-Barke et al. (2002) have observed that children with ADHD are more likely to have parents with ADHD, and this often interferes with the effectiveness of standard parenting interventions for this population. The *New Forest Parenting Program* (NFPP – Box 3.1) was therefore developed specifically to address the issues that can arise when both children and parents have ADHD.

As we discover more about how genetic and environmental factors interact, we learn more about the ways in which parenting interventions can target and counteract any potential adverse effects of genetically determined processes. For example, Belsky et al. (2007) have observed that children are **differentially susceptible** to environmental risks, meaning that some children require and benefit from good-quality parenting support more than others. To this end, Velderman et al. (2006) have observed that the VIPP attachment intervention (see next section) is more effective for highly reactive children than it is for moderately reactive children. There is also evidence to suggest that good-quality parenting support significantly reduces some of the genetically-based risks related to teenage drug and alcohol misuse (Brody et al. 2009). Collectively, these findings suggest that children benefit from nurturing parenting behaviors that are responsive to their individual needs at all stages of their development.

Attachment theory

John Bowlby

The roots of attachment theory can be traced to the work of British psychiatrist, John Bowlby (1907–1990), who believed that 'the propensity to make strong emotional bonds to particular individuals [is] a basic component of human nature' (Bowlby 1988: 3). This conclusion was based upon Bowlby's own observations of distressed children in the 'war nurseries' of World

---

Box 3.1: The *New Forest Parenting Program*

The *New Forest Parenting Program* (NFPP) is designed for parents of young children with moderate to severe symptoms of ADHD. The primary goal of the program is to increase parents' understanding of ADHD and improve children's behavior. Trained clinicians deliver NFPP to parents in their homes on a weekly basis over a period of eight weeks. During these visits, therapists use situations that regularly occur in families' homes to demonstrate and apply parenting strategies that will help parents teach their children how to regulate their attention on their own. Clinicians are also trained to respond to the mental health needs of parents, since parents of children with ADHD may be dealing with their own ADHD symptoms, as well as other mental difficulties. Two RCTs suggest that NFPP significantly reduces children's ADHD symptoms and increases parents' sense of wellbeing when implemented by appropriately trained clinicians (Sonuga-Barke et al. 2001, Thompson et al. 2009).

War II, as well as findings from ethological studies of animal parents and their young (van der Horst et al. 2007, 2008). Bowlby was especially impressed by the work of Konrad Lorenz (1903–1989), who observed that young goslings automatically 'imprinted' themselves onto their mothers by following and imitating them within a few hours of their birth. Bowlby was also influenced by Harry Harlow's (1905–1981) research with rhesus monkeys, which documented the extreme anxiety infant monkeys experienced when separated from their mothers. This monkey behavior was similar to what Bowlby had observed among toddlers who were separated from their parents during hospital stays and Bowlby theorized that these intense anxiety behaviors were infant survival mechanisms for keeping parents close by (Bowlby 1969). In particular, Bowlby believed that there were five infant behaviors that facilitated an attachment relationship between human infants and their caregivers: clinging, crying, smiling, sucking and following. Bowlby noted that, with the exception of following, all of these behaviors were present in early infancy and observed that they were usually effective in bringing and keeping the primary caregiver (most often the mother) near to the infant.

Mary Ainsworth and the 'strange situation'

Bowlby's colleague, Mary Ainsworth (1913–1999), empirically tested Bowlby's ideas by observing mothers and infants interacting in their homes during the infants' first year. From these studies, Ainsworth indentified three patterns of infant behavior: 1) infants who cried little and were content to explore their environment in their mother's presence, 2) infants who cried frequently and had difficulty exploring their environment even when their mother was close by and 3) infants who appeared not to be affected by the presence or absence of their mother. Ainsworth also observed that the mothers of the infants who cried little were more likely to sensitively and appropriately respond to their infants' bids for attention. Ainsworth theorized that this first group of infants were 'securely' attached and maintained that this security was supported by warm and sensitive parenting behaviors.

In order to further understand attachment security in low- and high-stress situations, Ainsworth drew from Harlow's observations of the anxiety exhibited by young rhesus monkeys when separated from their mothers. Ainsworth hypothesized that such separations activated the attachment system and was interested in understanding what human infants did when they were similarly stressed. In order to systematically consider individual differences in separation reactions, Ainsworth developed the now famous 'strange situation' laboratory condition to simulate the kinds of separations infants might typically experience in their everyday lives.

In this experiment, a mother and her 1-year-old child are introduced to a laboratory play room filled with toys. They are instructed to play together while they are joined by a 'stranger' who initially engages the mother and then plays with the child when the mother is asked to leave for a short period. After the mother returns, there is a second brief period of play with the mother and stranger, followed by a second separation, when both the stranger and mother leave. The 1-year-old is then left completely alone for a very short time, after which the mother returns once again and comforts her child.

Ainsworth and her colleagues identified three consistent patterns of mother–infant interaction during the 'strange situation' separation and reunion episodes (Ainsworth et al. 1978):[1]

* **Securely attached**: Approximately 70 per cent of the infants showed distress when their mother left the room, but were easily comforted and went back to play when the mother returned.

- **Avoidant-insecure**: Another 20 per cent avoided their mothers during reunion. Although these infants spent some time looking for their mother during separation, they did not appear as stressed as the others.
- **Ambivalent/resistant-insecure**: Another 10 per cent were very stressed when their mother left the room, but were surprisingly angry when she returned. While these infants wanted to be picked up, they were difficult to cuddle or soothe.

During the play session, Ainsworth also observed that securely attached children used their mothers as a **secure base** from which to explore the room and toys. Ainsworth and Bowlby believed that the ability to use caregivers as a secure base enables infants to mature into social and confident children. Ainsworth and Bowlby further believed that, through their interactions with their primary attachment figure, infants form expectations regarding the extent to which others can reliably meet their needs. Bowlby and Ainsworth called these expectations 'internal working models', or mental representations that inform children's global perspectives of themselves and others. If infants perceive their mothers as trustworthy, they are likely to expect others to be trustworthy as well and take these expectations with them into future relationships. Considered collectively, Bowlby's and Ainsworth's ideas suggest the following model of child development (Figure 3.4):

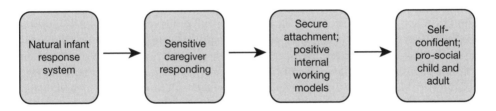

Figure 3.4 The influence of attachment security on child development

Attachment and human development

Mary Ainsworth made further advancements in the field of attachment by providing a 'secure base' for many of her graduate students who went on to test her original hypotheses. One of these students was Mary Main (1947–), who studied attachment patterns in adulthood and observed that the parents of securely attached children were able to provide clear and coherent accounts of their own childhood in interview situations, whereas those with insecurely attached children could not. These findings provided further evidence of the internal working model concept, suggesting that adult attachment security could be readily identified and that attachment status could be transmitted through generations (Main et al. 1985).

Mary Main and her students also identified a fourth, **disorganized/disoriented**, attachment category that characterized the attachment behaviors of approximately 5 per cent of all babies. The behaviors displayed by these 'D' babies often lacked any coherent organization, with babies frequently behaving as if they were confused or disoriented. Many disorganized infants also behaved as if they were frightened of their caregiver, frequently freezing or rocking when their mothers returned during the reunion phases of the 'strange situation'. These behaviors led Main and her colleagues to hypothesize that a disorganized attachment may be related to a history of abuse or neglect, or inconsistencies in parental sensitivity related to their own mental health problems (Main and Solomon 1986).

Another student of Mary Ainsworth's, Everett Waters (1951–), initiated the large-scale Minnesota Longitudinal Study of Parents and Children (MLSPC) with Alan Sroufe (1941–) at the University of Minnesota in the mid 1970s. Over the past 35 years, this study has carefully considered the various ways in which attachment security predicts a wide variety of developmental outcomes. Findings from this research consistently suggest that a secure attachment is highly predictive of greater self-confidence, mastery motivation, improved social skills and higher school achievement (Sroufe et al. 2005). These studies also suggest that a securely attached child will remain secure throughout childhood if his family and life circumstances remain consistently supportive. A child's attachment status is likely to change, however, if life circumstances change – especially if they change for the worse (Hamilton 2000, Waters et al. 2000). Securely attached infants are thus likely to be reclassified as insecure in adolescence and adulthood if they experience various childhood adversities, including a parental divorce, parental unemployment, or a parent with poor mental health, which may threaten their attachment security. Despite this malleability, research suggests that an early history of warm and loving parenting sets the stage for the development of healthy internal working models of the self and others (Waters et al. 2000).

Attachment-based interventions

Attachment research highlights the idea that a warm and sensitive caregiving environment is central to adaptive and competent child development. For this reason, numerous interventions have been developed to support the attachment relationship. However, relatively few target children's attachment security specifically (Bakermans-Kranenburg et al. 2003). This is because an insecure attachment is not considered to be a psychological disorder on its own, but instead a risk factor for the development of mental health problems as children mature (Greenberg 1999, Kobak et al. 2006, Sroufe et al. 2005). There is a growing consensus, however, that a disorganized attachment presents a particularly strong risk for future mental health problems (Lyons-Ruth and Jacobvitz 1999, Moss et al. 2005, Sroufe 2005 et al.). As noted previously, disorganized attachments are likely to be a result of abuse or neglect, or other parental dysfunction. For this reason, interventions aiming to change children's attachment status often specifically target children that would be categorized as disorganized (Berlin et al. 2005, Cicchetti et al. 2006. Hoffman et al. 2006).

Improving parental sensitivity

Interventions aiming to change children's attachment classification tend to fall into one of two categories: those which focus on improving maternal sensitivity exclusively and those which aim to change parents' internal representations of their child (Berlin 2005). Interventions which aim to improve parents' sensitivity are based on findings from a meta-analysis of attachment interventions conducted by Bakermans-Kranenburg et al. (2003) that found that short-term interventions focusing on parental sensitivity through the use of video-tapes were the most likely to improve maternal responsiveness and attachment security. Based on these findings, the authors developed the VIPP (*Video-feedback Intervention to promote Positive Parenting*) to increase parents' ability to respond sensitively to their 6-month-old infants' cues (Juffer et al. 2008). In a program delivered over a period of six weeks, mother and child pairs are video-taped as they interact naturally in their homes. The video-tapes are then viewed with the parents with the aim of reinforcing positive behaviors and correcting less sensitive responses. A series of recent RCTs suggest that the VIPP improves parental sensitivity and attachment security in both normal and at-risk samples (Juffer et al. 2005, Stein et al. 2006, Velderman et al. 2006).

Improving parental internal representations

Interventions which aim to alter internal representations are based on research suggesting that attachment security is more strongly associated with a parent's internal representations of their child than it is with their overall sensitivity (van IJzendoorn et al. 1995). These findings have contributed to the 'transmission model' of attachment that assumes that a parent's ability to respond sensitively to their child is influenced by the parent's own attachment history, as well as his or her internal working models (Figure 3.5).

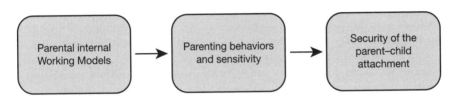

Figure 3.5 'Transmission model' of the relationship between parental internal working model and children's attachment security

According to the transmission model, parents who were securely attached during their own childhood are more likely to have developed positive representations of themselves and others. These positive representations allow parents to be receptive to the full range of their children's behaviors and respond to them more sensitively. By contrast, parents with an insecure attachment history have greater difficulty in appropriately interpreting their children's behaviors, since interactions with their child often trigger painful memories from their own childhood (Fraiberg et al. 1980 – see Chapter 4 for a full discussion). Parents with less positive internal working models are also more likely to distort or misrepresent their child's behavior and thus respond to their child in a negative or insensitive way (Bosquet and Egeland 2001, Cicchetti et al. 2006, Ensink and Mayes 2010, Fonagy et al. 1991, Fonagy 1997, George 1996, Suchman et al. 2008).

Interventions which aim to change parents' negative representations of their children often involve therapeutic sessions taking place on a weekly basis for over a year or more. During these sessions, the practitioner aims to 'correct' negative internal working models by providing the parent with a warm and supportive therapeutic environment (Berlin 2005). Infant–Parent Psychotherapy (IPP) and Child–Parent Psychotherapy (CPP – see Box 3.2) are examples of therapeutic interventions used to change mothers' representations of their children.

Evaluations of programs aimed at improving parental representations generally observe positive changes in parents' sensitivity, but relatively few have improved children's attachment security (Bakermans-Kranenburg et al. 2003, Egeland, 2009). However, a recent randomized controlled trial comparing IPP to a psycho-educational parenting intervention (PPI – based on the *Nurse–Family Partnership* model – see Box 1.2) found that both interventions were equally effective in improving maltreated children's attachment status when compared to community-based support (Cicchetti et al. 2006). This finding was surprising,

Box 3.2: *Child–Parent Psychotherapy*

Child–Parent Psychotherapy (CPP) and *Infant–Parent Psychotherapy* (IPP) are manualized therapeutic interventions delivered by Master's-qualified psychologists to mothers and children who may have experienced trauma or abuse (Lieberman 1991, 1992, Lieberman and Pawl 1988). Both interventions are delivered via weekly sessions for one year. Practitioners address mothers' concerns through empathic, non-didactic support which aims to help the mother reflect on her childhood experiences and differentiate them from her current relationship with her child. Sessions involving CPP also focus on parent and child interactions to support reciprocity and healthy coping behaviors. Parents also receive advice on child behavior management. During sessions involving IPP, the mother and practitioner jointly interact with the infant. This enables the practitioner to respond empathically to the child and suggest positive explanations for its behavior. As the therapeutic relationship develops, parents are able to dissociate negative childhood-related feelings from their interactions with their infant and appropriately interpret their infant's behaviors (Cicchetti et al. 2006).

A series of RCTs involving the use of CPP with mothers and children exposed to domestic violence suggest that it is an effective method for reducing trauma-related symptoms. Children receiving CPP treatment reported significantly less trauma-related stress and significantly improved behavior. Mothers also benefit from the intervention, reporting significantly less post-trauma stress and improved expectations for their relationship with their child (Lieberman et al. 2005, Lieberman, Briscoe-Smith et al. 2006, Lieberman, Ippen et al. 2006, Toth et al. 2002). Additional studies involving IPP suggest that the intervention is effective in improving children's attachment security (see main text).

given the difference between the two treatment models. While both treatments take place over the course of a year, the focus of IPP was primarily therapeutic, whereas PPI focused more on children's development and maternal life-management strategies. Although the PPI approach has been proven to be highly effective with first-time teenage mothers (through the NFP program), this was the first time it had been applied to maltreating mothers to improve the attachment relationship with their child.

Findings from the study suggested that both models resulted in dramatic improvements in the attachment security of disorganized infants. For IPP, the number of toddlers classified as secure increased from 3 to 60 per cent and those classified as disorganized decreased from 88 to 30 per cent. For PPI, the number of toddlers classified as secure rose from 0 to 54 per cent and the number classified as disorganized dropped from 81 to 44 per cent. By comparison, the rates of insecurely attached children remained relatively stable in the control group receiving community-based support.

Collectively, the above findings suggest that interventions which aim to increase maternal sensitivity (such as VIPP) and interventions which aim to alter maternal representation both have potential for improving the attachment relationship. Given the efficacy of both models, the question then becomes which model is better. Velderman et al. (2006) attempted to answer this question by comparing the standard VIPP to VIPP-R – a variation of the VIPP model which included additional therapeutic support altering parental representations. The study observed that both models were equally successful in improving mothers' sensitivity and improving the attachment security of highly reactive infants. It is worth noting, however, that the sample used for the Velderman et al. study, as well as other VIPP implementations, was not representative of mothers with a history of child maltreatment (Kalinauskiene et al. 2009). It may be that short-term interventions such as the VIPP are adequate for insecure attachment dyads that are not otherwise at risk and that more intensive therapies are necessary for parents who maltreat their children (Berlin 2005).

VIPP, IPP and PPI are all examples of attachment-based interventions underpinned by positive RCT evidence. Two other interventions which show promise in improving children's attachment security include *Watch, Wait and Wonder* (WWW) and *The Circle of Security* (COS). *Watch, Wait and Wonder* is described as an 'infant-led' psychotherapy delivered to mothers and toddlers (approximately 30 months) through weekly sessions for approximately five months. During the first half of the session, mothers are told to get down on the floor with their infant and interact with the infant only through his/her initiative. This is done to help the mother observe and reflect on her infant's behavior and encourage the infant to take the lead in interacting with their mother. During the second half of the session, mothers discuss their observations and experiences with the therapist. In a study involving a comparison group and some randomization, infants in the WWW group demonstrated a greater shift towards a secure attachment and improved emotion regulation. Mothers in the WWW group also reported less depression and greater satisfaction in their parenting role (Cohen et al. 1999).

COS has also shown promise in improving children's attachment security. Unlike VIPP, IPP, PPI and WWW, COS involves both group and individual therapeutic sessions. The program begins by developing an individualized treatment plan for mothers and infants enrolled in the program that identifies their most problematic interactions. After the individual treatment plan is completed, caregivers attend 20 weekly group sessions where they are helped to understand how their own caregiving history may be influencing their relationship with their child. Parents are also taught methods for increasing their empathy towards their child and responding more sensitively to his or her cues. COS is currently undergoing an RCT and preliminary findings are positive (Marvin, personal correspondence, 2010). Findings from a well-designed pre-/post-treatment study have also observed significant positive changes in observer ratings of children's attachment classification. By the end of the program, 70 per cent of those classified as disorganized were reclassified as secure (Hoffman et al. 2006).

Attachment-based interventions not supported by evidence

It should be noted that while many programs claim to be based on attachment theory, relatively few of them are evidence-based. While many programs borrow a few of Bowlby's ideas, they are often represented in ways that are not substantiated by research evidence and may even be considered as incompatible with attachment theory. In particular, 'holding therapies', including *Rebirthing, Rage Reduction, Attachment Therapy* or *Holding Therapy* use attachment principles in combination with distortions of psychoanalytic theory (e.g. ideas regarding rebirthing and rage reduction) to advocate the use of extreme holding techniques as a way of calming down disruptive children (Marvin 2000).

Holding therapies are typically endorsed in situations where children exhibit so-called 'reactive attachment disorders' which are characterized by extremely violent and angry behavior, which is often observed in children who have been abused or neglected. Some have argued that children who exhibit these extreme behaviors are enraged at a very deep and primitive level and may be at risk of becoming psychopaths. Proponents of holding therapies argue that holding methods are appropriate for these children because they are resistant to more commonly used therapies (Chaffin et al. 2006).

Investigations into these interventions suggest that, while they are endorsed by practitioners with good intentions, they have the potential to be harmful and in some cases life threatening. During the past 15 years a number of deaths have been attributed to parents, caregivers and foster caregivers who have engaged in holding techniques based on an attachment therapist's instructions. For this reason, the American Professional Society on the Abuse of Children (APSAC) has investigated attachment therapies and has issued a set of recommendations for their use. Some of their key points are described in Box 3.3.

Box 3.3: Advice regarding the use of holding techniques for treating attachment disorders (from Chaffin et al. 2006: 86–87)

- Treatment techniques or attachment parenting techniques involving physical coercion, psychologically or physically enforced holding, physical restraint, physical domination, provoked catharsis, ventilation of rage, age regression, humiliation, withholding or forcing food or water intake, prolonged social isolation, or assuming exaggerated levels of control and domination over a child are contraindicated because of risk of harm and absence of proven benefit and should not be used.
- Intervention models that portray young children in negative ways, including describing certain groups of young children as pervasively manipulative, cunning, or deceitful, are not conducive to good treatment and may promote abusive practices. In general, child maltreatment professionals should be skeptical of treatments that describe children in pejorative terms or that advocate aggressive techniques for breaking down children's defenses.
- State-of-the-art, goal-directed, evidence-based approaches that fit the main presenting problem should be considered when selecting a first-line of treatment. Where no evidence-based option exists or where evidence-based treatment options have been exhausted, alternative treatments with sound theoretical foundations and broad clinical acceptance are appropriate. Before attempting novel or highly unconventional treatments with untested benefits, the potential for psychological or physical harm should be carefully weighed.

Social learning theory

The Oregon Social Learning Centre

Most evidence-based parenting programs are informed by the research conducted by Gerald Patterson (1926–) and his team at the Oregon Social Learning Centre (OSLC). Patterson's work has its roots in operant conditioning and social learning theories, which suggest that human behavior is shaped by its consequences. Research involving operant conditioning has repeatedly demonstrated that behavior increases if it is rewarded and decreases if it is not (Skinner 1953, 1972, 1974 – see Chapter 4 for a more in-depth discussion). Social learning theory takes this idea one step further by suggesting that behavior does not have to be directly reinforced in order to increase (Bandura 1977, Bandura and Walters 1963). Rather, children will increase certain behaviors if they see others being rewarded for the same actions.

These ideas were originally supported in a series of classic experiments involving 'Bobo' the blow-up clown (Bandura et al. 1961, 1963). In these studies, children were exposed to various films or cartoons where a model aggressively punched Bobo. In some instances the model was rewarded for his behavior and in others he/she was not. After watching the film, the child participants were left alone in a room full of toys that included the same Bobo doll. The children's behavior was then filmed and in every instance the children imitated the model's aggressive behavior by punching the clown. In instances when the filmed model's actions were rewarded, the children's aggressive behavior was more intense and occurred for a longer period of time.

Patterson expanded Bandura's findings through a series of naturalistic observations of young children playing together in a preschool. These observations suggested that while all young children engaged in aggressive behavior, aggressive acts increased when they were rewarded or received attention, but decreased if they were ignored or properly sanctioned by the teacher (Patterson et al. 1967). These classroom observations led Patterson and his colleagues to conclude that aggressive behavior increased if it was reinforced. These observations also caused Patterson and his colleagues to question whether parents inadvertently rewarded their children's negative behavior at home.

'Coercive' parenting

Patterson and his colleagues thus initiated a series of studies that involved detailed observations of parents and children interacting with each other in their homes (Patterson 1976). In these investigations, Patterson and his team observed that negative child behaviors were indeed supported by 'coercive' exchanges between parents and children. During these interactions, parents reinforced aggressive child behavior either by fighting with them or by giving in to their angry demands in an attempt to get some short-term peace (Patterson et al. 1989).

A typical example of a coercive exchange involves a child demanding sweets in a grocery store. The mother says no, but the child asks again – this time in a more demanding way. The mother again says no, but the child responds by throwing a temper tantrum. At this stage, the mother feels as though the entire store is watching her, including the store manager. So she reluctantly gives in to her child's wishes and buys the sweets, but says to the child in a hushed tone, *Ok, here you go, you can shut up now*. In doing so, she quiets her child, but at the same time essentially 'trains' it to tantrum again, since the child's tantruming was ultimately rewarded with the desired sweets.

Patterson's team observed that coercive interactions between children and parents were evident in all families (Snyder 1995, Snyder et al. 2005). However, parents of children with conduct disorders were more likely to initiate coercive interactions and persist in them for longer periods of time than were parents who did not have aggressive children. Moreover, coercive interactions in homes with aggressive children were more likely to escalate into the use of physical punishment, with a typical coercive interaction between a parent and child proceeding like this:

1 Child is watching television when he should be doing his chores
2 Parent tells child to get off his 'bum' and start working
3 Child says he will do chores after show is over
4 Parent leaves child, but then asks child to do his chores again when the show is over
5 Child tells parent to shut up and starts watching another show
6 Parent calls child lazy and threatens to take away all television-watching privileges
7 Child sticks tongue out at parent
8 Parent becomes angry and comes toward child in a threatening manner
9 Child jumps up and runs away from parent, laughing

10   Parent chases child
11   Child runs into corner and picks up chair to fend off parent, still laughing
12   Parent tries to grab chair away, while child attempts to kick and trip parent, still laughing
13   Phone rings and parent goes to answer it
14   Child goes back to watching television.

Through these interactions, the parent promotes aggressive behavior by modeling it, but also by failing to *appropriately* respond to the child's negative behavior. Patterson and his colleagues also observed that parents of aggressive children failed to appropriately reward positive child behavior and, for this reason, children had less incentive to behave well (Patterson et al. 1989). Thus, over time, children from coercive families learned to use aggression as the primary way of getting their needs met, because 1) it was effective and 2) they had not had any opportunity to learn more mature strategies for managing their emotions and interacting with others.

Once coercive patterns are well established within families, Patterson's team observed that aggressive children frequently transfer coercive behaviors to other contexts, such as the playground or school. Within these external environments, aggressive children once again solicit aggressive responses from others and their negative behavior is further reinforced. As aggressive children mature, they do not learn to control immature emotional responses, such as temper tantrums, but instead transform them into more serious forms of misconduct, such as fighting and stealing (Granic and Patterson 2006, Patterson et al. 1989).

These patterns of child and parent behavior suggest the following theory of change for improving child outcomes: reductions in coercive or inappropriate parental responses to aggressive child behaviors will decrease child aggression, increase self-regulation and ultimately decrease the potential for conduct disorders and antisocial behavior (Figure 3.6).

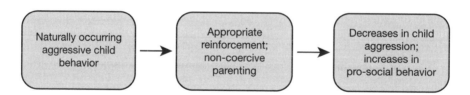

Figure 3.6 Parenting behaviors that decrease to child aggression

Parent management training

In order to stop coercive patterns between parents and children, Patterson and the OSLC team developed a parent training program aimed at reducing coercive parent–child interactions (Feldman and Kazdin 1995, Kazdin 2005). This 'training' starts with an extensive period of observation, where practitioners make detailed notes of coercive parent and child behaviors. Practitioners then use examples of the parents' own behavior to demonstrate its ineffectiveness. Parents are then taught to:

•   Not give in to coercive child demands
•   Not respond to children in a coercive way
•   Use **time out** as a way of appropriately sanctioning bad behavior and calming children down

- Establish a point system where children can exchange points for desirable consequences
- Stay alert for positive child behaviors and reward them appropriately.

Had these principles been applied to the child who refused to do his chores, the parent would have:

- Refrained from all coercive behaviors, including scolding, ridiculing and threatening
- Calmly turned off the television and provided an incentive for the child to do his chores, which might have included permission to watch television once the chores were complete or the promise of a point, if a point system had been established
- Used time out or docked points if the child's coercive behavior persisted.

Research involving the OSLC parent training model repeatedly suggests that both parents and children benefit by changing their coercive behavior (Brestan and Eyberg 1998, Dishion and Andrews 1995, Feldman and Kazdin 1995, Kazdin 2005). While the OSLC program was developed primarily for research purposes, its principles now form the basis for most of the evidence-based parenting programs, including the *Incredible Years*, *Triple P, Strengthening Families 10–14* and *Families and Schools Together* (FAST). It is also worth noting that Patterson's original parenting management training program, known as *Parent Management Training-Oregon* (see Box 3.4) is currently implemented nationally in Norway (Ogden et al. 2005).

Box 3.4: ***Parent Management Training–Oregon***

Parent Management Training-Oregon (PMTO) is designed for parents with children between the ages of 4 to 11 with behavioral problems, as well as other issues. PMTO reduces children's behavioral and emotional problems by reducing coercive interactions between the parent and child and providing parents with strategies for increasing their sensitivity and positively interacting with their children. Research evidence (including multiple RCTs) suggests that PMTO successfully improves parents' self-esteem, behavioral strategies, sensitivity and limit-setting behaviors in the short term. Longer-term child outcomes include reductions in conduct disorders and behavioral problems associated with ADHD, reductions in substance misuse, improvements in school achievement and increased self-esteem. Research findings have also observed reductions in parental depression and substance misusing behaviors (Weisz and Kazdin 2010).

Parenting styles

Four kinds of parenting styles

American psychologist Diana Baumrind's (1927–) research in parenting styles began with the assumption that children's behavior is strongly influenced by their parents' childrearing practices (Maccoby 1980). Like Patterson and Ainsworth, Baumrind's ideas were informed by natural observations of parents and children interacting during dinner and bed times. These studies suggested that parents' behaviors typically varied in terms of the level of control they exerted over their children, as well as the amount of affection and warmth they displayed.

Through further research, Baumrind (1978) and her team at the University of California, Berkeley identified three styles of childrearing behaviors:

- **Authoritarian**: Parents within this classification are likely to control and evaluate the behavior and attitudes of their children within the context of absolute standards. Authoritarian parents value hard work and respect for authority, can be highly critical and are likely to use harsh discipline.
- **Authoritative parents**: These parents are more likely to adopt a 'democratic' approach towards parenting. Authoritative parents expect that children will conform to their requirements, but within a context that respects the rights of both parents and children. Authoritative parents set high standards and expect children to achieve them, but with adequate parental support.
- **Permissive parents**: Permissive parents are likely to be highly accepting of their children's impulses, desires and actions. They frequently use little punishment and make few demands on their children in terms of their time, behavior or family responsibilities. They allow their children to regulate their own activities and impose few standards for behavior or achievement.

The above descriptions suggest that while the authoritative approach places high demands upon the child, it is fundamentally child-centered, as it recognizes the child as a valued contributor to the family. These practices contrast sharply to those of authoritarian parents, who also place high demands on their children, but from their own, parent-centered perspective. An authoritarian style of parenting is characterized by less warmth and considerably less verbal give and take. Permissive parents, on the other hand, are much more accepting and positive towards their children, but set relatively few, if any, limits or standards for their children's behavior. Instead, their approach is entirely child-centered and has been characterized by some as indulgent, since permissive parents allow their children to set their own standards and regulate their own behavior (Maccoby 1980, Scarr et al. 1986). It is worth noting that in a reworking of Baumrind's ideas, Maccoby and Martin (1983) have added a fourth parenting style – **neglecting**. These parents are typically uninvolved in their children's lives and have been characterized by some as abusive.

Maccoby and Martin additionally provide a helpful framework for considering the four parenting styles in terms of increasing levels of parental control and warmth.

As Figure 3.7 suggests, authoritarian and authoritative parents both are characterized by high levels of control. However, authoritative parents combine this control with high levels of warmth. It is likely that high levels of warmth combined with high levels of control – in terms of maintaining high standards for behavior and responsibility – contribute to a variety of positive child outcomes, as described below.

Parenting styles and child behavior

Baumrind (1971, 1978) observed that parenting styles reliably predict child behavior. For example, children with authoritarian or permissive parents often lack confidence and independence, and those with permissive parents are less likely to take responsibility for their own behavior. Children with authoritative parents, however, are more likely to be self-confident, pro-social and socially responsible. Over the last 30 years, hundreds of studies have confirmed these findings, suggesting that authoritative parenting is consistently related to the following positive child and adolescent outcomes:

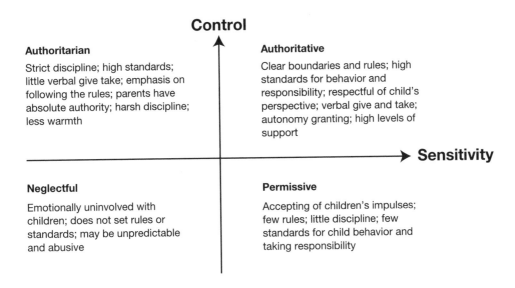

Control

Authoritarian

Strict discipline; high standards; little verbal give take; emphasis on following the rules; parents have absolute authority; harsh discipline; less warmth

Authoritative

Clear boundaries and rules; high standards for behavior and responsibility; respectful of child's perspective; verbal give and take; autonomy granting; high levels of support

Sensitivity

Neglectful

Emotionally uninvolved with children; does not set rules or standards; may be unpredictable and abusive

Permissive

Accepting of children's impulses; few rules; little discipline; few standards for child behavior and taking responsibility

Figure 3.7   Parenting styles within the context of parental control and sensitivity

- **A secure identity**. Research has shown that parents who are warm and accepting and create an atmosphere where it is easy to express one's feelings are more likely to have children who have a strong ego identity, are able to solve problems flexibly and are empathic to others (Hauser et al. 1984, Powers et al. 1983).
- **Higher self-esteem**. Buri et al. (1988) observed that young people who are allowed to contribute to family decisions and feel valued in this role are more likely to rate themselves higher on standardized assessments of self-esteem. Adolescents who perceive their parents as authoritarian, however, consistently rate their self-esteem lower than others. Permissive parenting styles are not linked to teenagers' ratings of self-esteem.
- **Greater autonomy**. Research suggests that authoritative parenting, particularly with respect to shared decision making, is linked to higher levels of autonomous functioning amongst young people – i.e. the ability to hold and express their own views (Allen et al. 1994, Collins and Laursen 2004, Fuhrman and Holmbeck 1995, Lamborn and Steinberg 1993, Steinberg et al. 1994, 1991, Weiss and Schwarz 1996).
- **Higher levels of morality, social responsibility and pro-social behavior**. Parents who model high standards for behavior and communicate their expectations clearly within the context of a warm and loving relationship are more likely to have teenagers who maintain pro-social values and engage in higher levels of moral reasoning (Eisenberg 1990, Eisenberg et al. 2004, Grotevant and Cooper 1998, Walker et al. 2000, Walker and Taylor 1991).
- **Higher achievement and school competence**. Research repeatedly demonstrates that authoritative parents are more likely to be involved in their children's education. This involvement (in the form of high levels of acceptance, supervision and 'autonomy granting') in turn leads to higher levels of school engagement and school achievement (Baumrind 1991, Brody et al. 2002, Connell et al. 1994, Steinberg et al.

1992). Conversely, authoritarian and permissive parenting are significantly related to lower levels of academic performance (Dornbusch et al. 1987, Pittman and Chase-Lansdale 2001).

- **Greater resistance to peer pressure**. Research consistently suggests that peer influence is moderated by the parent–child relationship, demonstrating that a positive relationship with one's parents significantly reduces the likelihood of a teenager engaging in negative behavior endorsed by their peers (Steinberg 1986, 1987, Steinberg and Silverberg 1986). Conversely, authoritarian parenting appears to increase the likelihood that teenagers will rely on their peers for advice and support. For example, Fuligni and Eccles (1993) found that peer reliance was greatest amongst young people who lived in households where they believed their parents to be overly strict and had few opportunities to participate in the decision-making process. Authoritative parenting has also been linked to improved social ties with peers and other significant adults, such as teachers (Cui et al. 2002).
- **Less risk of mental health problems**. A US-based survey of over 12,000 adolescents in grades 9–12 found that perceived parental warmth was significantly linked to less emotional distress, fewer suicidal thoughts and a lower interest in violence (Resnick et al. 1997). Conversely, a poor relationship with parents has been consistently linked to higher levels of adolescent psychopathology, including suicide (Brody et al. 1988, Steinhausen et al. 2006).
- **Later onset of sexual behavior**. The above study (Resnick et al. 1997) also found that teenagers were less likely to engage in risky sexual behavior and more likely to postpone intercourse if they had a supportive relationship with their parents. This finding is consistent with other studies that demonstrate that strong parental disapproval towards sexual activity, communicated within the context of an otherwise warm and supportive relationship, significantly postpones the timing of teenage girls' sexual debut (Meschke et al. 2002, Rodgers 1999). However, teenage girls who feel less connected to their mothers are more likely to engage in sexually risky behavior at an earlier age, whether or not their mothers approve of it (Ford et al. 2005, Pittman and Chase-Lansdale 2001, Sieverding et al. 2005, Sieving et al. 2000, Woodward et al. 2001).
- **Resistance to substance use and abuse**. Parents who set clear expectations regarding drug and alcohol use (as well as sexual behavior – see above) within the context of an authoritative relationship are significantly more likely to have teenagers who comply with these expectations and refrain from using these substances, as well as exhibit greater overall self-control (Baumrind 1991, Brody et al. 2000, Brody et al. 2002, Cleveland et al. 2005, Resnick et al. 1997, Weiss and Schwarz 1996, Whitaker and Miller 2000).

It should be noted that an authoritative parenting style is associated with positive child behaviors, regardless of culture, parental education, economic wealth or family structure (Steinberg 1990, 2001). While Baumrind (1978) originally maintained that authoritative parenting was likely to be most effective for middle-class 'protestant ethic' families, research now tells us that this is not the case. A growing body of international research suggests that, despite cultural differences, authoritative parenting practices are evident in most societies and that children and young people do much better when their parents adopt this style of child rearing (Dmitrieva et al. 2004, Steinberg 1990, 2001, Vazsonyi et al. 2003).

How do parenting styles influence child development?

It is clear that an authoritative style of parenting serves to protect children from many of the developmental risks they face, but why might this be the case? Youniss and Smollar (1985) have noted that as children mature, the parental role shifts from one of unilateral authority to mutuality. Through this process, parents must relinquish some of their power and 'grant' their child a certain degree of autonomy by allowing him or her to enter what Maccoby (1992) calls a 'system of reciprocity'. In this respect, key authoritative practices, such as mutual trust and open communication, enable young people to think for themselves, trust their judgment and take risks (Figure 3.8). Conversely, authoritarian and permissive parenting styles do not foster independent thinking and personal agency and this may interfere with optimal child development.

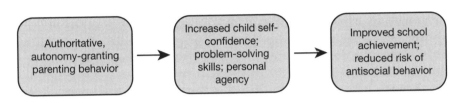

Figure 3.8 The influence of parenting styles on child development

For this reason, most evidence-based parenting programs encourage an authoritative style of parenting. While there are no parenting programs based solely upon Baumrind's theories, most endorse and promote the following authoritative parenting behaviors:

- High levels of parental acceptance
- High parental warmth
- An open style of communication
- Democratic decision making
- Mutual respect
- Mutual trust
- Personal agency and responsibility
- Independence and autonomy.

Evidence-based parenting programs that draw from Baumrind's parenting styles theory include the *Incredible Years*, *Triple P*, *FAST* and *Strengthening Families 10–14* (See Box 3.5).

Model of human ecology

Nested systems

Most large-scale community-based initiatives aimed at children and their families have their roots in Urie Bronfenbrenner's model of human ecology (also known as the ecological systems theory). As a Russian emigrant living in the United States, Bronfenbrenner believed that good schooling on its own does not guarantee positive outcomes for children. Rather, all environments – including children's homes, schools, neighborhoods and communities – must work together to support children's development. Bronfenbrenner also believed that parental

Box 3.5: The *Strengthening Families 10–14 Program*

The *Strengthening Families Program for Parents and Youth 10–14* (SF 10–14) is a universal, family-based intervention which aims to protect children from the risks leading to substance misuse by encouraging democratic family interactions. Parents and their children (aged 10 to 14) attend seven weekly sessions which use video-tapes to teach parents how to utilize appropriate and consistent discipline techniques, manage strong emotions concerning their children and develop effective communication skills. At the same time, children learn peer resistance and refusal techniques, personal and social interaction skills and stress and emotion management. Each session also includes a period where parents and children work together to practice conflict resolution and communication skills through activities designed to increase family cohesiveness. A series of RCTs suggest that SF 10–14 significantly reduces the risks associated with adolescent substance misuse (Spoth et al. 2001, 2006) and improves school achievement (Spoth et al. 2008).

involvement in children's education was crucial for it to have a lasting impact. These ideas were used by the Johnson administration in the development of the *Head Start* program to mandate that parents be involved in the delivery and development of each local program (see Box 2.1).

Bronfenbrenner also led the evaluation of *Head Start* during the early 1970s. This research, along with Bronfenbrenner's cross-cultural comparisons of childrearing practices in the US and Soviet Union, led to the publication of the groundbreaking book *The Ecology of Human Development* (Bronfenbrenner 1979, Bronfenbrenner et al. 1970), which has since transformed the way children are studied. Drawing from the theories of Piaget and Lewin, Bronfenbrenner's **ecological model** suggests that child development is influenced by children's interactions with adults and peers in the contexts of the home, school, community, culture and society. Like nested Russian dolls, Bronfenbrenner asserted that each environment exerts its influence on the other and it is the combined effect of these environments (as opposed to any single one) that determines each child's developmental path. Figure 3.9 provides an overview of the ways in which the ecological systems are nested, demonstrating how elements within each system influence the other systems surrounding it.

The ecological perspective begins with the child as the 'engine' of his or her own development. This development is directly influenced by each child's **microsystem** – i.e. the immediate environment in which interactions with parents, caregivers and friends take place. Within the microsystem, the child actively influences his or her family and neighborhood, while these environments simultaneously influence him or her. Individual child characteristics, such as child temperament and physical health, influence and interact with parenting factors such as childrearing practices and family structure, to determine immediate developmental outcomes.

Family interactions are then further influenced by the **mesosystem**, which involves the family and community, including each family's relationship with its schools, churches, neighborhoods and civic bodies. Children's interactions with peers also take place at the level of the mesosystem. The mesosystem is then further influenced by the **exosystem**, which affects family life through parents' employment and access to community resources, such as parks, libraries and government bodies. The exosystem is, in turn, surrounded by

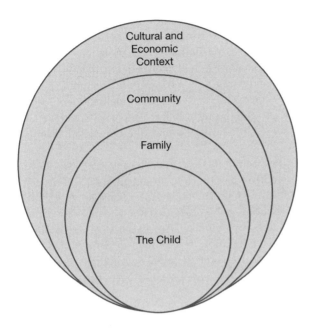

Figure 3.9   Bronfenbrenner's ecological model of child development

the **macrosystem**, which includes each child's religion, culture and race, as well as socio-historical events, such as wars and economic downturns. In this respect, the beliefs, values and societal rules that constitute the macrosystem provide the 'top down' governance that determines how children, families, schools and communities interact.

Bronfenbrenner argued that attention must be paid to all ecological systems in order to ensure the wellbeing of children and their families. Bronfenbrenner also emphasized that while child development was influenced by the quality of these systems, it was also determined by the connections between them. Thus, the quality of the relationships between children and parents, parents and schools and schools and communities are all important. For example, an excellent support service for families would have little or no effect if it were difficult to access (e.g. remote from the community) or did not make efforts to engage parents and children.

Risk and protective factors

A second related model proposes that, throughout childhood, a variety of biological and environmental factors (existing at all four ecological levels) often protect or put children at risk for undesirable developmental outcomes, such as antisocial behavior, low achievement, poor mental health and child abuse. 'Risk' factors include any individual characteristic or circumstance that increases the likelihood of negative developmental outcomes, whereas 'protective' factors are processes that buffer or reduce the chances of adverse outcomes occurring in the first place.

For example, research in the area of child maltreatment suggests that the likelihood of parents abusing their children is determined by a variety of factors existing at the individual, community and societal levels (Cicchetti and Lynch 1993, Cicchetti and Rizley 1981, Rutter 1985, 2000). Research suggests that it is unlikely that child maltreatment is caused by any single risk factor, but by multiple risk factors occurring at multiple ecological levels (Loeber 1990, Rutter 1979, 1985, 2000). For example, Sidebotham et al. (2006) have observed that a wide range of parental stressors are correlated with child maltreatment, but the strongest risks are from socio-economic deprivation and parents' own background, including poor mental health. Community-level risk factors consistently linked to child maltreatment include lack of social support, neighborhood poverty and the accessibility of alcohol (Coulton et al. 1995, 1999, 2007, Garbarino and Crouter 1978, Garbarino and Sherman 1980, Korbin et al. 1998, Molnar et al. 2003).

It is important to note that protective factors also exist at each ecological level. Key protective factors include a warm and supportive parenting environment, a lack of abuse-related stress and strong neighborhood cohesion (Collishaw et al. 2007, Jaffee et al. 2007). Recent findings from the Chicago Longitudinal Study also observe that attendance in a community-based nursery school may protect children from future child maltreatment (Mersky et al. 2009).

Because families are often exposed to multiple risks, many evidence-based parenting programs seek to help parents manage or overcome these risks at multiple ecological levels. Examples of such programs include *Communities That Care*, the *Nurse–Family Partnership* and *Families and Schools Together* (FAST, see Box 3.6).

Coparenting theory

Coparenting theory recognizes the impact of parents' coordination with each other (or lack thereof) on family functioning and children's development (Belsky et al. 1995, Feinberg 2003, McHale et al. 2004). Coparenting theory has its roots in family systems theory (see Chapter 4 for a complete discussion), which considers family functioning in terms of multiple subsystems. Family systems include the couple subsystem, the parenting subsystem, the sibling subsystem and various combinations of parent and child subsystems. While these systems most often involve the child's biological father and mother, they may also include the child's mother and grandmother, a parent and paid caregiver, or other members close to the family. Thus, coparents do not have to be a couple or live together, nor must they always be the child's father and mother. Rather, coparenting refers to the ways in which childcare duties are divided and coordinated between the adults who perform a parenting role in a child's life.

The coparent system is typically formed during the transition to parenthood. As couples become parents they must learn how to work together as co-managers of the wider family system (Minuchin 1974). In this respect, the term 'coparent' applies only to the way in which parents work together as parents – not to their interaction as a romantic couple. While the quality of the couple system often influences the quality of the coparental subsystem (Carlson et al. 2009), the two are treated as discrete systems within the parenting literature (Belsky et al. 1995, McBride and Rane 1998, McHale et al. 2004, Van Egeren 2004). It is therefore theoretically possible for parents to have a well-functioning couple system but a poorly functioning coparenting system. Alternatively, mothers and fathers may coparent well, but interact poorly with each other. This is sometimes the case with separated or divorced couples who have learned to look past their personal differences to develop effective strategies for jointly parenting their children. Research suggests that the quality of the coparenting system is more strongly linked to child developmental outcomes than the quality of the couple system (Carlson et al. 2009, McHale and Rasmussen, 1998, Schoppe-Sullivan et al. 2009).

Box 3.6: *Families and Schools Together* (FAST)

Families and Schools Together (FAST) aims to reduce the risks associated with substance misuse and antisocial behavior by promoting protective links within the family, school and community (McDonald and Sayger 1998). This is done through a group-based after-school program delivered to parents and their children that promotes the following seven protective factors:

- **Parent-to-child bond**: Parents are encouraged to follow their children's lead through one-to-one play sessions.
- **Parent-to-parent bond**: Couples are coached in methods for reducing conflict and improving their coparenting skills (see next section and Chapter 4). Single parents are encouraged to form coparenting bonds with other adults who play a supportive role in their children's lives.
- **Cohesive family unit**: Family cohesion is encouraged through the use of family meals and family fun times, which take place during the sessions. During these activities, families receive coaching on how to interact with one another and build their strength as a family.
- **Parent self-help support group**: This includes activities to help parents develop their own informal social networks.
- **Parent–school affiliation**: This includes activities which encourage parents to become more actively involved in their children's school.
- **Parent to community agency connections**: These help parents to gain access to community-based resources by providing information on community services and by facilitating problem-solving discussions with parents on how to better access support.
- **Parent empowerment**: Parents' sense of self-efficacy and self-esteem is encouraged through positive feedback and opportunities for parents to share positive experiences with one another. During the course of the program, each parent wins a cash lottery. Parents are then encouraged to give back to the group by cooking a meal for it.

FAST is delivered by a team of practitioners that includes representatives from the school and community, as well as other parents. FAST groups initially meet for eight weeks and then carry on as monthly parents' meetings. The FAST program has undergone several RCTs, all demonstrating significant reductions in antisocial behavior and improvements in children's psychological wellbeing. Two follow-up evaluations suggest that the effects have been maintained for up to two years (Kratochwill et al. 2004, 2009, McDonald et al. 2006). Increases in parents' willingness to volunteer and be active in their communities have also been observed (Crozier et al. 2010).

Feinberg (2003) asserts that the coparenting system consists of the four key elements illustrated in Figure 3.10: 1) childrearing agreement, 2) division of the child-related labor, 3) the extent to which parents support or undermine each other in their coparental role and 4) the way the parents jointly manage family interactions.

The childrearing agreement refers to the degree to which parents agree on child-related topics, including their disciplinary practices, educational standards, family priorities, safety issues, peer associations and responses to children's emotional needs. Childrearing attitudes

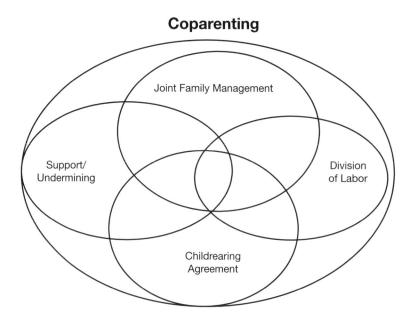

Figure 3.10 Feinberg's coparenting model (reprinted with permission from Feinberg 2003)

are, in turn, influenced by the parents' own developmental history, as well as their cultural and educational values and their knowledge of child development. While parents often disagree on a variety of childrearing issues, this disagreement does not always impair the coparenting system (Ehrenberg et al. 2001, Feinberg 2002). Parents who can successfully 'agree to disagree' are still able to effectively parent together, as long as they do not try to undermine one another. However, if these disagreements become hostile or overly critical, they may lead to inter-parental conflict that can interfere with parents' ability to effectively manage their children (Belsky et al. 1995).

The second component of the coparenting relationship involves the ways in which parents divide the duties and responsibilities pertaining to housework and childcare. Although the term 'coparent' implies a sharing of duties, it does not necessarily mean that parental roles are or should be equal in authority or responsibility (Ehrenberg et al. 2001). Authority and responsibility within the coparent system is something that is negotiated between parents in response to the wider ecological needs of the family (Feinberg 2003, McHale et al. 2004). In many families, the coparenting relationship is often more complementary than comparable. While fathers often have influence and control related to their breadwinning status, mothers generally have greater coparenting influence in their role as primary caregiver (McHale et al. 2002).

The third component of the coparenting subsystem is the extent to which parents support one another in the parenting role. In other words, do parenting partners uphold each other's parenting decisions and respect each other's contribution, or does one parent undermine the other through critical or competitive behaviors? Research consistently suggests that mutually supportive coparenting behaviors may be the most significant aspect of an effective coparenting alliance (Schoppe-Sullivan et al. 2004). For example, statements such as 'I think you are a terrific mother/father' significantly predict each parent's sense of closeness to their child, when an equitable and flexible approach to shared family work does not (Ehrenberg et al. 2001). Research also suggests that undermining and competitive parenting interactions contribute to problems with children's behavior, including conduct disorders (Davis and Cummings 1998, Floyd and Zmich 1991, Belsky et al. 1996, Schoppe et al. 2001, Schoppe-Sullivan et al. 2009). In particular, Webster-Stratton and Hammond (1999) have observed that negative marital interactions predict critical parenting behaviors in mothers and overly punitive behaviors in fathers.

The fourth component of the coparenting subsystem involves the ways in which the parents jointly manage the family. Joint family management involves three distinct processes: 1) the quality of the communication between the parents, 2) the ways in which parents create boundaries between themselves and other family members and 3) the extent to which both parents are accessible and contribute to the family system. Research consistently suggests that the quality of communication between parents is predictive of children's emotional and behavioral problems. High levels of inter-parental conflict may interfere with children's ability to self-regulate and increase the likelihood of an insecure attachment (Cummings et al. 1994, Davies et al. 2002, Frosch et al. 2000, Laurent et al. 2008). For example, Owen and Cox (1997) observed that inter-parental conflict at 3 months predicts a disorganized infant attachment at 1 year, even if the parents are warm and sensitive during their interactions with their child. In extreme cases, inter-parental conflict can significantly interfere with parents' ability to appropriately support their children's physical and emotional needs (Feinberg 2003).

Many evidence-based parenting programs, including *Incredible Years* (Box 1.7) and *Triple P* (Box 1.3), include elements that help parents learn how to coparent more successfully. Programs that place an emphasis on coparenting interactions frequently target parents during the transition to parenting or parents when they are divorcing or separating. *Family Foundations* (see Box 3.7) is an example of a universally accessible parenting course for expectant parents. *New Beginnings* (Box 5.1) and *Dads for Life* (Box 3.8) target coparenting issues for divorcing couples.

Box 3.7: The *Family Foundations Program*

Family Foundations is a prevention-based program embedded within an eight-session childbirth education group. Unlike other prenatal classes, four of the sessions focus on parenting skills that are likely to enhance the coparenting relationship. This focus includes information on how parenthood might strain the couple relationship, ways of overcoming this strain and the use of parenting skills to foster the attachment relationship. Observational findings from the program's first randomized controlled trial suggest that mothers and fathers attending *Family Foundations* were less likely to demonstrate competitive or undermining parenting behaviors and demonstrated more positive parenting skills, including improved sensitivity and positive affect towards their infant 12 months after attending the program. Findings from a second follow-up when children were aged 3 observed that *Family Foundation* parents experienced less parental stress and depression, exhibited improved coparenting skills and reported using less physical punishment than parents in the comparison group. Program effects were particularly pronounced for families with boys, who exhibited significantly fewer behavioral problems (Feinberg and Kan 2008, Feinberg et al. 2010).

Box 3.8: *Dads for Life*

Dads for Life is an intervention targeted at separated fathers only. It aims to improve outcomes for divorcing fathers and their children by improving the quantity and quality of time nonresident fathers spend with their children and reducing the amount of conflict separated fathers have with their ex-wives. These 'distal' goals are supported by 1) increasing fathers' commitment to the parenting role, 2) improving fathers' parenting skills, 3) improving motivation and conflict management skills and 4) increasing perceived control of the divorce process. The program is delivered via eight group sessions and two individual sessions via trained Master's-level psychologists. Half of the sessions focus on the father–child relationship and the other half concentrate on improving cooperation between fathers and their ex-partners.

Two RCTs of the program demonstrate positive outcomes for both fathers and their children. Father participants were significantly more likely to report decreased levels of conflict with their ex-partner at the two-year follow-up and their children were less likely to report internalizing problems. Moreover, mothers interviewed as part of the evaluation (not participating in the program) also reported decreased levels of conflict with their ex-partner as well as higher levels of satisfaction with the coparenting relationship. Although it is surprising that mothers were more likely to perceive improvements in the coparenting relationship than fathers were, findings from both *Dads for Life* evaluations provide good evidence that coparenting skills can be improved for parents no longer involved in a romantic couple relationship (Braver et al. 2005; Cookston et al. 2006).

Evidence-based theories do not equal an evidence-based parenting intervention

This chapter provides an overview of the key theories of parenting and child development that underpin most evidence-based parenting programs. While there are many other theories that could have been included in this chapter, the six presented here are supported by an extremely robust evidence base involving research conducted in both naturalistic and laboratory settings. Those commissioning and delivering parenting support should take efforts to ensure that the interventions they offer are informed by sound theories of parenting practice that are underpinned by solid research evidence.

This task should be undertaken with a word of caution, however. There are literally thousands of books, magazines, television shows and parenting programs claiming to be informed by scientific theories of child development. Many are very popular and are usually quick to pop up on the search engine screen. Some are even endorsed by celebrities and television shows. And many use the theories described in this chapter as proof of their evidence base. This does not mean that their methods are evidence-based, however, as the example involving holding therapies suggests.

An evidence-based parenting program should be grounded in solid theories *and* experimental research. A program that claims to be grounded in attachment or parenting-styles theory is not necessarily evidence-based if its specific methods have not yet been tested. As described in Chapter 2 and elaborated in further chapters, rigorously tested theories and practices include a well-articulated theory of change that demonstrates how specific parenting behaviors are linked to improved child outcomes. These links should be tested through rigorous evaluations that ideally include one randomized controlled trial and, at the very least, standardized pre- and post-measures demonstrating positive change. In other words, a good parenting program should be able back up its claims with actual (not theorized) scientific evidence.

Those working with parents should therefore be wary of interventions that do not have a program of research attached to them. Ideally, this research should be published in well-respected journals, rather than books. While books are often an excellent source of information (especially edited volumes of scientific studies), they are not subject to the same level of scrutiny that academic journal articles are. This is because the information in them has not undergone **peer review** and thus the methods for testing their theories and claims may not have been rigorously examined. In many instances, books are published because they have widespread appeal and profitability, not because they are scientifically-sound. A PhD or similar qualifications are no guarantee that the author's ideas are evidence-based. And testimonials that endorse a book or program are nothing more than testimonials.[2] They are not scientific evidence and should not be used as proof that a specific method or program works.

While the theories endorsed in this chapter are indeed evidence-based, they are frequently used to substantiate the opinions, beliefs and values of individuals and organizations. Being an evidence-based practitioner means knowing how to discriminate real evidence from social ideals and political agendas. For this reason, practitioners should maintain a healthy skepticism regarding claims that popular parenting practices are, in fact, evidence-based.

Box 3.9: Key points

- An infant's attachment to their adult caregiver is a natural part of child development.
- Evidence from the neurosciences suggests that brain development is extremely malleable to environmental influences during the first three years of development.
- During the first three years, brain cell development undergoes a period of synaptic overproduction, which is followed by a period of synaptic pruning. Synaptic overproduction increases the brain's potential to learn a wide variety of things. Synaptic pruning then improves the brain's ability to efficiently process information.
- Neurological processes that are genetically determined and 'environmentally expected' appear to take place within limited time frames, also known as critical periods.
- Neurological processes that are 'environmentally dependent', including processes that contribute to the development of memory, appear to be less subject to critical periods.
- A second period of synaptic overproduction takes place during puberty. This is followed by a second period of synaptic pruning that lasts until the mid 20s.
- Research from the neurosciences suggests that good-quality parenting support is important during all stages of a child's development.
- A child's attachment security is based upon how sensitively parents respond to their needs.
- Mental representations of the attachment relationship formed during infancy are carried into relationships with friends and other adults as children mature.
- A secure attachment in infancy and toddlerhood predicts positive behaviors when children are older if life circumstances remain stable.

- Unstable life circumstances can alter children's attachment status, especially if these circumstances are negative.
- Evidence-based parenting programs have now been developed to improve maternal sensitivity.
- Inappropriate parental responses to aggressive child behavior promote poor child self-regulation and antisocial behavior.
- Parent management training programs that teach parents to respond appropriately to their children's aggressive behavior consistently result in improved outcomes for children and parents.
- Parenting behaviors are classified into four different styles – authoritarian, authoritative, permissive and neglecting.
- An authoritative style of parenting, characterized by high levels of warmth, high standards and high supervision is strongly related to positive child outcomes.
- Authoritative parenting is effective because it encourages children to think for themselves and promotes self-confidence.
- Child development is influenced by many factors that exist at the individual, family, school, community and societal levels.
- Some factors place children at risk for negative developmental outcomes, whereas others protect them and foster resilience.
- Parenting programs that address risk and protective factors at multiple ecological levels have consistently demonstrated positive long-term benefits.
- Parents' ability to coparent their child effectively significantly contributes to improved child outcomes.
- The coparenting relationship is characterized by four components: 1) childrearing agreement, 2) division of the child-related labor, 3) the extent to which parents support or undermine each other in their coparental role and 4) the way the parents jointly manage family interactions.
- Evidence-based parenting programs are underpinned by evidence-based theories, although evidence-based theories are no guarantee that a parenting intervention will be effective.

Notes

1   These figures represent the distributions originally observed in Ainsworth's 'standard' American sample. In a cross-cultural study by van IJzendoorn and Kroonenberg (1988), significant variations across cultures were observed, although the American figures still represent the 'average' distribution across attachment categories.

2   In fact, the APSAC Task Force advises that client testimonials not be used to market treatments, because there is potential for exploitation.

4 Evidence-based therapies used in parenting interventions

Introduction

Parents' ability to adequately care for their children is influenced by a variety of factors, including their knowledge of effective childrearing strategies, their life circumstances and their physical and mental health. The most effective parenting interventions (used in both individual and group work) include methods for considering parents' psychological well-being, as well as improving their parenting skills. Methods for addressing the psychological needs of parents should be informed by empirically supported theories of personality, as well as rigorously tested therapeutic practices. This section provides an overview of the therapies and theories used in evidence-based parenting interventions that address parents' psychological needs.

Psychodynamic theory

The id, ego and super-ego

Psychodynamic theory begins with the ideas of Austrian psychiatrist Sigmund Freud (1856–1939), who is widely credited with establishing the practice of psychoanalysis. Although most of Freud's ideas were based on case studies and were not empirically tested, they are worth discussing here, since they provide the starting point for many therapeutic practices that are underpinned by scientific evidence.

Freud believed that human personality is organized into three basic parts: the id, the ego and the super-ego (Freud 1933). Freud identified the id as the primary force behind all human activity, involving both inherited and instinctual behaviors, including sex and aggression. Freud believed that infants come into the world in an 'id-ridden' state, where behavior is determined by unconscious drives and impulses, rather than logical thoughts or feelings. Freud asserted that instinctual drives operate off of a pleasure principle that seeks immediate gratification, with no consideration of what the longer-term consequences of pleasure-seeking behavior might be (Freud 1940, 1948).

Freud also noted that infants quickly learn that immediate gratification is not always possible. In order to compensate for this, Freud theorized that young children form internal representations of objects associated with the reduction of their id-related drives in an attempt to gain some short-term satisfaction. For example, a hungry infant may conjure up an image of his or her mother's breast in an attempt to relieve the tension created by the hunger. Freud called this activity wish fulfillment and asserted that it primarily takes place at an unconscious level, in the form of dreams and hallucinations.

Freud called the use of images to reduce id-related tensions primary process thinking. He noted that while representations provide partial gratification of id-related drives, they do not reduce these tensions entirely. The ego thus develops in response to the need for id-related gratification within realistic limits. In this respect, the ego acts according to the reality principle, which requires individuals to test reality and delay gratification until the appropriate environmental conditions are found. Freud believed that the ego operates through secondary process thinking, which involves the use of realistic, logical thought processes, including planning and decision making, to appropriately manage the impulses of the id. While most id-related thoughts are unconscious, individuals are totally aware of their conscious, ego-related thoughts.

Freud's third mental structure is the super-ego (Freud 1933). The super-ego develops through children's interactions with their parents and contributes to their ability to self-regulate behavior. Super-ego processes involve judgments of right and wrong and good and bad, informed by the morals and standards of parents and society. Whereas the id seeks pleasure and the ego tests reality, the super-ego seeks perfection. Super-ego thoughts are sometimes repressed to the unconscious, but are usually accessible through preconscious thinking, which involves unconscious memories that can easily be accessed.

According to Freud, the ego is constantly trying to reconcile the demands of the id and the super-ego with the requirements and restrictions of the external world. Its task is to realistically balance pressures from primitive id-related drives with the high standards of the super-ego. Mental health is thus characterized by a well-functioning ego that is capable of keeping the id and the super-ego in check.

Psychopathology occurs when ego processes become unbalanced and the id is either under- or over-controlled (Freud 1933). For example, Freud believed that anxiety stems from people's perceived inability to appropriately manage id-related impulses or the exceedingly high demands created by the super-ego. Freud identified neurotic anxiety as stemming from a fear of being overwhelmed by id-related impulses. Individuals who feel that they are constantly on the cusp of losing their temper, their rationality or even their mind suffer from neurotic anxiety. Moral anxiety, on the other hand, stems from an inability to manage feelings of shame or guilt caused by an over-involved super-ego. Morally anxious individuals often feel paralyzed because they are afraid that they may be punished for the things they think and do.

Freud acknowledged that all fears and anxieties are not unrealistic or irrational. In this respect, mentally healthy individuals must occasionally cope with realistic anxiety, where they are appropriately afraid of realistic threats that could occur in their daily lives. Realistic anxieties include concerns that one's home might be burgled when no one is there, or the fear of being robbed in a dark alley, late at night. While such fears can also become out of control, they are often managed when people take the appropriate precautions.

Freud additionally observed that individuals manage perceived and unconscious threats through a variety of coping processes that he referred to as defense mechanisms (Freud 1924). Table 4.1 provides an overview of some of the more common defenses. Freud believed that defense mechanisms were primitive responses to perceived threats that also contribute to various forms of neurosis and maladaptive behavior. An extreme form of neurotic behavior involves hysteria, which is characterized by functional blindness, paralyses or deafness when there is no underlying physical cause. Freud observed that hysteria occurred as a defense against difficult feelings created by the inability to adaptively regulate sexual impulses.

Freud developed his psychoanalytic treatment as a way of reducing neurotic conflict by helping clients to uncover difficult feelings that might be repressed, denied or distorted. Because

Table 4.1 Common defense mechanismsw

Defense mechanism	Definition	Example
Level I: Level I defense mechanisms are considered to be the most severe. These defenses enable individuals to cope with a perceived threat by reorganizing external realities. In extreme cases, Level I defenses characterize 'psychotic' behavior. When exhibited by children or represented in dreams, they may be considered a healthy form of coping.		
Denial	Refusing to perceive or consciously acknowledge anxiety-provoking information.	An unemployed father purchases extravagant toys for his children even though he cannot afford them.
Distortion	Grossly reshaping external reality to better meet internal needs.	A depressed student interprets her teacher's critique of her essay as an indication that the teacher thinks she is stupid.
Delusional projection	Harboring false and often extreme impressions about external reality via projection (see below).	A single mother imagines that that all of her friends and family are conspiring to take her children away from her.
Level II: People use Level II defenses to cope with threatening situations or people. They are often seen in severe depression and personality disorders. However, they are considered as a normal part of adolescent coping. For this reason, they are often referred to as 'immature' defense mechanisms.		
Fantasy	Retreating into imagined situations in order to avoid inner and outer conflict.	A teenager exaggerates his parents' wealth to create a sense of security to himself or others.
Projection	Attributing one's own attitudes, feelings or desires that have been internally judged as unacceptable to someone or something else.	A child who is resentful of her new baby brother 'projects' these feelings by saying that the baby hates her.
Hypochondriasis	Transforming negative feelings towards other people or situations into physical symptoms of illness.	Constant worry that one is sick or about to die.
Passive aggression	Indirectly exhibiting aggression by not complying with the wishes of others.	A husband agrees to take out the trash week after week but never does it.
Acting out	Directly expressing an impulse without conscious awareness of the driving emotion.	A child who is sad about his parents' separation behaves aggressively at school.
Idealization	Perceiving another individual as having more positive qualities than he or she may actually have.	A little girl thinks of her friend's older sister as the perfect individual and a person she would like to be when she gets older.

Defense mechanism	Definition	Example
Level III: These mechanisms are fairly common in adults. They often have short-term advantages in coping, but can result in long-term problems in personal and professional relationships.		
Displacement	Shifting impulses to a less threatening or otherwise more acceptable target.	A father yells at his son when he is angry with his wife.
Dissociation	Modifying one's usual behavior to avoid or postpone emotional distress.	A woman is calm in the hospital when she hears that her father has terminal cancer.
Isolation	Separating feelings from ideas and events.	A young girl has been abused by a family member for years. She recounts the details of her abuse without apparent distress.
Intellectualization	Concentrating on the intellectual aspects of a situation and distancing the emotional components.	A teenager has been coming home most nights drunk. Her father is unconcerned because he read a newspaper article that describes adolescence as a time for rebelling against authority and pushing boundaries.
Reaction formation	Converting unacceptable impulses into their opposites.	An aunt is jealous and resentful of a baby who has consumed the attention of her sister. She goes out of her way to celebrate and adore the child.
Repression	Pushing painful or dangerous thoughts into the unconscious.	An abused women represses her feelings of pain, but has difficulty forming relationships with others.
Regression	Reverting patterns of thought or behavior to an earlier stage of development.	A 12-year-old is having trouble making friends at her new school. She starts spending more time playing dolls with her younger sister.
Rationalization	Using false reasoning to convince oneself that one's behavior is more acceptable than it really is.	A substance misusing woman rationalizes that her behavior is not problematic because she does not misuse substances when at work.

these feelings are often unconscious, the aim of therapy is to provide a safe environment in which feelings can be exposed and explored. Freud did this by asking his clients to rest on a couch, discuss their dreams and **free associate** ideas (Freud 1911). Freud believed that these methods relaxed the ego's defense mechanisms and allowed access to unconscious thoughts and feelings that may be repressed. Freud and his followers believed, however, that defenses still worked to distort the content of dreams. An expert opinion of the therapist was therefore required to accurately interpret the significance of dreams and other unconscious associations.

Freud believed that throughout treatment the therapist should deliberately reveal little about him- or herself in order to facilitate the development of a **transference** relationship (Freud 1940). Transference occurs when the client responds to the therapist as if he or she were the client's father, mother or some other important childhood figure. Transference allows the client to revisit past conflicts that may be distorted or repressed, with the support and advice of the therapist. Once repressed conflicts are explored in a non-threatening context, the client is in a better position to understand and resolve them.

Object relations theory

Freud's ideas were hugely influential during his lifetime and have since been applied to a wide variety of mental health disorders by his many followers. Theories from the **object relations**[1] school of psychotherapy are of particular interest to those working with parents, as they directly address how parenting behaviors influence children's development. The term 'object relations' was first coined by British psychologist Ronald Fairbairn (1889–1964), who departed from Freud in assuming that child behavior is driven not by pleasure-seeking activities, but by object-seeking desires (Fairbairn 1952–1986).

The term 'object' refers to the child's first love object – the parent. Fairbairn noted that as the infant interacts with his or her parents, a strong and enduring bond is formed. Within the context of this bond, children develop expectations of their parents that are then transferred to their future relationships with others. Fairbairn believed that positive parenting behaviors socialize children to behave in a positive, outward way towards others. When parents fail to meet their children's needs, however, children compensate by fantasizing false relationships with internalized others.

Donald Winnicott (1896–1971) was a contemporary of Fairbairn's and shared his belief that object relations were a primary force in children's development. Winnicott noted that the quality of the interaction between the mother and child was so intense that 'there [was] no such thing as a baby – only a nursing couple' (Winnicott 1960). By this he meant infant development is inextricably linked to maternal care. Winnicott also noted that early motherhood was marked by a period of **primary maternal preoccupation** that enables mothers to intuitively identify with their infants in order to meet their physical and emotional needs (Winnicott 1958).

Winnicott believed that appropriate maternal responses were key in providing the infant with a sense of control (also referred to as **subjective omnipotence**) related to healthy ego development. In this respect, mothers did not need to be perfect, but they needed to be 'good enough'. In fact, Winnicott believed that perfectly responding to an infant's every need could actually impair its development. Instead, a good-enough mother instinctively allowed some time before she met her child's demands. As Winnicott stated: 'The good-enough mother ... starts off with an almost complete adaptation to her infant's needs, and as time proceeds she adapts less and less completely, gradually, according to the infant's growing ability to deal with her failure' (Winnicott 2005: 14).

Winnicott believed that this gradual lessening of maternal responsivity allows the child to learn how to self-regulate his or her emotional and physical states. Through this process, the infant also gains a sense of control, as it learns how to predict its mother's behavior. The final phase of this process provides the infant with a sense of independence, which is never absolute since the child is never completely isolated from the mother. The mother's role is thus to first create the illusion of **undifferentiated symbiosis** that is associated with safety and security, which is then followed by a gradual sense of disillusion that separates the child from the mother and introduces it to the social world. Winnicott believed that healthy ego development takes place when the child recognizes that the mother is neither all good nor all bad, but instead a separate individual with valid needs and wants of her own.

Although Winnicott never scientifically tested his ideas, they were extremely popular during his lifetime and remain influential in parenting work today. Like Bowlby's theory of attachment, Winnicott highlights the importance of the quality of the interactions between the parent and child in determining the child's early emotional development. However, Winnicott's work additionally observes that a primary task of early development is the psychological separation of the infant from the mother. Winnicott asserts that this separation process is most successful when the mother is able to balance and negotiate her needs with those of the infant's. In this respect, Winnicott is generally perceived as highly sympathetic towards mothers and is regarded by many as one of the first parenting practitioners.

In the 1940s, Winnicott did a series of radio shows dedicated to the 'ordinary mother' that offered advice on a variety of issues ranging from thumb sucking to toilet training. His messages highlighted maternal strengths rather than weaknesses and, to this end, Winnicott advocated the use of brief parenting interventions that aimed to empower mothers rather than analyze their behavior. He and his wife Clare were also pioneers in the field of British social work, where they established good practice standards for individuals working with emotionally deprived children and their parents.

Selma Fraiberg – ghosts in the nursery

Selma Fraiberg (1918–1981) is another psychodynamic therapist whose ideas remain highly influential in the fields of parenting and social work. As a clinical social worker, Fraiberg observed that difficulties in the parent–infant relationship were often rooted in problems that happened during parents' own childhoods. In a paper entitled 'Ghosts in the Nursery' Fraiberg and her colleagues (Fraiberg et al. 1980) noted that parents who experienced pain and rejection from their own parents were often less able to empathize with their infants' needs. In particular, the authors observed that the parenting difficulties exhibited in their clinic were frequently similar to the parents' reports of problematic interactions occurring in their own childhoods. This led Fraiberg and her colleagues to conclude that maladaptive parent and child interactions are often repeated across generations.

Fraiberg also believed that parents who rejected their children did so because caregiving activities brought back painful memories, or 'ghosts' from their pasts. In an effort to repress these memories, parents suppress a variety of feelings and this process interferes with their ability to empathize and appropriately respond to their children. Fraiberg and her colleagues also noted that many of the parents in their clinic had difficulty developing trusting relationships with others, including their therapists. Fraiberg and her team therefore hypothesized that these parents would not be able to respond appropriately to their infants until their own psychological needs were met (Shapiro and Gisynski 1989).

In order to meet the psychological needs of the parents visiting their clinic, Fraiberg and her colleagues developed a four-stage family intervention model that included: 1) crisis intervention (when necessary), 2) family support (including attention to each family's housing, safety and nutrition), 3) guidance about child development and 4) infant–parent psychotherapy. After going through these four steps, the parents appeared better able to trust their therapists and make use of the support offered to them. The psychotherapy also provided them with the opportunity to reflect upon their early histories with their own parents and consider how their pasts might be influencing their present relationship with their child. Within this supportive environment, the mothers became better able to empathize with their children and realistically interpret their needs. More importantly, the parents were able to openly acknowledge that they did not want to repeat their own painful histories and appropriately altered their behavior so that negative patterns were not repeated. As the parents did this, they observed their children responding more positively to them and became more confident about themselves as parents.

Although Fraiberg did not empirically test her ideas during her lifetime, a series of studies since her death have confirmed that dysfunctional parenting behaviors are related to negative childhood experiences (Fonagy et al. 1993, Wakschlag et al.1996). Her treatment methods have also had widespread appeal, especially in the field of social work, where they have been incorporated into much of mainstream practice (Shapiro 2009). Fraiberg's influence is also evident in the therapeutic work aimed at changing parents' representations of their infants in an effort to improve their sensitivity towards them and increase attachment security (see Chapter 3 for a more in-depth discussion). The Nurse–Family Partnership (NFP) program also uses her framework to develop trust with parents who may have difficulty forming positive relationships with others (Olds et al. 1997).

Client-centered therapy

Basic assumptions

As a founder of the humanistic psychology movement, Carl Rogers (1902–1987) based his system of client-centered therapy[2] on several core assumptions regarding human nature (Rogers 1951):

1   All people are essentially good and psychologically healthy
2   Psychological maladjustment occurs because of an **incongruence** between the real and ideal self
3   Each individual has a unique, subjective 'internal frame of reference' of his or her reality, making each person the world's best expert on him- or herself
4   All humans have a natural **actualizing tendency** to become mature, socially adjusted and independent individuals.

First articulated in the mid 1940s, these ideas were a significant departure from the more diagnostic understanding of human behavior advocated by Freud and his followers. In particular, Rogers emphasized the individual's own capacity for self-understanding and asserted that the purpose of therapy was to provide a supportive and non-judgmental setting in which the client could manage his or her own therapeutic change. Within this safe context, the client is then able to examine his or her own behavior and determine appropriate changes without any specific expertise or direction from the therapist (Rogers 1946).

Rogers felt that the following three therapist behaviors were necessary to create a sufficiently supportive therapeutic environment (Rogers 1957):

1   **Congruence** – genuineness, transparency and honesty with the client
2   **Empathy** – the ability to feel and connect with what the client feels
3   **Respect** – expressed through acceptance and **unconditional positive regard** towards the client.

Rogers believed these three behaviors facilitate the development of a fully accepting and unconditional relationship between the therapist and client. Within the context of this supportive relationship, the client is then able to explore uncomfortable feelings and experiences, including those which may have previously been denied or distorted. Once the individual is able to accept these distortions, a re-organization of the self structure should take place, allowing the client to achieve greater **congruence** and self-actualization.

Rogers asserted that these three therapist behaviors are *necessary* and *sufficient* for positive therapeutic change to occur. In other words, if the therapist demonstrates congruence, empathy and respect, the client will naturally improve on his or her own, even if no other special techniques are used. During therapy, the therapist should not provide advice or interpret behavior, but instead take the role of an **active listener**, who listens deeply to what the client says and then mirrors or **reflects** back key phrases and ideas. At no point should the therapist make suggestions for how the client might wish to change (Rogers 1957).

The effectiveness of client-centered therapies

Rogers was an early advocate of evidence-based treatments and therefore established a program of research alongside his clinical practice. While his research methods were not as rigorous as those used today, Rogers demonstrated that his non-directive approach typically achieved positive results in less time than did more traditional, psychodynamically oriented therapies. More rigorous randomized controlled trials have since found that a client-centered approach is more effective than no therapy at all and is comparable to other therapies, including Cognitive Behavioral Therapy (CBT, see following section, this chapter), in treating anxieties and depression (Bower et al. 2003, Cuijpers et al. 2008, Elliott et al. 2004, Ward et al. 2000). These studies suggest, however, that client-centered approaches, which allow some therapist-initiated direction,[3] are more effective than those that are entirely non-directive (Elliott et al. 2004). For example, Rollnick and Miller (1995 – see Box 4.1) observe that a non-directive approach is not as effective for treating substance misuse disorders.

When it comes to parenting interventions, Kazdin and his colleagues have observed that while an emotionally supportive environment may be necessary for engaging and motivating parents, it is probably *not* sufficient for improving parenting skills (Kazdin et al. 2005, 2006). Instead, it is likely that the learning of key parenting principles and skills (such as those associated with social learning theory) improve parent and child outcomes, although a positive therapeutic relationship is likely to improve the chances that this learning will take place (see Chapter 5 for further discussion).

Parent Effectiveness Training

One of Rogers's graduate students, Thomas Gordon (1918–2002), applied Rogers's client-centered principles to the parent–child relationship in what is widely considered to be the first parenting training program – PET (*Parent Effectiveness Training*). Findings from a series of PET evaluations illustrate why a warm and supportive environment may be necessary, but not sufficient for improving child outcomes.

Box 4.1: Motivational interviewing: a directive, client-centered approach to counseling

Rollnick and Miller define **motivational interviewing** as 'a directive, client-centered counseling style for eliciting behavior change by helping clients to explore and resolve ambivalence' (Rollnick and Miller 1995: 325). It is supported by over 80 RCTs conducted across a range of populations and settings and is particularly effective with those struggling with a drug or alcohol dependency (Rubak et al. 2005). The primary aim of motivational interviewing is to resolve feelings of ambivalence towards changes that may help individuals overcome their addictions. Motivational interviewing begins by asking the client what he or she wants from treatment and then links this to the client's overall goals and dreams. Throughout the treatment, the therapist uses questions (rather than comments) to improve the client's awareness of the potential problems caused by their dependency, as well as identify areas where changes in behavior could improve their current circumstances.

Like Rogers, Gordon believed that all children are born with the natural desire to self-actualize. From this perspective, children are not bad or mischievous; they simply behave in ways that satisfy their needs at any given moment. For example, a baby cries because he is hungry, a 4-year-old may hit another child to gain access to a desired toy, and a teenager might stay out past his curfew in order to spend more time with his or her friends. While children have a right to have these needs met, their parents have needs too – and from Gordon's perspective, this is where parent–child conflict begins. According to Gordon, the best way to resolve these issues is for parents to come up with ways of meeting both their own and their children's needs. In particular, Gordon believed that a warm and supportive parenting environment reduced the likelihood of conflict and promoted children's psychological growth. Hence, PET encourages parents to actively listen to their children, provide them with unconditional positive regard (referred to as unconditional love) and involve them in democratic (i.e. authoritative) family decision-making processes.

While PET covers some principles regarding positive reinforcement (such as the use of praise), it places a stronger emphasis on the use of communication and problem-solving skills for reducing negative child behavior. For example, in a situation where a 3-year-old child is jumping on his family's new sofa, PET principles advocate that parents interpret this behavior as the child fulfilling a need (perhaps to get exercise, explore the new furniture, etc.), rather than as any sort of misbehavior. Instead of using incentives to stop the behavior, PET encourages the parent to explain why he or she wants the child to change it. Thus, the parent should not use an incentive or distraction technique to get their child off the sofa; the parent should instead explain why it is not a good idea to jump on the furniture (i.e. it's not safe, could break the furniture, etc). The PET program suggests that this be done through **I-messages**, which enable parents to emphasize what they want without assigning blame. An I-message is a direct statement where the individual affirms clearly what he or she wants. Thus, the command *I am afraid you will get hurt when you jump on the sofa. I want you to get off now* is preferable to the accusation *Why on earth are you jumping on the sofa?*

Through the use of I-messages, parents can appropriately confront negative child behavior without attacking the child. Because they do not imply any blame, they reduce resistance and encourage cooperation. Once the child is off the sofa, the parent can then explore solutions with him or her that will meet both of their needs (e.g. jumping outside or on an old mattress). Gordon believed that these problem-solving skills were preferable to the use of rewards, because they encourage the development of empathy and self-discipline. From Gordon's perspective, children will change their behavior because they understand their parents' needs – not because they fear them or hope to get some kind of reward.

A number of evaluations of PET suggest that while the program effectively improves parenting skills and attitudes, consistent improvements in children's behavior have not been observed (Dembo et al. 1985, Gerris et al. 1998). Some believe that this lack of change is related to the fact that PET does not advocate the use of behavior modification systems for sanctioning negative child behavior and argue that a positive and nurturing parenting environment may not be sufficient for dealing with aggressive or disruptive acts (Bandura 1977, Taylor and Biglan 1998). Nevertheless, the PET program advocates a democratic/authoritative style of parenting that *is* consistently associated with better child outcomes (see Chapter 3). For this reason, many evidence-based parenting programs, including the *Incredible Years* and *Triple P*, combine social learning principles with key PET concepts (including the use of I-messages and active listening) to improve parents' interactions with their children.

Personal Construct Theory

A postulate and eleven corollaries

George Kelly's (1905–1967) Personal Construct Theory (PCT) begins with what he referred to as a 'fruitful metaphor'. Kelly was working as a clinical psychologist in rural Kansas when he noticed a similarity between the ordinary farm people he treated and the scientists he worked with when he was in graduate school. Kelly observed that his clients interpreted (or construed) their experiences and actions through mental **constructs** much in the same way that scientists use theories to explain various events and phenomena. Just as scientists test their theories through hypotheses and experiments, ordinary people test their constructs against what actually happens in their day-to-day lives. People also refine and **re-construe** their constructs when their experiences do not match expectations, much in the same way that scientists alter their theories to explain the results of their experiments.

Figure 4.1 provides an overview of Kelly's general theory, which he organized into a fundamental postulate and eleven corollaries. The **fundamental postulate** states 'A person's processes are psychologically channelized by the ways in which he interprets events' (Kelly 1963: 46). By this, Kelly means that an individual's activities (processes) are informed by the constructs he or she uses to anticipate and/or explain what happens in their day-to-day lives.

While Kelly believed that there is only one true reality, people experience this reality differently through their individual **constructions**. He called this **constructive alternativism**, as alternative constructs can always be provided to explain the same behaviors and events. Take the example of James, a 6-year-old boy who cannot sit still at his desk at school. Although his teacher, his mother and father all agree that James has difficulty sitting still, they all have different theories for why this happens and what should be done about it. James's teacher, who has years of experience with 'boys like him', thinks that his behavior reflects a lack of respect for authority and believes that it would improve if his parents used better discipline at home. She has come to this conclusion because of several constructs she holds regarding the nature of children and her role as a teacher:

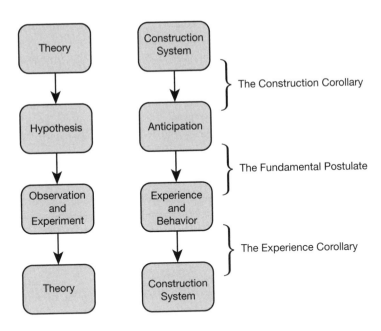

Figure 4.1   George Kelly's Personal Construct Theory

1   She is a good teacher. The majority of her students sit still in her class, listen to her lessons and do well at school.
2   Children should automatically respect teachers' authority and teachers should not have to do anything to earn this respect.
3   A child's disobedience reflects a deficit in character reinforced by poor discipline at home.
4   Children's behavior cannot be explained by neurologically-based conditions such as ADHD. ADHD is a concept invented by the pharmaceutical companies to make money from parents who are looking for an easy way out.

For these reasons, James's teacher does not believe there is any need to change her teaching style because of James's inability to sit still in her class. James's mother, on the other hand, does not agree with the teacher's conclusions. She thinks that James is a nice boy who would not do anything purposively to disrespect the teacher. She also perceives herself as an effective disciplinarian at home, since she has no serious problems with the behavior of her other children. She does notice, however, that James has trouble sitting still and paying attention and wonders whether he might have ADHD. She is nevertheless skeptical about neurological explanations of children's behavior and believes that James's teacher could do more to help him pay better attention at school.

   James's father provides a third explanation of James's behavior. Unlike James's teacher and mother, James's father does not think that his difficulty sitting still is a problem. Instead, he believes that James is 'just like he was' when he was younger and considers his behavior as evidence that James is actually smarter than his fellow classmates. James's father believes that James's impulsivity reflects the fact that he is bored at school and it will stop once he is appropriately challenged. James's father questions whether the teacher is any good, and wishes that she would deliver more imaginative lessons. However, James's father shares the teacher's belief that ADHD is a 'phantom disorder' created by the medical community and therefore believes that there is no point in having James assessed.

Thus, James's teacher, mother and father all have different and distinct constructs that inform their understanding of why James behaves the way that he does. This understanding, in turn, informs their expectations of James, as well as their behavior towards him. James's teacher does not change her behavior because she does not believe that her teaching style has anything to do with James's difficulty sitting still. James's father does not change his attitudes or actions, because he does not think anything is wrong with James's behavior. James's mother wonders if she should do something to find out more about why James can't sit still, but refrains because she shares constructs similar to James's father and hopes that James's behavior will improve on its own.

Kelly's eleven corollaries can be understood through the above example. The first corollary, known as the **construction corollary**, states that 'a person anticipates events by construing their replications' (Kelly 1963: 50). This is exemplified by the fact that all three adults developed a construction of James's behavior based upon their previous experience with him. Note, however, that each adult had a different construct. This fact illustrates Kelly's second corollary, the **individual corollary**, which states that 'Persons differ from each other in their construction of events' (Kelly 1963: 55). As the above example suggests, these differences occurred because the adults' constructs were developed through their unique histories with James, as well as their past experiences with other children and adults (e.g. other pupils, James's uncle, etc.). These differing constructions were also informed by the adults' individual understanding of themselves, as well as their beliefs about human nature in general.

Kelly's **organization corollary** asserts that 'Each person characteristically evolves, for his convenience in anticipating events, a construction system embracing ordinal relationships between constructs' (Kelly 1963: 56). By this, Kelly means that constructs are organized in terms of subordinate and super-ordinate constructs. Applying this corollary to the teacher's construct of James's behavior, the teacher may already have a construct of 'disobedience' organized around specific child behaviors, which may include impulsive or restless actions. However, the teacher does not view James's behavior as leafy, juicy or technical. This is because some constructs are subordinate to others. For example, impulsive could be considered subordinate to 'disobedient', but leafy, juicy and technical could not be. Instead, these adjectives are related to entirely different constructs – such as trees, fruit and microscopes.

This last point illustrates Kelly's **range corollary**, which stipulates that people's constructs are limited in their range of applications. For example, many constructs are fairly limited in their scope – thus, 'leafy' is generally limited to the description of plants and 'technical' is most often reserved for items of a scientific or mechanical nature. Other constructs have a much broader range of applications, however – such as big versus small, good versus bad and smart versus stupid. Kelly noted that people tend to organize these broader constructs in dichotomous dimensions and referred to this as the **dichotomy corollary**. Kelly believed that people tend to think in dichotomous dimensions because it is too difficult to assign objects and actions to discrete categories. If something can be big, then something can also be small – i.e. you cannot have the concept of big without the concept of small. In addition, these dichotomous categories tend to be quite broad. Hence, James's teacher saw his behavior as falling in the dimension of bad versus good, whereas his father organized it in terms of smart versus stupid.

According to Kelly, people use their dichotomized constructs when choosing one course of action over another. Kelly called this the **choice corollary** and, when applying it to the above example, we see that the father's dichotomized concept – 'James is smart' – resulted in his choice of not doing anything further to improve James's behavior. Kelly noted that people are not always conscious of making these choices and tend to choose actions that they perceive as open. In this instance, James's mother likely chose to do nothing further because she perceived this as the most open option.

Going forward with the example of James, we find that his teacher and father maintain their constructions of his impulsivity, with the teacher viewing his behavior through her construct of 'disobedient child' and his father perceiving him as 'smart boy who is under-challenged'. The mother's construct begins to change, however, after watching a documentary on television that proposes that ADHD may be a genetic disorder. She remembers that her brother had similar behavioral problems when he was younger and wonders if it is possible that James has inherited his difficulties, as his behavior appears to be getting worse. While she still does not think that James is purposively naughty and believes him to be smart, she does start to think there is a problem. She personally wonders if James should receive an educational assessment, but continues to share her husband's skepticism regarding the diagnosis of ADHD.

The mother's attitudes exemplify three additional corollaries. The first of these, the **fragmentation corollary**, states that individuals often maintain construction subsystems which are seemingly incompatible with one another. In this instance, the mother has two somewhat incompatible constructs. As James's mother, she has first-hand knowledge about how his behavior differs from her other children's and wonders if this is normal. However, she shares her husband's views of the psychological community and is not sure whether she would accept the results of a professional assessment that may confirm her concerns about her son.

The mother's behavior also exemplifies Kelly's **sociality corollary**, which states that 'to the extent that one person construes the construction processes of another, he may play a role in a social process involving another person' (Kelly 1963: 95). In this case, the mother and father share similar opinions of their son's behavior because of their ability to relate to each other's construct system. Kelly also observed, however, that two individuals need not know each other in order to share similar constructs. Kelly referred to this as the **commonality corollary**, which is exemplified by the fact that the teacher, mother and father all share a mutual disregard for the psychological community. This may be related to the fact that all three adults share common values and beliefs, based upon a similar upbringing and culture.

In the above example, the teacher and father maintained their constructs as long as James's behavior remained the same. The mother's construct began to change, however, after she watched the television documentary. This is the main point of Kelly's **experience corollary**, which states that 'A person's construction system varies as he successively construes the replication of events' (Kelly 1963: 72). The extent to which individuals re-interpret or re-construe behavior is related to how **permeable** their construct systems are. In this instance, the mother's construct system of James's behavior was relatively more permeable than the teacher's. Kelly referred to this as the **modulation corollary**, which states that some constructs are more permeable than others.

So which construct is correct? In terms of reality, any one of them may be correct and, according to the construction, experience and modulation corollaries, each adult's construct will remain intact, depending upon the consistency in James's behavior and the permeability of their construct system. Taking the above example one step farther, James's situation finally resolves itself after his mother takes him to their GP for a bacterial infection. The GP notices that James has difficulty sitting still during his examination and refraining from playing with the medical instruments. The GP discusses his observations with James's mother and she shares with him her concern that James might have ADHD. The GP recommends that James be assessed for the disorder and this suggestion is sufficient for James's mother to begin to permanently alter the constructs she uses to interpret her son's behavior.

The assessment indicates that James has ADHD. The psychologist recommends that he take stimulant medication and that his parents attend an evidence-based parenting course to learn how to better manage his behavior. After James has been on medication for some weeks and his parents have completed their training, both the teacher and the parents see that James has less difficulty sitting still and paying attention. Is this now enough of a change for the three adults to alter their construct systems?

Depending on the permeability of their constructs, they may be either challenged *or* reinforced. In this case, James's improvement reinforced some of the adults' constructs, but changed others. For example, James's mother's constructions of ADHD and the medical community completely changed as a result of James's improved behavior. She now firmly believes that ADHD is an inherited disorder and is convinced that her brother has it as well. Her construction regarding her parenting skills has not changed, however. While she is happy about the new approaches learned in the training program, she still thinks her original strategies were effective – just not with her son, who requires a different style of parenting that must be learned. Her constructions about James have not changed either, as she continues to see him as a nice boy, albeit one with ADHD.

James's father also changes some of his constructions, but maintains others. The positive change in James's behavior has also motivated him to alter his views about the medical community. However, he is now more convinced than ever that his son is a genius. Since his diagnosis, James's father has started reading more about ADHD and has learned that Einstein might have had the disorder. He thus becomes extremely optimistic that his son has a similarly bright future in front of him and double-checks his savings options to make sure that there will be sufficient funds for James's university education.

None of the teacher's constructs changes, however. While she admits that James's classroom behavior has improved, she attributes this to changes in his parents' disciplinary strategies. She also continues to believe that ADHD is a myth and wonders whether stimulant medication could damage James's health. This concern makes her additionally doubt James's parents' ability to appropriately care for their child. At no point does James's teacher think that his behavior is in any way connected to her style of teaching or the taking of stimulant medication.

Thus, despite the improvements in James's behavior, not all of the adults' constructs were changed. In particular, the constructs most closely linked to their sense of self were the most resistant. The mother continued to view her parenting skills as effective, the father continued to consider himself as smart and the teacher continued to think that she was a good teacher. Kelly asserted that constructs that are core to one's role structure – i.e. central to one's sense of self and integrity – are often the least likely to change. This is because **core constructs** are most often integral to one's experience of his or her 'true' self. While people experience a variety of roles in their day-to-day lives, there are some that are more central to their sense of self than others. In this respect, the father's skepticism regarding the medical community may have been a firmly rooted conviction, but more malleable to change than his belief that he and his son were smart. In this respect, the father used the information gained from his son's assessment to reinforce his core concept of 'self as smart' and adapted his beliefs about the diagnostic process. This enabled him to refine his construction system without threatening his **core role structure**.

The use of PCT in parenting interventions

Kelly's theory has a number of important implications for parenting work. First is the understanding that each individual interprets his or her daily experiences through a unique construct system. This means that the interactions between parents and practitioners will be influenced by their individual constructs of each other. For this reason, practitioners should continually reflect on their personal constructs and consider how they might influence their interpretation of the parents that they work with. Practitioners should also recognize that interactions with parents will be dictated by parents' own construct systems, which are likely to be informed by their previous experience with helping professionals, as well as their reasons for seeking help in the first place. In some cases, parents may maintain negative constructs about parenting interventions and the individuals who deliver them. Practitioners should consider how these feelings might influence parents' willingness to accept their support.

Practitioners should also recognize that parents' construct systems inform their understanding of themselves as parents, as well as of their children's behavior. Kelly observed that psychological disorders occur when individuals maintain constructs that are consistently invalidated through their day-to-day experiences. While the majority of parents are not mentally ill, it is not uncommon for them to consistently misconstrue their children's behavior because of a lack of understanding of what is developmentally appropriate or because they are projecting suppressed feelings of their own onto their child. For example, a mother might attribute a 2-year-old's angry cries to anxiety, because the mother herself is anxious. In a similar vein, James's father projected his perception of himself as intelligent onto his son when explaining James's impulsive behavior. While this belief helped the father to maintain positive feelings towards his son, it kept him from being open minded about possible treatments. Hence, a common goal of parenting work is to help parents change their constructions of their children's behavior so that their expectations and beliefs are more realistic (Davis et al. 2002).

As the example of James suggests, changing personal construct systems is not always easy. This is especially true of parents, as their understanding of their parenting efficacy is often integral to their own core role structure. For example, James's mother refused to see her original parenting strategies as ineffective, because her understanding of herself as a good mother was core to her sense of self. In order to help parents examine their personal constructs, Davis et al. (2002) suggest that practitioners demonstrate the qualities identified by Rogers – congruence, empathy and respect – so that parents feel safe to challenge their own firmly held beliefs. When parents feel that they are not being judged, they are likely to become more willing to change their constructs of their children's behavior, as well as their own.

Kelly believed that therapeutic change takes place when people are able to understand and re-enact the roles of others. Kelly therefore encouraged his clients to engage in **role play** during therapy, as he believed this helped them to understand how others might view them and make changes when appropriate. Through role play, parents can be encouraged to empathize with their children's feelings, as well as examine the efficacy of their parenting behaviors from their children's perspective. Role play also enables parents to practice new perspectives and behaviors in a way that facilitates positive and lasting changes in their own construct systems. For this reason, many evidence-based parenting programs use role play as a way of helping parents improve their parenting strategies.

Cognitive Behavioral Therapy

Cognitive Behavioral Therapy (CBT) is an umbrella term for a collection of therapeutic methods that share the same basic premise: that people's feelings and behaviors are influenced by their thinking patterns. The aim of most CBT techniques is therefore to help people change their thinking patterns in order to improve their psychological wellbeing. Numerous RCTs suggest that CBT techniques significantly reduce psychological symptoms in the short term and also prevent them from re-occurring in the future. For this reason, NICE recommends CBT as the treatment of choice for a number of mental health disorders, including post-traumatic stress disorder, obsessive compulsive disorder, bulimia and clinical depression. CBT methods originated in the theories of behaviorism and cognitive theory, which are both summarized below.

Behaviorism

Behaviorism has its roots in the experiments of Russian psychologist Ivan Pavlov (1849–1936), who demonstrated that behavioral responses could be conditioned (or learned) through associations with various stimuli. In his classic experiments with animals, Pavlov observed that dogs naturally salivate (unconditioned response) in the presence of food (the unconditioned stimulus) in anticipation of eating. Pavlov rang a bell (conditioned stimulus) every time he fed the dogs and found that the dogs soon came to associate the bell ringing with the arrival of food. Pavlov also rang the bell when the food was not present and found that the dogs still salivated (conditioned response) in anticipation of the food. Through this experiment Pavlov demonstrated that neutral stimuli (e.g. the ringing of the bell) can stimulate or 'condition' natural, physiological responses.

In the United States, John Watson (1878–1958) similarly observed that neutral stimuli could easily condition strong emotional responses in humans. In his infamous 'Little Albert' experiment, Watson conditioned an 11-month-old toddler to become frightened of rabbits and other furry objects. After a control period in which Albert was allowed to play with a white rat, Watson paired its presence with a loud, jarring noise caused by the clanging of two pipes behind little Albert's head. As the trials progressed, Albert began showing signs of distress at the sight of the rat, even when unaccompanied by the frightening noise. Albert then generalized this fear to other similar objects, including toys that where white and fluffy, a white rabbit, a fur coat and John Watson dressed up as Santa Claus. Although the ethics of this study have since been questioned, most agree that Watson's 'Little Albert' experiment demonstrated how strong emotions, such as fear, can easily become associated with relatively harmless stimuli.

During this same time period, American psychologist Edward Thorndike (1874–1949) observed that cause-and-effect associations are often learned through trial and error. Thorndike demonstrated this by placing cats in puzzle boxes and motivating them to escape by placing a smelly fish outside of the box. Escape was only possible if they pushed a lever inside the box. When first placed in the box, the cats tried to escape by moving about frantically and only opened the box when they pushed the lever by accident. With experience, however, the cats learned to associate the pushing of the lever with successful escape. Thorndike called this association the **Law of Effect**, and theorized that successful responses were 'stamped in' by satisfying results and unsuccessful responses were 'stamped out' because the cats learned they did not work. In short, Thorndike demonstrated how satisfying consequences strengthen behavior, while non-satisfying results weaken it.

B. F. Skinner (1904–1990) was influenced by all three of these experiments when developing his ideas regarding **operant conditioning**. Operant conditioning is distinguished from Pavlovian conditioning (or classical conditioning) in that it deals with the modification of voluntary or 'operant' behaviors. Starting with Thorndike's Law of Effect, Skinner observed that operant behaviors (voluntary actions like the cat pressing the lever) will increase when reinforced and decrease if punished or ignored. Skinner originally conceptualized reinforcements as either 'positive' or 'negative'. **Positive reinforcement** involves the use of rewards, whereas **negative reinforcement** involves the removal of negative or aversive stimuli. In Skinner's box experiments, rats learned that the pressing of a certain lever would keep them from receiving electric shocks. The ceasing of the shocks hence became a negative reinforcement that increased the rats' lever-pushing behavior.

Skinner believed that punishments could also be 'positive' or 'negative'. An example of a **positive punishment** might be the use of an aversive stimulus (such as spanking or smacking) to stop a behavior, whereas a **negative punishment** involves removing something positive – such as a privilege or a toy. **Extinction** occurs when a behavior (i.e. response) that had previously been reinforced is no longer rewarded. Extinction is exemplified in Skinner's experiments by rats first receiving a food pellet after pushing a lever and then never receiving a food pellet again – no matter how many times the lever was pushed.

Through these concepts, Skinner demonstrated how various patterns of reinforcement, punishment and extinction could teach or **shape** new animal behaviors. Through **successive approximation** Skinner demonstrated how successive rewards could teach animals new behaviors that were not in their natural repertoire. Successive approximation is illustrated through the methods used to teach a dog to roll over. At first, reinforcements (i.e. treats) are given whenever the dog naturally does something that is part of the rolling over process – like lying down. Treats are then withheld until the dog does something that more closely approximates rolling over – like lying on its side. Movements are then selectively reinforced until the dog finally rolls over.

Skinner also demonstrated how varying schedules of reinforcement variably increased response rates. For example, **variable schedules** of reinforcement are less vulnerable to extinction than are **fixed-ratio schedules**. Fishing and gambling are both examples of activities that operate on a variable rate of reinforcement. Although the rewards of these activities are fairly infrequent, the fact that they can occur at any time serves to increase fishing or gambling behavior.

Skinner's operant conditioning principles were highly influential during his lifetime and have since been incorporated into a wide variety of therapeutic interventions used today. As discussed in Chapter 3, operant conditioning principles underpin most parent management training programs, by teaching parents to reward positive child behaviors and ignore or sanction negative ones. Operant and classical (i.e. Pavlovian) conditioning principles have also been successfully applied to the treatment of anxieties and phobias through the use of **systematic desensitization** (Wolpe 1958).

Phobias occur when relatively neutral objects and activities (including heights, spaces, animals and associated activities such as flying), become irrationally associated (i.e. conditioned) with strong emotions and fears. In order to overcome these fears, individuals are asked to establish their own hierarchy of fearful situations. For example, a spider-phobic individual is likely to rate a picture of spiders as less fear inducing than actually touching one. Phobic individuals are then taught relaxation techniques and asked to apply them to successively more frightening situations. In the case of spider phobia, the phobic individual is taught to use relaxation techniques when looking at a picture of a spider until he or she feels completely at ease. The individual is then exposed to increasingly threatening situations (seeing a larger picture, looking at a spider in a box, etc.) in combination with relaxation techniques until he or she feels completely comfortable holding a spider. Through these experiences, the phobic individual comes to realize that the threat is imaginary and the fear is eventually extinguished.

Albert Ellis and Rational Emotive Theory

Albert Ellis's (1913–2007) Rational Emotive Theory (RET) uses operant and classical conditioning principles to explain human behavior, but emphasizes the role of thoughts and beliefs in determining people's emotional responses to events. Like Kelly, Ellis believed that humans interpret their experiences through cognitive representations and individual belief systems (Ellis 1989). Ellis explained this through his 'ABC' model, with **A** standing for **Activating Events** that are interpreted through **B** – specific **Beliefs** – which in turn determine the **Emotional Consequences** (**C**) (i.e. the response) of the event (Figure 4.2).

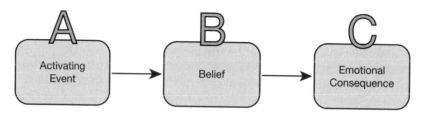

Figure 4.2 Albert Ellis's ABC model of behavior

While the ABC model treats beliefs and emotional consequences as separate entities, Ellis said that this was done for conceptual purposes only, stating that:

> human thinking, emotion, and action are not really separate or disparate processes, but all significantly overlap and are rarely experienced in a pure state. Much of what we call emotion is nothing more, nor less than a certain kind – a biased, prejudiced, or strongly evaluative kind – of thought. But emotions and behaviors significantly influence and affect thinking, just as thinking significantly influences what we call emotions and behaviors.
>
> (Ellis 2003: 221)

Ellis also believed that many emotional and behavioral responses are unconsciously established early in people's lives. As people grow older, they are more likely to find ways to re-affirm these ideas rather than challenge them, even if they have little evidence to support them. Like Kelly, Ellis believed that people had a tendency towards dichotomous thinking and categorized behavior into 'shoulds' and 'musts' rather than 'coulds' or 'maybes'. Ellis felt that this kind of thinking was maladaptive, since rigid belief systems often create self-defeating emotional consequences which are often precursors to more serious, psychopathological problems. Box 4.2 provides an overview of eleven common irrational beliefs that Ellis identified as contributing to negative emotional consequences and psychopathological thinking (from Mischel 1986).

Box 4.2: Eleven common beliefs identified by Ellis as irrational

1   It is an absolute necessity for adult humans to be loved or approved by virtually every significant other person in their life.
2   One absolutely must be competent, adequate and achieving in all important respects or else one is an inadequate, worthless person.
3   People absolutely must act considerately and fairly and they are damnable villains if they do not. They *are* their bad acts.
4   It is awful and terrible when things are not the way one would very much like them to be.
5   Emotional disturbance is mainly externally caused and people have little or no ability to increase or decrease their dysfunctional feelings and behaviors.
6   If something is or may be dangerous or fearsome, then one should be constantly and excessively concerned about it and should keep dwelling on the possibility of it occurring.
7   One cannot and must not face life's responsibilities and difficulties and it is easier to avoid them.
8   One must be quite dependent on others and need them and one cannot mainly run one's own life.
9   One's past history is an all-important determiner of one's present behavior and because something once strongly affected one's life, it should indefinitely have a similar effect.
10 Other people's disturbances are horrible and one must feel upset about them.
11 There is invariably a right, precise and perfect solution to human problems and it is awful if this perfect solution is not found.

Ellis observed that individuals often respond to the above thoughts through a variety of maladaptive feelings including self-blame and self-pity, as well as over-reactive forms of hurt, guilt, shame, depression and anxiety. Maladaptive behavioral responses to such feelings often include procrastination, over-compulsiveness, avoidance, addiction and withdrawal as ways of coping with or avoiding unwanted emotional consequences. However, Ellis also observed that humans are capable of mastering belief systems which are positive, open-minded and flexible. Ellis believed that flexible thinking often enables more constructive and self-promoting beliefs and behaviors and therefore theorized that if individuals learned to change their self-defeating interpretations of events, they could successfully avoid the irrational feelings related to self-destructive behaviors.

Thus, a main objective of Ellis's Rational Emotive Behavioral Therapy (REBT) is to help clients understand that they can choose how they interpret activating events. The therapist's role in this process is to help clients examine their belief systems and consider the extent to which they are rational, beneficial and necessary. Therapists can then help clients to choose and learn new thinking patterns that are more flexible and positive.

Ellis called this process **cognitive restructuring** and believed that this was a difficult process that could not be achieved through self-reflection alone. Instead, clients must actively question their irrational thoughts by challenging their beliefs and feelings. Ellis believed that the therapist's role in this process is to systematically confront clients' ideas and assumptions and make suggestions for alternative ways of viewing things. While therapists should actively listen, they should also actively question their clients' assumptions and conclusions.

Ellis believed that this was best accomplished through a **Socratic** method of questioning, as well as homework assignments that provided clients with opportunities to test their beliefs and practice more adaptive emotional responses.

Aaron Beck and cognitive therapy

Ellis's ideas were highly controversial when he first introduced them in the mid 1950s. By the mid 1960s and early 1970s, however, they had revolutionized therapeutic practice. This was due to the widespread appeal of best-selling books, such as *How to Live with a Neurotic* and *Sex without Guilt*, as well as scientifically based research that demonstrated the efficacy of his ideas. During this same time period, Aaron Beck (1921–) was applying similar principles to the treatment of depression and was finding that his cognitive techniques were much more effective than behavioral or psychodynamic approaches. Ellis contacted Beck in 1963 after reading an article Beck had published on the cognitive treatment of depression and the two established a professional relationship that remained until Ellis's death in 2007 (Weishaar 2002).

Like Ellis, Beck believed that emotional responses, including depression, were driven by firmly established maladaptive thinking patterns, which he referred to as **negative automatic thoughts**. Beck observed that such thoughts are often learned observationally within dysfunctional families, where parents cannot successfully cope with stressful experiences or traumatic events. Negative thinking also occurs because of a lack of opportunity to practice adaptive thinking and coping skills.

Beck also observed that depressed individuals over-generalize the quality of their lives, by magnifying the negative aspects and minimizing the positive. Beck asserted that this typically happens because of three main dysfunctional belief systems (or 'schemas'): 1) I am defective or inadequate, 2) all of my experiences result in defeats or failures and 3) the future is hopeless. Beck calls these three schemas the **Negative Cognitive Triad** and developed the **Beck Depression Inventory** as a way of determining their presence in depressed clients.

Like Ellis, Beck believed that depressive symptoms are most often caused by negative, maladaptive thoughts and not by any specific event on its own. Beck's treatment of depression therefore focuses on challenging these negative schemas and replacing them with positive ones. In doing so, his cognitive therapy helps clients to monitor and change their thinking in five basic steps (taken from Mischel 1986):

1   Clients are first taught to recognize and monitor their negative thoughts. These thoughts are 'dysfunctional' (i.e. ineffective) and often lead to serious psychological dilemmas.
2   Clients are taught to recognize the connections between these negative thoughts (i.e. cognitions), the emotions they create and their own actions.
3   Clients learn to examine the evidence for and against their distorted thoughts.
4   They learn to substitute these distorted negative thoughts with more realistic interpretations.
5   Clients are taught to identify and change the inappropriate assumptions that predisposed them to distort their experiences.

In order to test the effectiveness of this therapeutic approach, Beck launched a series of rigorously conducted RCTs. Through these investigations, he found that his methods not only reduced his clients' depressive symptoms but also prevented them from happening again (Hollon and Beck 2004). These findings have led Beck and others to assert that cognitive therapy not only effectively treats depressive symptoms; it teaches clients new coping skills that keep the symptoms from occurring again. Beck has applied his cognitive techniques to the treatment of anxiety disorders, substance misuse and post-traumatic stress disorder and has achieved similar positive results.

Cognitive behavioral techniques

As noted previously, CBT, as we know it today, is an umbrella term for a wide variety of behavioral and cognitive techniques. CBT methods range from activities that require clients to hyperfocus on their irrational thoughts (most often through **self-monitoring** methods) to distraction methods, such as imagery work, that help clients to relax and keep them from dwelling on unpleasant ideas. Despite the diversity of these approaches, they all share the same fundamental aim: to alter thinking patterns in an effort to improve emotional responses (Creer et al. 2004). Box 4.3 provides an overview of CBT techniques commonly used in therapeutic practice today.

Box 4.3: Cognitive behavioral techniques

Self-monitoring consists of self-observing and reflecting upon one's behaviors and the recording of the observed findings. Self-monitoring is the single most important component of many cognitive behavioral interventions. An example of self-monitoring applied to an eating disorder would be to keep a record of what one eats during the day.

Self-statements are statements people make to themselves to guide their feelings, thoughts and behavior. Self-statements can be combined with other procedures as a way of controlling feelings and actions. Examples of self-statements include positive, self-affirming remarks aimed at improving mood or confidence.

Self-statements plus distraction refers to the combination of self-statements with the following three distraction techniques to change behavior:

- **External distraction:** One attempts to divert one's attention away from a situation by focusing on a stimulus in one's immediate environment.
- **Internal distraction:** One attempts to divert one's attention away from a situation by focusing on other thoughts or physical sensations. Internal distraction is a feature of mindfulness techniques.
- **Imagery:** One attempts to control thinking or behavior by picturing a possible negative or positive outcome.

Reperception of situation involves taking a new perspective on stimuli that formerly controlled one's behavior. One may manage a situation by refusing to follow one's old pattern of response to a stimulus. For example, an alcoholic may crave alcohol every time he passes the pub next to his office. Reperception involves consciously replacing these feelings with alternative ways of thinking – such as purposively listing all of the reason he should not have alcohol.

Thought stopping is used when negative thoughts, worries or compulsions enter consciousness, and mental techniques are used to literally stop the ideas. Methods include snapping a rubber band around the wrist, or stating 'halt' either externally or internally. *Thought substitution*, or taking on a desired thought in place of an undesired thought, is linked to thought stopping.

Relaxation involves relaxing on self-cue in the face of a stimulus or situation one finds aversive. One may follow a set of established relaxation exercises, such as deep breathing or muscle relaxation.

Meditation involves deep concentration that accentuates detachment from physical states and from feelings and thoughts. Continually repeating a word or saying a prayer can induce a meditative state.

Imagery involves picturing a scene in one's mind. Imagery may be used with other behavioral techniques. There are three recommended types of imagery:

Receptive imagery: Consists of relaxing, creating an ambiguous scene, asking a question and waiting for a response.

Programmed imagery: Consists of generating an image complete with everything that might be present in visualizing the scene.

Guided visualization: Imagining a scene or procedure in detail.

Mindfulness techniques are a form of cognitive therapy that emphasizes an awareness of what is happening in the present moment in order to reduce the negative thinking associated with depression and substance misuse (Linehan 1993).

CBT and parenting work

Although there are some forms of CBT that take place through group work, the majority of CBT treatments are delivered to parents on an individual basis. CBT treatments are especially appropriate for situations where a parent is suffering from anxiety or depression. For example, Murray et al. (2003) report some success in reducing the symptoms of postnatally depressed mothers and their infants with a home visiting service that combines active listening methods with cognitive behavioral techniques to improve mothers' sensitivity towards their infants.

Self-efficacy theory

Consider the behavior of two 4-year-old girls in a typical preschool class. The teacher has asked the class to work quietly and independently on jigsaw puzzles. The students are allowed to choose the puzzles they work on. Two of the girls are particularly excited because they get to choose from some new puzzles picturing kittens and puppies. Both appear pleased with the activity and eager to start the task.

The puzzles are challenging, but not beyond the girls' competence level. The first girl works diligently and patiently. When one piece does not fit, she searches for another. When she runs into difficulty, she uses a strategy to make the task easier by grouping pieces of a similar color. When the puzzle ultimately becomes too hard, the girl asks for her teacher for help. The girl carries on doing this until the final piece is in place. At this point, she is visibly proud and claps her hands as she exclaims 'I did it!'

The second child also works diligently when she receives the puzzle. However, when it becomes clear to her that it is difficult, she begins to lose interest. When the teacher sees that she is stuck, she kindly offers some assistance. Instead of taking up the teacher's offer of help, the girl whines and knocks some of the pieces to the floor. The girl then moves to another part of the room and sulks until the classroom starts another activity.

Why have these two young girls behaved so differently? From a behaviorist standpoint, their actions should be the same. They both had exactly the same reinforcement – the completion of a jigsaw puzzle with an attractive picture on it. Both puzzles were also of the same difficulty level. Yet one girl persisted until she completed it and the other gave up.

Albert Bandura (1925–) believed that such differences can be explained by variations in how people perceive their own efficacy. According to Bandura, **self-efficacy** is the belief that one can personally master a particular task or activity. This is not the same as self-esteem, which is related to how good people feel about themselves. Individuals can have relatively high self-esteem, but nevertheless believe themselves to have low efficacy when it comes to performing specific tasks.

Perceptions of self-efficacy influence the kind of goals people choose, and determine whether they persist in difficult situations. Going back to the example of the two 4-year-old girls, it is likely that the first girl believed that she was capable of completing the puzzle. Even when it became clear to her that the puzzle was too difficult to finish on her own, she remained calm and thought about strategies for simplifying it until she ultimately asked her teacher for help. The second girl, however, gave up as soon as the puzzle became tricky. This is likely because she perceived the puzzle as being too hard and interpreted her efforts as ineffective. These self-defeating beliefs, in turn, started off a **vicious cycle** that reduced her motivation and ultimately interfered with her ability to think of new strategies. The end effect was her inability to complete the puzzle, which likely reinforced her low expectations of herself and her inability to complete the task.

Bandura demonstrated a clear and measurable link between one's perceptions of self-efficacy and one's resulting behavior. In articulating his ideas, Bandura combined principles from social learning theory with his own research in observational learning. In order to understand Bandura's ideas and their application in parenting work, it is useful to first review a few key concepts from social learning theory, which are briefly described below.

Social learning theory

Julian Rotter (1916–) is often credited as the founder of social learning theory. In developing his ideas, Rotter believed that an understanding of personality required an understanding of human motivation (Rotter 1954). Rotter believed that Freud's drive theory was inadequate in this respect and instead preferred Thorndike's Law of Effect for explaining motivation. Recall from the previous section that this 'law' assumes that individuals are motivated to seek positive reinforcements and avoid unpleasant ones. When applying this principle to humans, Rotter believed that goals and positive consequences were greater motivators of human behavior than were punishments or negative outcomes.

Like his colleague George Kelly, Rotter also believed that humans formed constructs about their own behavior and the behavior of others. However, Rotter felt that personal constructs were limited in their explanation of human motivation. Like his professor Kurt Lewin[4] (1890–1947), Rotter believed that environment-specific reinforcements also determine human behavior and emotional responses. In this respect, some environmental situations are much more influential than others in determining human behavior.

Take, for example, a typical airplane flight. All of the passengers come with different expectations of the flight, based upon their understanding of mechanics of air flight and their past experience with airplanes. Some people may be excited, others fearful, others uncomfortable, and for some it will be a routine part of their life. However, all of the passengers are likely to behave more or less in the same way. They will sit still in their seats and try to distract themselves until the plane flight is over. Almost all of these people would likely become frightened, however, if the airplane suddenly lost altitude, no matter what their constructs were about planes and flying. Unless they had specific training in altitude loss, the environmental aspects of the situation would determine the passengers' fear response.

In a less dramatic but similar vein, Rotter observed that various situations encouraged similar behaviors among people, despite differences in their personalities and personal constructs. In particular, Rotter observed that various educational and work environments were more likely to elicit competitive behaviors through the use of **extrinsic rewards**, versus other environments which motivated people through more **intrinsic** means. In these instances, competitive behaviors were less evident.

In articulating these ideas, Rotter shared Lewin's notion[5] that human behavior is determined by both person characteristics (i.e. capabilities, beliefs and thoughts) *and* key aspects of the environment. From Rotter's perspective, personality remains stable only to the extent that individual beliefs and the environment are stable. Change the way the person thinks *or* change the environment, and the behavior will also change. Personality is thus not a fixed set of traits, although Rotter acknowledged that the longer one lives with a set of beliefs and attitudes, the more difficult it is to change them.

In further articulating his social learning theory, Rotter believed that human behavior could be predicted by four main components: behavior potential, expectancy, reinforcement value and the psychological situation.

*   **Behavior potential** is the potential to engage in a particular behavior in a given environment. In every situation, there are multiple behaviors one can engage in. What is the potential of an individual choosing one action over another?
*   **Expectancy** is an individual's perception that a specific behavior will lead to a specific outcome. Having 'high' expectations means that the individual believes that his or her behavior will achieve the desired outcome. Like Kelly, Rotter believed that expectations are based on past experiences.
*   **Reinforcement value** refers to the desirability of the consequences for specific behaviors. Things we want to happen or are attracted to have a high reinforcement value. Things we do not want to happen, that we dislike or wish to avoid, have a low reinforcement value. Rotter believed that individuals differ strongly in terms of the reinforcements they personally value.
*   **Psychological situation:** Rotter believed that there are strong, subjective differences between people in their interpretations of environments. These are based upon their previous experiences, as well as their personal values. In this respect, a situation is never completely objective and always prone to individual interpretation.

In explaining the relationship between the above components, Rotter developed a new formula for understanding why people behave the way they do:

$$BP = f(E \ \& \ RV)$$

Stated in simple terms, the above equation means that behavioral potential (BP) is a function of the individual's expectancy (E) of being successful and the reinforcement value (RV) for the behavior. In other words, an individual is more likely to engage in an activity if they 1) have high expectations that their behavior will be effective (i.e. they *can* do it) AND that 2) the outcome will be personally rewarding (i.e. they *want* the end result). If either the expectancy or reinforcement value is low, the behavior potential will also be low. Although not in the equation, it is important to remember that expectations and reinforcement values are **subjectively** determined. So it does not matter if the individual can actually perform a task. What matters is whether the individual *thinks* that he or she can perform the task. Subjective values also determine the extent to which someone will want the end result.

Locus of control

Rotter is perhaps most famous for developing the concept of **locus of control**. Locus of control refers to people's very general, cross-situational beliefs regarding the extent to which external and internal forces determine day-to-day outcomes. An internal locus of control refers to the belief that positive and/or negative consequences are determined by one's actions and are therefore under one's personal control. Conversely, an external locus of control assumes that positive and negative events are entirely unrelated to one's behavior. Rotter believed that humans varied on a continuum of internal versus external beliefs and developed a scale for measuring this (Rotter 1966).

When explaining human behavior, Rotter observed that a high internal locus of control – i.e. the belief that one's life consequences are self-determined – predicts improved persistence and higher achievement motivation. Conversely, the belief that outcomes are externally driven – by luck, powerful others (i.e. favoritism) or difficult circumstances (such as an 'impossible' situation) – predicts a lack of persistence, since increased efforts are unlikely to produce a positive result. An external locus of control has been linked to a variety of **learned helpless** behaviors, including those related to clinical depression (Benassi et al. 1988).

Bandura's model of social learning

Albert Bandura took Rotter's ideas several steps further. Through his own research involving observational learning, Bandura found that people form expectations about their environments by watching how the behavior of others is reinforced:

> Most human behavior is learned observationally through modeling: from observing others, one forms an idea of how new behaviors are performed, and on later occasions this coded information serves as a guide for action.
>
> (Bandura 1986: 22)

Bandura also observed that people do not always repeat what they see. In order to learn and repeat a new behavior, the following four elements must be in place:

1 **Attention**: People need to pay attention to what they see. Characteristics of both the model and the witness determine the extent to which attention is paid. Model characteristics include the distinctiveness of its behavior, its affect (happy, sad, mad), the complexity of the behavior and how frequently it occurs. Characteristics of the witness include their arousal level, their attention span, their cognitive level and their sensory capacity.

2 **Retention:** People need to remember what they paid attention to. Memory is also influenced by how distinctive the model's behavior was, its complexity, etc. It is also influenced by how important the information is to the witness and their memory skills.

3   **Reproduction**: People need to be physically capable of reproducing the observed behavior. Clearly, there is much behavior we observe that people do not reproduce because they do not have the skill, or the proper equipment.
5   **Motivation:** People are unlikely to model behavior if they are not motivated to reproduce it. Motives are determined by how the behavior is reinforced and whether or not the witness values the reinforcement.

Like Rotter, Bandura believed that both individual and environmental factors determine behavior. However, Bandura also asserted that while environments determine behavior, behaviors, in turn, determine environments. Bandura called this phenomenon **reciprocal determinism** and noted that this process takes place in families where the behaviors of all members reciprocally influence the behaviors of others (Figure 4.3). These reciprocal behaviors ultimately create a family environment that all members experience.

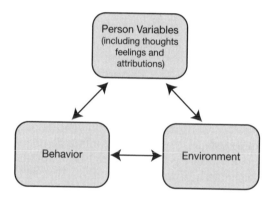

Figure 4.3 Bandura's model of reciprocal determinism

Reciprocal determinism can be exemplified by family members' mutual feeding and eating patterns. For example, a 2-year-old girl might be very picky about the food she eats. While her mother offers her a variety of nutritious foods, the daughter refuses almost everything except 'Winnie the Pooh' yoghurt. Because the mother is worried that her daughter is not eating enough, she allows her to eat more yoghurt and less of other foods. As the daughter's behavior continues to influence the behaviors of the mother, her eating patterns eventually get her to the point where she is eating 'Winnie the Pooh' yoghurt only at the times she wants. Through the reciprocal behaviors between the mother and daughter, the 2-year-old girl has essentially determined her own nutritional environment.

Self-efficacy theory

Bandura's theory of self-efficacy combines his understanding of reciprocal determinism with Thorndike's original Law of Effect and Julian Rotter's behavioral equation (Figure 4.4, adapted from Bandura 1977):

Bandura's model is similar to Rotter's, in that expectations and one's subjective value of the outcome determine the extent to which one will engage in any particular activity. However, Bandura's model provides a more complete explanation as to why some people persist under difficult circumstances and others do not. According to Bandura, people take

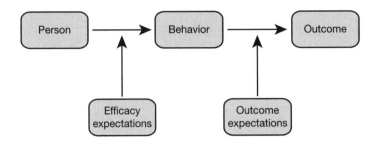

Figure 4.4 Bandura's model of self-efficacy

note of their effectiveness while engaging in activities. Going back to the puzzle example, both girls thought they would successfully complete them at the time they started to work on them. This was their efficacy expectation. The first girl's expectation was that she would be able to successfully complete the puzzle and did not see her initial difficulty as evidence of her lack of ability. As the second girl persisted, however, her lack of immediate success caused her to view the task as beyond her skill level and she subsequently gave up. Had the puzzle remained easy, it is likely that she would have completed it. The girls' persistence was therefore determined not by their actual behaviors, but by their interpretation of their behaviors in light of their ongoing success or failure.

Bandura also believed that efficacy expectations are influenced by four sources of information: the individual's own personal previous accomplishments, vicarious experience (i.e. observations of others' relative success or failure in completing a given task), verbal persuasion (this includes encouragement from others) and emotional arousal – i.e. the extent to which engaging in the activity results in a positive or negative emotional state.

Bandura believed that verbal persuasion was limited in its ability to enhance one's sense of efficacy because it can easily be contradicted through personal experience. However, Bandura was curious as to how vicarious experience (i.e. observational learning) influenced self-efficacy expectations. In order to better understand the extent to which vicarious experiences informed self-efficacy attributes, Bandura asked snake-phobic individuals to participate in a task aimed at reducing their fear of snakes.

Using Wolpe's method of systematic desensitization (see previous section), Bandura randomly assigned highly snake-phobic individuals to a control group and one of two treatment groups. In the first treatment group, the phobic individuals were exposed to a 'participant modeling' treatment session with a live boa constrictor. Under this condition, participants were successively and rapidly exposed to increasingly more threatening situations involving the snake – progressing from looking at the snake, touching it, holding it and letting it move around the room before chasing it and picking it up. This was done with the assistance of a model who broke the snake-handling behaviors down into small steps. This model first demonstrated snake-handling behaviors and then allowed the participant to try the behavior until he or she had mastered it while doing relaxation exercises. Once the participants felt they had comfortably completed a step, they moved on to a progressively more difficult one.

In the second treatment group, the participants were exposed to an observation of the model doing the same tasks, with no opportunity to practice the actions themselves. The control group received no treatment. One week after the experiment, the three treatment groups were asked to rate their self-efficacy in their ability to comfortably handle a snake. They then participated in second 'similar' session where they repeated the same tasks with the original snake, as well as a third 'dissimilar' session with a corn snake.

At the end of the experiment no change was observed in the control group. However, participants from both treatment groups demonstrated significant improvements in their ability to manage their fear in the presence of snakes. Both groups also reported significant improvements in their perceived self-efficacy in managing their emotions whilst handling the snake. More importantly, there was a strong correlation between the participants' self-efficacy attributions and their subsequent snake-handling behavior. In other words, those who reported having high self-efficacy before handling the snake were also the most likely to demonstrate comfort in picking up the snake during 'similar' and 'dissimilar' sessions. In addition, those who were assigned to the participant modeling group were the most likely to have strong self-efficacy beliefs regarding their ability to handle the snakes. When comparing the pre- and post-test measures, perceived self-efficacy rather than previous snake-handling success best predicted who would best manage the post-treatment session with the corn snake. In this respect, Bandura demonstrated that behavior is more influenced by one's perception of one's efficacy, rather than one's actual efficacy.

The results of Bandura's snake experiment have several implications for how self-efficacy affects cognitive, motivational and affective processes (Bandura 1994). First, Bandura asserts that self-efficacy beliefs determine an individual's understanding of what constitutes success and how this is best achieved. Those who have a high sense of self-efficacy focus their attention on what a successful outcome looks and feels like and concentrate their thinking on performance-related behaviors that are likely to contribute to their success. Alternatively, individuals with a low sense of self-efficacy are likely to envision outcomes in terms of their potential failure and dwell on things that could potentially interfere with their success.

Self-efficacy beliefs are also related to people's motivation, especially in terms of expectations, goals and causal attributions. Bandura observed that people who believe themselves to be highly efficacious are more likely to attribute their failures to insufficient effort, whereas those with a low self-efficacy are more likely to attribute their failures to their lack of ability. Bandura additionally noted that individuals with low self-efficacy are at greater risk of stress and depression. Because these individuals do not feel as though they can control the events in their lives, they are more likely to dwell on their coping deficiencies. Bandura observed that in this respect, individuals can maintain both an internal locus of control and perceptions of low self-efficacy. These individuals are particularly vulnerable to depression, for they believe that while most people are able to control the events in their lives, they (for whatever reason) cannot.

Self-efficacy theory applied to parenting work

When applying his ideas to the treatment of mental health disorders, Bandura, believed that maladaptive behavior occurs because of unreasonably high expectations and/or inadequate learning experiences. For this reason, clients do not need to have their mental illness 'cured', but do need opportunities to learn new coping skills and assistance in choosing more achievable goals. In this respect, the role of the practitioner is not one of an expert or advocate, but one of a teacher who breaks down long-range goals into realistic and achievable subtasks. By doing this, practitioners create opportunities for clients to obtain a sense of mastery and, over time, their sense of efficacy should improve.

When applying Bandura's ideas to work with parents, the primary aim is to help parents achieve a greater sense of self-efficacy in the parenting role. The NFP model provides a good example of how this can be done (Olds et al. 1997; see Box 1.2). In their first randomized controlled trial of the program, the developers observed that the women participating in the program appeared to have little control over their own lives. In order to help them improve their sense of control, several self-efficacy-related elements were introduced into the model:

* Mothers are educated in how to improve their health-related behaviors. Health-related goals (like giving up smoking) are broken down into small, achievable steps.
* Practitioners model positive child-caring behaviors and then give mothers opportunities to practice them. Practitioners reward positive care-giving behaviors with praise and positive regard.
* Mothers are asked to identify specific problems. The practitioner and mother then set small, realistic goals for overcoming these problems. The practitioner then helps the mother to come up with a plan for monitoring her progress towards these goals.
* Solution-focused methods are introduced that emphasize family members' strengths in order to enhance their sense of efficacy.

NFP program developers believe that a self-efficacy-based approach has improved the effectiveness of the program. However, they also believe that the extreme adversity experienced by the majority of the mothers makes this work especially challenging. In particular, the program developers feel that self-efficacy methods are inadequate for helping parents cope with aspects of their personal histories that may be impacting upon their parenting skills. For this reason, NFP also includes methods developed by Selma Fraiberg (see previous section) in combination with self-efficacy exercises.

Family systems theory

Systems theory

General systems theory is the study of complex systems in nature, society and science. The field, as we know it today, originated in the work of Ludwig von Bertalanffy (1901–1972) in the mid 1920s and has since been informed by research in the fields of biology, **cybernetics** and the social sciences. Systems theory is a framework for understanding how the individual components of complex systems interact with each other to produce an end result. The term 'system' can be applied to a single organism, organization, society or technological process.

Family systems theory involves the application of systems theory principles to the study of families. It draws from Bertalanffy's original ideas as well as the work of Gregory Bateson (1904–1980), who studied maladaptive patterns of interaction within families of schizophrenics. Family systems theory also includes ideas from social learning theory, object relations theory, attachment theory and the model of human ecology. Psychologists who pioneered the application of general systems family work include Salvador Minuchin (1921–) and Virginia Satir (1916–1988). Systems theory principles core to family research and therapy include the following (Broderick 1993, Minuchin 1985):

1   **Family systems are open systems**. As Bronfenbrenner observed, family systems exist within larger systems, including the community and society. Families, by their very nature, need to be open to the influences of these wider systems in order to survive.

Communication between the family and its wider environment takes place through **input** and **output** processes. Input and output processes are managed by boundaries that are selectively and adaptively permeable. Permeable boundaries allow the family to access resources essential for its survival, yet protect it from outside dangers. These boundaries also enable the family to establish its own sense of identity through values and goals shared by all family members.

2   **Family systems are complete systems. Each member within the system is a necessarily interdependent part of the greater whole**. From this perspective, the behavior of an individual family member reflects processes within the entire family. An individual family member is thus never truly independent and can be fully understood only within the context of the family. For this reason, family therapists focus on interactions between members rather than the behavior of any one individual.

3   **Patterns of behavior between families are circular rather than linear**. Going back to Bandura's concept of reciprocal determinism, uni-directional models of causality (e.g. A → B) are not adequate for explaining patterns of interaction within families. Family therapists instead prefer to conceptualize family interactions in terms of feedback loops and spirals rather than linear processes. For this reason, therapists concentrate on relationships between family members, rather than the behavior of any one individual. This is precisely what Winnicott meant when he said that there is no such thing as a baby, just a nursing couple. It is the reciprocal pattern of behaviors between the mother and child that influence the course of the child's development – not the behaviors of the mother or child separately.

4   **Family systems are homeostatic, self-regulating systems**. This means that the interactions between family members are stable and predictable and that family members engage in behaviors that keep them that way. Behaviors that potentially disrupt the equilibrium within the system are frequently controlled via corrective feedback loops used by all family members. In healthy families, corrective and self-regulating processes are adaptive. In dysfunctional families, corrective processes are rigid and interfere with the family's ability to adapt to the changing needs of its members and environment.

5   **Family systems are ongoing and evolving**. All families have a past, present and future. Broderick (1993) observes that the lifecycle of the family is linked to the developmental stage of the children. At earlier stages, the family is focused on having and raising children. At later stages, the family must launch the children from the family system. Families must adaptively respond to the requirements of each developmental transition in order to meet their children's psychological and physical needs, as well as the demands of society (i.e. school, work). Change happens when there is a 'perturbation' that disrupts established patterns within the system. This forces the family into a period of disequilibrium, where new patterns emerge and shift until a new equilibrium is established. Less healthy families have difficulty coping with change and the role of the therapist is often to help them manage the change process.

6   **Family systems are goal-seeking systems**. Children's developmental progression defines some family goals, as do health- and employment-related factors. Within these broader goal structures there is a high degree of variation between families, however. Some families are very goal oriented, whereas others appear to be less committed to any predefined direction.

7　**Family systems are complex systems, composed of subsystems**. At the most basic level, each individual is a family subsystem. However, subsystems between family members also exist. Common subsystems include the spousal, coparent, sibling and extended family subsystems. A common goal of family therapy is to understand each family member's participation within these subsystems and the interaction between them.

8　**Subsystems within the larger family system are separated by boundaries**. Interactions across these boundaries are governed by implicit rules and patterns. Each subsystem has its own integrity as a system, guided by a unique set of rules. For example, adult parents have their own rules for interacting as a couple, which are different and separate from the rules established for interacting with their children as coparents. Boundaries exist between these subsystems that are maintained by **bonds** between subsystem members. Bonds keep some members psychologically close, while **buffering** others from entering in. Healthy families have clear boundaries between subsystems, whereas less healthy families have difficulty maintaining these boundaries. A common example of boundary blurring occurs in families where one parent misuses substances. In these instances, it is not uncommon for the other, non-misusing parent to blur the parent–child boundary by relying on the child for adult emotional support.

Understanding family systems through genograms

Family therapists often use **genograms** to understand subsystems and record the quality of the relationships between family members. Genograms can be used to represent historic and emotional relationships and patterns of communication. Figure 4.5 provides an example of a genogram. Figure 4.6 provides examples of various genogram symbols and Figure 4.7 shows how emotional relationships are depicted. A variety of software packages for producing genograms are available for purchase. More information about the design and use of genograms can also be found at http://www.genograms.org/index.html.

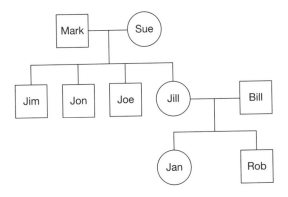

Figure 4.5 An example of a simple genogram

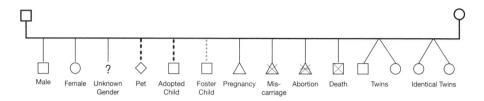

Figure 4.6 Typical genogram symbols

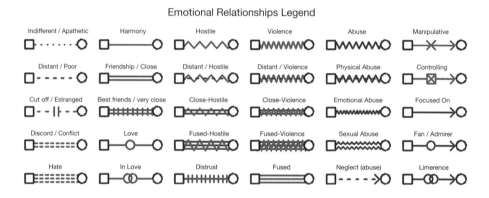

Figure 4.7 Genogram symbols typically used to depict the quality of relationships

Structural family theory

Argentinean physician Salvador Minuchin (1921–) developed his model of structural family therapy[6] during the mid 1960s through his research and therapeutic work with delinquent boys at the Wiltwyck School in New York. The term 'structural' refers to the idea that families organize themselves around an implicit set of structures and rules which determine how each member relates to the other. Family structures determine the interactions that take place between family members, their subsystems and the family's interface with the outside world. Minuchin observed that some structures are better than others in helping families adapt to change and crises.

Minuchin noted that subsystems may be temporary or permanent, depending upon their function within the family. Family members are likely to belong to more than one subsystem and their roles within these systems are likely to differ, depending upon the role of the subsystem. Minuchin identified the spousal, parent and sibling subsystems as the primary subsystems within families.

- The **spousal subsystem** entails the relationship between parents. Interactions within this subsystem involve the adults' mutual need for affection, support and shared decision making. The spousal subsystem is considered the primary mediator between the family and the outside world.

- The **parental subsystem** (or coparent system, also discussed in Chapter 3) maintains the authority for ensuring the care and safety of the children. When parents share this responsibility, it is important that they work together as a team and negotiate conflicting interests. In order to work effectively, parents should be aligned on key issues such as discipline and educational achievement. The parental subsystem must also be able to adapt to the developmental needs of the children.
- The **parent–child subsystem** provides children with enough care and nurturance to allow them to develop and gain autonomy within the parent–child relationship.
- The **sibling subsystem** provides the context within which children learn to cooperate, compete and prepare for peer-related activities and friendships as they develop.

Minuchin believed that clearly defined hierarchical relationships between the parent and child subsystems improved the functionality of families. This means that parents should have clear authority over their children and that older siblings have greater privileges over younger ones. Minuchin also believed that clear boundaries between family subsystems were necessary for adaptive family functioning. Minuchin noted that boundaries existed on a continuum ranging from **rigid** to **diffuse**. Healthy boundaries exist in the middle of this continuum, containing both rigid and diffuse elements. Boundaries that are either too rigid or too diffuse significantly reduce a family's ability to effectively adapt to change and cope with their environment.

Minuchin observed that within and across these boundaries, family interactions are organized via **power**, **alignments** and **coalitions**. Power is related to each member's level of authority (i.e. their decision-making power) and responsibility (who carries out the decision). Minuchin believed that adults should have power over children, although this should be used responsibly. Alignments are defined by the way family members join or oppose one another in carrying out specific activities. Alignments can be functional or dysfunctional, depending on the demands of the task. Good alignment between parents in shared childrearing duties is considered highly functional. An alignment between a parent and child in opposing the other parent (also referred to as **triangulation**) is considered to be dysfunctional, however. Triangulation often occurs when parents are not able to resolve conflicts on their own and one parent draws a child into the conflict in an attempt to gain control over the other. While these situations sometimes provide children with greater power within the system, they ultimately place the child in a no-win situation, as the child becomes vulnerable to attack from the excluded parent.

Coalitions are enduring alliances that occur between specific family members against a single member. **Detouring** takes place when a coalition holds an excluded member responsible for problems occurring within the coalition. For example, adult parents may use a child's antisocial behavior as an excuse for problems occurring between them. This detouring of the problem may be temporarily beneficial for their spousal relationship (since it keeps the partners from blaming each other), but it is highly detrimental to the development of the child and the family's overall ability to function effectively.

Minuchin identified five common dysfunctional family structures: enmeshed, disengaged, families with a peripheral parent, under-involved parents and families with juvenile parents.

- **Enmeshed** family members are overly involved in each other's lives and do not maintain clear boundaries.
- **Disengaged** families have members who function autonomously, but with little or no loyalty to each other.

- In families with a **peripheral parent**, one parent maintains a role exterior to the others. When this parent re-enters the family system, he or she often does so in an authoritarian or abusive manner.
- **Uninvolved parents** are indifferent about their children and show very little emotion towards them.
- **Juvenile parents** act immaturely in relation to their children, often placing the children in the parenting role.

Minuchin believed that individual behavior or mental health problems are frequently a 'symptom' of dysfunction within the entire family system. Minuchin further noted that such symptoms (also referred to as the **presenting problem**, see Satir, next section) are implicitly reinforced by other members because they often serve a maladaptive purpose for them. This is exemplified by detouring behaviors, which enable coalitions to shift the focus or blame from their issues onto a specific individual. Presenting problems are also often an indication that the family is having difficulty adapting to developmental transitions. A young child's refusal to feed him- or herself is frequently a sign that the parents are reluctant to allow the child to mature. Minuchin additionally observed that presenting problems may be an indication of dysfunctional patterns that have been passed down from generation to generation. Through his work with poor families in New York and Philadelphia, Minuchin noted that living in a hostile and impoverished environment commonly interferes with families' ability to adapt and cope with change. Minuchin believed that adaptability – i.e. the family's ability to access and execute alternative interactional patterns – is the 'master trait' that determines how well a family handles stressful life events.

Structural family therapy

The primary aim of structural family therapy is to help families adapt to change and alter dysfunctional patterns of interaction. Once families are able to appropriately adapt to their circumstances, individual members' symptoms should stop and the family's overall functioning should improve. In order to accomplish this, all family members must undergo a **conceptual shift** that restructures the family's previous organization. Restructuring involves changes in family rules, and realignments, breaking down and rebuilding boundaries and disabling patterns of interaction that support the maladaptive behavior of individual members.

Minuchin used **family mapping** as a way to understand areas where the family functions well, as well as areas of dysfunction. A family map is a genogram that places a particular emphasis on family boundaries, coalitions and detouring behaviors. Family mapping also allows the therapist to understand how the family is hierarchically organized. A primary goal of structural family therapy is to make sure that parents are in charge of the family system and that there is a clear boundary between the parent and child subsystems. However, family therapists also work to ensure that the parental subsystem is flexible enough to adapt to the developmental needs of the children. This means making sure that parents provide children with opportunities to share in family decision-making processes and grant them increasing autonomy as they become older.

During structural family therapy, the role of the therapist is to actively disrupt dysfunctional patterns so that they can be replaced by improved processes for interaction. The therapist does this by encouraging family members to use their personal strengths to generate new and more adaptive responses to each other within a safe, therapeutic environment.

Once individual family members begin to change, their behavior reciprocally influences the behavior of others, including the member with the 'presenting problem'.

Minuchin's therapeutic style has been described as that of a 'conductor' (Goldenberg and Goldenberg 1996) who actively places him- or herself in the centre of the family and makes suggestions for change. This might involve interrupting disputes, rearranging family members' preferred seating patterns and challenging implicit rules for communication. Minuchin did not believe that the therapist should assume this role as an expert, however. Instead, Minuchin believed that the best way to lead was by following. In this respect, the therapist should **join** the family as a 'distant relative' who respectively **accommodates** to its style of interaction. This is accomplished through **mimesis**, a term Minuchin coined from the Greek word for copy. By mimesis, Minuchin meant that the therapist should subtly mimic the style and manner of communication within the family, as well as share his or her personal experiences that may be similar to what the family has experienced.

Once the therapist has entered the family system, he or she becomes able to understand the **family's narrative**, including its values, beliefs, myths and realities. The therapist should also begin to understand the trauma that some family members may be experiencing. As the therapist joins and accommodates, he or she should gain an understanding of the family's structure and develop hypotheses (often shared with the family) about the boundaries that exist and the ways in which they can be changed. One of the ways in which the therapist alters family structures is by physically rearranging them. Thus, if a triangulated parent and child are seated opposite to the excluded parent, the therapist may physically change the way they are seated. By manipulating structures, the therapist is able to test systems that are more rigid, as well as those that are more flexible to change.

Additional therapeutic techniques developed by Minuchin are tracking, enactment and reframing. **Tracking** involves the therapist actively tracking family-relevant themes, stories, metaphors and words that repeatedly surface during the course of the therapy. For example, the therapist may hear a mother describe something that happened to her when she was small. At a later point, the therapist may observe a similar theme during an interaction between the mother and her own child. The therapist should then 'track' that theme by making a connection between the mother's past experience and her present behavior. This tracking then introduces opportunities for considering how the past may be influencing the present.

Enactments are an important feature of family therapy. During an enactment, the therapist asks family members to literally re-enact a conflict that may have recently occurred between them. While watching the enactment, the therapist can observe how family members behave towards each other and draw conclusions about the structure of the family. During the enactment, the therapist may also attempt to alter existing patterns and encourage members to try more functional responses to each other.

Reframing (Watzlawick et al. 1974) takes place when the therapist offers an alternative interpretation of the meaning of an event or behavior. This is done so that family members can adopt a more constructive understanding of what might be occurring. For example, a teenage son shouting at his mother is likely to be interpreted as belligerent and rebellious by other family members. The therapist may offer an alternative interpretation, however, by reframing the young person's behavior as expressing hurt and fear. This gives the young man 'permission' to express his hurt, rather than anger, and also improves the other family members' ability to understand and listen.

At some point in the therapy, family members may resist the change introduced by the therapist in order to maintain the familiar comfort that homeostasis represents within the system. This often takes place when the symptom bearer exhibits his or her maladaptive behavior, which is then reinforced by other family members. At this point, the therapist may want to suggest new behaviors and perspectives to the family members, although it is likely that members will initially resist and/or reject these alternative responses. Reframing techniques are often an effective way of helping family members overcome this resistance and understand that the symptom bearer's behavior is an expression of problems that belong to the entire family – not just the individual with the presenting problem. This new understanding should then enable family members to change their behaviors and resolve the underlying issues that underpin the behavior of the individual with the presenting problem.

Virginia Satir

A human validation process model

> Feelings of worth can flourish only in an atmosphere where individual differences are appreciated, mistakes are tolerated, communication is open, and rules are flexible – the kind of atmosphere that is found in a nurturing family.
>
> (Satir 1972: 13)

American therapist Virginia Satir (1916–1988) asserted that positive self-worth is the cornerstone of all individual and family mental health. Like Rogers, Satir believed that every individual strives towards healthy growth and development and that each person possesses the resources necessary to fulfill his or her potential. Moreover, Satir believed that every individual's intentions are positive, no matter how difficult their behavior might be. Satir asserted that difficult behavior, which she referred to as the 'presenting problem', was, in fact, not the real problem. Instead, it is how people *cope* with the problem that *creates* the problem (Satir 1982).

Satir viewed families as systems that were constantly seeking balance and homeostasis. Satir observed that problems are often created when family members sacrifice individual needs in order to maintain balance within the family system. In particular, Satir observed that each member must 'pay' a personal 'price' to keep the family unit balanced. Individual symptoms often indicate a blockage towards growth within a family as it struggles to maintain balance. According to Satir (1982), the rules that determine the family's balance are related to how parents achieve and maintain their own self-esteem. These rules, in turn, determine how children grow and develop their own sense of self-worth.

Satir's *Human Validation Process Model* is based on the premise that an individual's behavior is a representation of what he or she has learned up to any given point in time. Satir believed that a child's experiences within the **primary survival triad** (i.e. the father, mother and child) are particularly influential in determining how the child comes to know him- or herself (Satir and Baldwin 1983). Within the primary survival triad, the child learns to decipher parental messages that are communicated not just through words, but through body language, tone, touch and looks. The child's understanding of these messages, in turn, influences how the child perceives him- or herself, as well as how he or she communicates with others.

Satir believed that communication systems within families are a reflection of each individual member's sense of self-worth. Dysfunctional communication (including indirect, incomplete, unclear, inaccurate, distorted and inappropriate messages) is a characteristic of a dysfunctional family system. Satir (1972) identified four dysfunctional communication stances:

- The **placater** is weak, tentative and self-effacing. This individual always agrees, is quick to apologize and tries to please.
- The **blamer** dominates, finds fault with others and behaves self-righteously.
- The **super-reasonable person** over-intellectualizes things, is often rigid, tries to be calm and cool, keeps an emotional distance, but tries to maintain intellectual control.
- An **irrelevant person** attempts to distract others and is unable to relate to what is going on.

Satir observed that various combinations of these communication stances take place in most families. Satir asserted that these stances are used because some family members lack the self-esteem that provides them with the confidence to genuinely express their feelings. The above communication stances therefore keep people from exposing their true feelings and are often used when individuals are stressed. Satir asserted that people can learn to express their feelings more effectively, however, through a **congruent** communication stance. Whether stressed or not, an individual who is congruent with him- or herself should feel secure enough to communicate in a manner that is genuine and straightforward, as well as take responsibility for what has been said.

In explaining human relationships, Satir believed that individuals consider their interactions with each other from one of two contrasting perspectives: the 'threat and reward' model and the 'seed' model (Goldenberg and Goldenberg 1996). The 'threat and reward' model is based upon a hierarchical understanding of relationships where those in a higher position define the rules and those in a lower position follow them. From this perspective, it is each family member's role, not their individuality, which defines the nature of the relationship. Although those in a position of authority may not necessarily behave in a manner that is malevolent or self-serving, 'threat and reward' relationships tend to encourage feelings of helplessness and discourage a positive sense of self-esteem in others.

The 'seed' model, on the other hand, places an emphasis on the person, rather than the role, in determining relationships and one's identity. The seed model emphasizes each individual's potential and change is viewed as an opportunity for growth. While roles and status exist, Satir believed that they should be used to define relationships within a certain context and not determine roles outside of this context. Satir strongly advocated the seed model and believed that children, like seedlings, can grow into healthy adults when they are given the proper support and encouragement.

Satir's approach to therapy

Satir's therapeutic techniques are based upon her belief that change is always possible and that all people have the resources to cope and grow (Banmen 2002). Since most people prefer the familiarity of homeostasis over the discomfort of change, therapy should try to reduce this discomfort so that family members feel safe to change. Satir also believed that individual family members frequently need to resolve personal, intra-psychic issues before they are able to improve their interaction patterns with others. Hence, Satir's therapeutic model aims to support individual growth at the same time that it supports family change. In doing this, a primary goal of Satir's emotion-focused model is to help individual family members build a positive sense of self-worth, which should, in turn, improve the functionality of the entire family (Bandler et al. 1976). As part of this process, Satir used four overarching, meta-goals to help clients develop individual goals for positive change (Banmen 2002):

1   **Raise the client's self-esteem**. Self-esteem is considered as one's own judgment or experience of one's personal worth.
2   **Help clients to be their own choice makers**. Satir encouraged family members to make their own choices and did this by asking people to consider at least three options in any given situation. Satir purposely did this to keep people from viewing situations in terms of polar opposites. Rather than view choices as 'either/or,' Satir actively encouraged individuals and families to explore multiple possibilities.
3   **Help clients take responsibility**. Satir advocated that clients be responsible for both their behavior and their feelings. This means being in charge of one's feelings, managing them, and enjoying them. Satir helped clients accomplish this by encouraging them to reflect deeply upon their own feelings and actions.
4   **Help clients become congruent**. Achieving congruence was an ultimate goal of Satir's therapy, in terms both of one's feelings and style of communication. Satir believed that true congruence is achieved when the individual is not controlled or triggered negatively by the outside world, but responds to the world from a state of internal harmony and self-acceptance. Satir believed that it was important that therapists model congruence for their clients.

When working with families, Satir adopted the role of a teacher who taught families new forms of communication. Like Minuchin, she often interjected herself into the middle of family issues, to both block dysfunctional styles of communication and teach more effective methods of interacting. Satir also felt that body language and tone were particularly important forms of interaction and took efforts to make sure that family members' body language reflected what they said and meant. When doing this, she insisted that family members communicate with each other literally at each other's level. This meant that parents were encouraged to squat down when talking to their children and children were raised up (on chairs) to talk to their parents.

Satir was also interested in helping families understand and achieve their ideal family life. When doing this, she encouraged family members to take a problem-solving approach to identifying family strengths that could, in turn, be used to initiate positive change. Satir believed that in order for this to happen, families needed to trust each other and be open and unambiguous in their communication. As a way of encouraging open and trusting attitudes, Satir felt that it was necessary for therapists to model openness and trust with their clients. This meant showing parents and children how to get in touch with their own feelings, how to listen to others, how to ask for clarification and how to ask for what they wanted. In doing this, Satir encouraged family members to clearly state their needs through I-messages (see Gordon and Rogers, previous section), by beginning sentences with *I want, I think* or *I feel* (Satir 1972). She then required parents to carefully listen to their children and children to carefully listen to their parents. Satir believed that, within time, these feedback processes helped family members to replace dysfunctional patterns of communication with more congruent styles of interaction.

In order to help family members reflect upon their family functioning, Satir frequently asked members to jointly create a **family life chronology** (1967). A family life chronology (often accompanied by a family map or genogram) describes the history of the family, beginning with when the parents met, decided to marry and have children. When explaining their history, parents are asked to recount their relationship with their own parents and siblings, as well as to describe their own parents' parenting styles. As parents do this, parents are encouraged to think about the ways in which their upbringing is currently influencing their present relationship with their own children. Satir believed that when family members have properly examined their past, they become better able to understand their current difficulties and explore ways in which problems can be solved.

Change model

In order to help families better understand their own change processes, Satir et al. (1991) developed her own five-stage change model to describe the effects of change on people's feelings, thinking, behavior and physiology (Figure 4.8).

Satir's model of change begins with the **old status quo**. The old status quo is characteristic of a fairly stable system (individual or group) where family life is predictable, familiar and comfortable (Sayles 2002). This may mean that things are working well, but it more frequently means that family members are using familiar solutions (for better or worse) for common problems. For most families, the status quo does represent some level of success and balance, although some members may have to pay different prices to maintain this balance. For example, a child may refuse to eat at the table as a way of keeping his parents from arguing with each other. The child accomplishes this by uniting the parents over his problem and reduces the stress created by the arguing.

At some point, however, the old status quo is challenged through the introduction of a **foreign element** that acts as a catalyst towards change. This may be introduced internally by a family member who envisages an improved family life or externally by an unexpected event (e.g. a parent loses a job or there is a family illness), an expected event (the birth of a new child or a child's entry into school) or difficulty with the authorities (e.g. a child or a parent has done something illegal). This foreign element requires the family to change

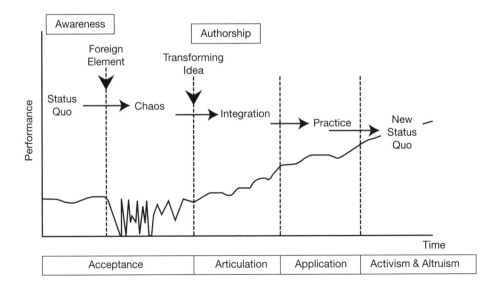

Figure 4.8 Virgina Satir's change model

and threatens the stability of familiar power structures. Initially, most family members resist this change by denying the validity of the foreign element, avoiding the issues it creates or blaming each other for it.

If the foreign element is strong enough to defend itself against the family's resistance, family members enter the second stage in the change model: **chaos**. At this time, family members realize the status quo is no longer achievable and begin to lose their sense of control. Some family members may feel frightened and vulnerable, whereas others may become angry and stressed. During this time, dysfunctional communication stances come to the surface. This provides the therapist with an opportunity to challenge these dysfunctional methods of coping and replace them with more adaptive forms of communication. From this perspective, chaos is an extremely important part of the change process.

As family members struggle to cope with the chaos, emotions are felt and acknowledged at a deeper level than what was experienced before. This shift often brings individual family members to their core self, which can be a very scary place for some. Through this process, individuals also discover new inner resources and strengths that they previously were not aware of. This provides family members with a new sense of hope and a willingness to learn new coping skills. During this process, family members often undergo a **transformation** where they realize how their specific behaviors contributed to previous problems. This understanding enables them to make choices about their behavior that will keep them from returning to the old status quo and enable them to go forward in the process of change.

Initially, family members may feel strange and awkward with the feelings brought forward during the transformation process. However, as time goes by, family members become more comfortable with their new feelings (Satir et al. 1991). The role of the therapist at this stage is to **integrate** these new feelings in family members' perceptions, beliefs and behaviors by providing them with opportunities to safely **practice** them. Another way the therapist supports this process is by helping family members make positive decisions without making the decisions for them (Satir and Baldwin 1983). Once the decision is made, the therapist should then support the choice and positively reinforce the members' willingness to take the risks involved in making this decision. This further reinforces the outcome of the transformation. Once the transformation has been fully practiced and integrated, the family will have achieved the fifth stage of Satir's change model, a **new status quo** where members can feel heard and more fully acknowledged. At this point, all family members should feel an increased sense of trust and hope, as well as a higher sense of self-esteem (Satir et al. 1991).

While Virginia Satir's change model was originally developed through her work with families, it has since been applied to a variety of contexts, including organizational change. Satir's principles are also a cornerstone of the evidence-based FAST program, which uses 'I want, I think, I feel' drawing exercises to improve communication between parents and children (see Box 3.6 for a program overview).

Evidence-based models of family therapy

A growing body of research suggests that specific forms of family therapy are an effective treatment for a wide variety of child and adolescent mental health problems. For example, evidence consistently suggests that family therapy is an effective method for treating anorexia nervosa in adolescent girls, especially when it includes work with the adolescent (including the use of CBT) and the parents individually (Bulik et al. 2007, Eisler et al. 2007). Various models of family therapy are also effective in treating adolescent substance-misuse problems and issues related to antisocial behavior. *Multisystemic Therapy* (MST – see Box 4.4) and

Box 4.4: *Multisystemic Therapy*

Multisystemic Therapy (MST) is an evidence-based program targeting the multiple determinants of serious antisocial behavior and youth offending. MST assumes that problematic youth behavior is determined by a variety of risks existing within systems at
the individual, family, peer, school and community level. MST aims to reduce these
risks by using strengths within each system to facilitate family and youth change. MST
accomplishes this through a combination of cognitive behavioral therapy (CBT) and
family therapy which is delivered to parents and youths in their homes. The MST
therapist is available to families 24 hours a day and provides several hours of treatment
per week that combine individual and family sessions. Work with the parents aims to
provide them with the skills and resources to independently address the difficulties
arising with their teenager. Work with the young person focuses on skills which will
allow him/her to cope with family- peer-, school- and community-based pressures.
The average duration of treatment is 60 hours delivered over a period of four months.

   MST has undergone multiple RCTs demonstrating the following positive youth
outcomes (Henggeler et al. 1998):

- 25–75 per cent reductions in long-term rates of re-arrest
- 47–64 per cent reductions in out-of-home placements
- Extensive improvements in family functioning
- Decreased mental health problems for serious juvenile offenders.

   A recent benefit–cost analysis of MST suggests that, when properly implemented,
the program saves the taxpayer $9.50 for every $1 spent. This estimate is considered
conservative, however, since it was calculated by taking into account re-arrest rates.
When actual crime rates are taken into account (with the understanding that not all
recidivists are arrested for the crimes they commit) the potential benefit cost of MST
then rises to $23.60 for every $1 invested in program costs (Klietz et al. 2010).

Functional Family Therapy (FFT – described in this section) are two models that have been
particularly successful in improving adolescent outcomes and reducing crime.

Functional Family Therapy

Developed by James Alexander and his colleagues at the University of Utah, the FFT model
asserts that problematic adolescent behavior (i.e. the presenting problem) is a reflection of
dysfunction at the ecological levels of the individual, family and community and the interaction between these multiple systems (Sexton et al. 2004). While the program focuses on the
family as the unit of treatment, it uses the adolescent with the presenting problem as the
primary source for understanding how the family functions (Sexton et al. 2004, Sexton and
Alexander 2003).

   By combining principles from social learning theory, family systems theory, cognitive theory
and the ecological model, the program aims to improve family members' understanding of
how their behavior plays a functional role in their relationships with others (Alexander and
Parsons 1982, Sexton and Alexander 2003). Within this model, no specific behavior is identified as 'wrong', since functional family therapists believe that all behavioral patterns perform

an adaptive function within the family. Once family members understand the functional reasons behind specific behaviors, they are then in a better position to change them.

This is more easily said than done, however, as family members are initially likely to label behaviors as good or bad or interpret them as an example of a parent's or child's character flaws. For example, a mother might perceive her son's untidy room as a sign of his laziness or a father might interpret his daughter's back-talk has an indication that she is inconsiderate. FFT therapists strive not to assign a value to these behaviors, but instead interpret them within the context of the individual family member as a whole person. A key feature of the intervention is to help family members identify and re-label such behaviors in terms of the function they might be serving.

Alexander (Alexander and Parsons 1982) believed that most behaviors – positive or negative – can be interpreted as an effort to achieve one of three interpersonal states: **merging** (seeking contact or closeness), **separating** (seeking distance or independence) or **midpointing**, which includes elements of being close and independent (Sexton and Alexander 2003). Alexander believes that all of these behaviors serve an adaptive function within the system, although their outcome may be maladaptive. For example, a father who 'rejects' his teenage son may do so in order to maintain a sense of separateness from the family. His son may, in turn, feel a need to act out in order to gain the attention of his father so that he can feel connected to him (Sexton and Alexander 2003). Both of these behaviors serve a function within the system, yet both have undesirable outcomes. The father's behavior provides him with a sense of autonomy and the son's behavior reconnects him to the family. A primary goal of FFT is to thus help family members understand the function their behaviors are performing within the system and identify areas where behaviors can be changed. This is done with the understanding that positive changes in the young person's and parents' behavior will be sustained only for as long as their environment (i.e. other family members) supports these changes.

FFT's principles of change

Alexander and his colleagues (Sexton et al. 2004, Sexton and Alexander 2003) assert that positive change within dysfunctional families is predicted by four therapeutic processes: 1) alliance-based motivation, 2) reframing techniques, 3) appropriate and obtainable behavioral change goals and 4) matching the therapist and the therapy to the unique characteristics of the family.

Alliance-based motivation refers to the use of empowerment techniques aimed at helping resistant and unmotivated family members to become more open to change. The therapist accomplishes this by developing a positive alliance between him- or herself and each family member, as well as supporting positive alliances between the family members themselves. In this respect, a first goal of the therapy is to motivate the family members to work together.

Reframing is a technique developed by communication theorists (Watzlawick et al. 1974) and used frequently in structural family therapy (Goldenberg and Goldenberg 1996). In FFT it is used to help redefine the meaning of events and redirect negative emotionality. Sexton and Alexander (2003) also believe that reframing behaviors help to improve the alliance between family members and the therapist, as they serve to reduce negativity and blaming behaviors.

Within the context of FFT, reframing is a three-step process. First, the therapist validates the client's original perspective. The therapist then re-attributes meaning to the event by providing an alternative explanation. With feedback from other family members, the therapist then adjusts and more fully reformulates the meaning, the behavior or events. Box 4.5 provides an example of how reframing techniques can be used to help family members stop blaming each other and re-attribute meaning to the issues at hand. In this example, a mother is concerned about her 16-year-old daughter Alisha's ongoing dishonesty. On several occasions, the mother has discovered that Alisha has been out drinking with friends when she told her mother she was working the evening shift at a local fast-food restaurant. Alisha's mother is concerned about this behavior and raises it during a therapy session.

Box 4.5: An example of reframing techniques used in family therapy

Mother: (to therapist and family) I'm not really in the mood to talk today because I'm still angry about what happened last night.

Therapist: Well, maybe this would be a good time to discuss why you're angry.

Mother: (long pause) Well, we've discovered *yet again* that my daughter has been lying to me (sigh, pause – then to Alisha, almost yelling). How do you think I felt last night when I thought I'd pick you up at Burger King, just to find out that you weren't working a shift?

Alisha: (sits with arms crossed, says nothing and looks away).

Mother: I mean – I used to think you were a good kid. But look at you now. You're nothing but a lying brat! God only knows what you were doing last night (folds arms and turns away from daughter in disgust).

Alisha: (glares at mother) Mum, I told you – I just met up with my friends to have a few drinks.

Mother: Yeah, that's just great. Not only are you a liar, you're also a drunk. (Turns to therapist) See, this is what I was talking about last week – I have to put up with this sort of thing just about every night.

Therapist: I can see why you would really be bothered by this kind of behavior. I remember when my brother lied to me about something last year. I was really upset when I found out he wasn't telling the truth, because I thought we had a pretty good relationship.

Mother: Exactly. I used to think she was a good kid, but now it's clear that she isn't.

Therapist: Yeah, I used to think my brother was a good brother. I was pretty angry when he lied, but after we worked through it – I found out that he's still a pretty good brother, although a good brother who sometimes lies. Is there any other reason why you think Alisha lied to you?

Mother: What do you mean? She doesn't care how I feel and she'd rather be drinking with her mates than stay at home and be a responsible kid.

Therapist: OK – so she'd rather be with her friends. (To Alisha) Is this true? Do you care about how your mother feels OR would you rather be with your friends?

Alisha: Well, I do want to be with my friends (pause), but I also care about how my mum feels. (Gives her mother a sideways glance) I knew it would make her angry if I told her I wanted to go out.

Therapist: OK – so I'm hearing several explanations for Alisha's behavior. (To mother) You're worried that Alisha's untruthfulness about being at work last night means that she is becoming a dishonest person. (Mother nods) I also get the sense you're worried that she doesn't care about you.

Mother: (slowly nods) Yeah, sort of.

Therapist: (to Alisha) And I think I'm hearing from you that you wanted to be with your friends last night (pauses as Alisha nods), but that you do care about your mum's feelings.

Alisha: Yeah.

Therapist: (to Alisha) So did you lie as a way of not hurting her?

Alisha: Yeah – I knew she'd be upset if I wanted to go out, so I thought it would be better if I didn't tell her.

Mother: (still angry) That doesn't justify a lie.

Therapist: No – it doesn't justify a lie. But it might explain it. (Turning towards mother) I can see why you're upset about Alisha lying and it clearly was not the best thing for her to do. But can you think of a reason for lying that isn't all bad?

Mother: (calming down) Well – she said she wanted to be with her friends. When I was her age, I liked doing things with my friends, too. But not to the extent I had to lie about it.

Therapist: Why do you think Alisha wanted to lie about it?

Mother: (sighing) Because she knew it would make me angry and I would try to stop her.

Therapist: (to Alisha) OK – can we agree that lying is not a good thing to do, but might serve a purpose?

Alisha: (says nothing).

Therapist: (to mother) Can we also agree that it's sometimes OK to want to do things with your friends?

Mother: (smiles) Yeah.

Therapist: And can we also agree that it's sometimes OK not to want to make your mother angry?

(Both mother and Alisha smile and laugh.)

In the example provided in Box 4.5, the original problem, 'Alisha is a lying brat', has been reformulated to 'Alisha wants to spend time with her friends'. The therapist accomplishes this by first validating the mother's feelings by telling her he knows how it feels to be lied to. After letting the mother vent a little further, he then attempts to gradually re-attribute the focus from Alisha's dishonesty to the reasons why she might have wanted to lie. Note that he does not sanction Alisha's lying, but does re-attribute it to performing a function within the mother–daughter relationship. The therapist then checks with Alisha and her mother to see if his re-attribution makes any sense. The reframing process is completed when the therapist reformulates Alisha's dishonest behavior as expressing an appropriate need for independence and a willingness to remain connected by not hurting her mother's feelings.

Within the FFT model, change is also achieved by the therapist and family members setting small **obtainable change goals**. Sexton and Alexander (2003) assert that these goals should be specific, easy to achieve and relevant to the family. In the above example, a small and obtainable change goal might be the mother agreeing in principle that it is alright for her daughter to go out with her friends. Although this does not constitute a major therapeutic breakthrough it should curtail her emotionally abusive statements. It is also a small but achievable step that can be mastered before the therapist addresses more difficult issues, such as the poor communication between the mother and daughter, or the daughter's underage drinking. Sexton and Alexander assert that once family members become successful at these small and obtainable goals, the family's overall functioning gradually begins to improve. These small accomplishments also provide family members with a sense of empowerment and improve their willingness to work together towards positive change.

A fourth principle of change in the FFT model is the therapist's use of **matching** behaviors. Similar to Minuchin's notion of joining and accommodating, FFT therapists adopt a 'matching to' approach that ensures that the therapeutic methods and goals are relevant to the family. Matching behaviors aim to work with family members on 'their own terms' in a manner that is respectful of their culture, race, religion and gender-based values. FFT therapists strive not to impose their own values on the family and instead take efforts to make sure that the goals of the therapy make sense within the family's context.

Sexton and Alexander (2003) describe the FFT model as 'phasic', involving three distinct phases of intervention:

- **Phase 1: Engagement and motivation**. The primary goals of this phase are alliance building, negativity reduction, blame reduction and developing a shared family focus. This is accomplished by reframing techniques, which are used to alter dysfunctional perceptions, beliefs and emotions. Through this process it is expected that families will become less resistant to change and more motivated to work together.
- **Phase 2: Behavior change**. The primary aim of this phase is to set goals for behavioral change. The therapist should make sure that these goals are appropriate within the culture and the context of the family. Behavioral goals often include improved parenting and communication strategies, as well as new problem-solving skills.
- **Phase 3: Generalization**. This phase focuses on helping the family maintain and generalize the skills and strategies learned in the previous phase. The focus shifts from the problem that brought the family to therapy in the first place to methods for anticipating and coping with future issues. If a family member is recovering from a substance-misuse problem, this phase also covers relapse-prevention techniques. During this time, the therapist also helps the family to access community resources that may further strengthen their functioning.

The first RCT of FFT showed that adolescents whose families participated in FFT therapy had half the recidivism rates in comparison with the control group during the 18-month period following treatment (Alexander and Parsons 1973). These findings have been replicated through multiple RCTs over the past 30 years, suggesting that the model is also a highly cost-effective method of reducing crimes within communities, resulting in a potential saving of $28 for every $1 invested in the program (Aos et al. 2001, Aos et al. 1998). Evaluation findings also suggest that parents participating in the program are significantly more likely to show improvements in their parenting skills and knowledge that can be applied to their other children (Gordon 2000).

Bringing it all together: four basic assumptions

This chapter presents six different theoretical frameworks for understanding human behavior and improving psychological wellbeing. In a systematic review of therapies aimed at improving psychological outcomes for parents, Barlow et al. (2001, 2002) observed that all of the therapeutic approaches described in this chapter have a proven track record in reducing parents' anxiety and depression and increasing their self-esteem. Because all of the therapies achieved similar positive outcomes, the authors tentatively concluded that there may be a set of effective therapeutic processes that are common to most parenting interventions. A lack of a detailed description of the therapeutic models made it difficult for the authors to identify what these processes might be, however.

While this chapter has not identified a core set of processes, it has identified four assumptions common to most evidence-based parenting support. First is the need for interventions to provide parents with a warm and supportive therapeutic environment. While Rogers's humanistic approach places an emphasis on the need to create a safe psychological environment, all of the approaches described in this chapter require practitioners to treat parents in a manner that is genuine and empathic and values them as a person. Even Freud's expert-driven model assumes that positive change will take place only after the client feels that he or she has been heard and understood. For this reason, all evidence-based parenting intervention models begin with the assumption that therapeutic change will occur only if parents and their problems are treated in a manner that is respectful and non-judgmental and that parents feel psychologically safe.

A second assumption shared by most evidence-based parenting programs is the understanding that the past affects the present. This point was originally emphasized in Freud's psychodynamic theory and further developed by the object relations psychologists who observed that 'good-enough' parenting is passed down through the generations. This is why many evidence-based parenting interventions have methods for considering how parents' previous negative experiences affect the quality of their current relationship with their children. Once parents have had an opportunity to explore unresolved issues left over from their pasts, they are then in a better position to respond sensitively to their children's needs.

A third assumption shared by most evidence-based parenting programs is that parents' behavior is influenced by how they think and feel about their experiences and circumstances. This means that parents' behavior is based upon their subjective understanding of their environment, their constructions of causality, their associations between events and feelings, the extent to which they value certain outcomes and their perceptions of their personal efficacy. For this reason, many evidence-based parenting interventions aim to improve the way parents interpret their children's behavior, manage their own thought processes and perceive their sense of efficacy.

A fourth assumption held by most evidence-based intervention models is that parent and child behaviors are reciprocally determined between family members and reflect the overall functionality of the family system. For this reason, many programs focus on patterns of interaction between parents and children, rather than the individual behaviors of the parent or child. In doing so, most parenting interventions aim to improve communication within the family system and provide family members with a sense of connectedness.

Box 4.6: Key points

- Parents' ability to provide their children with love and support is related to their mental health and feelings of efficacy and self-worth.
- Many evidence-based parenting interventions include therapeutic methods aimed at improving parents' psychological wellbeing.
- These methods are underpinned by a variety of therapeutic models, including Freudian psychodynamic theory, Rogers's client-centered approach, Kelly's personal construct theory, the cognitive behavioral approaches of Ellis and Beck, Bandura's model of self-efficacy and family systems theory.

- Psychodynamic theory begins with the premise that human behavior is determined by the id, the ego and the super-ego. The id involves instinctual behaviors related to the fulfillment of physical needs, including sex and aggression. The super-ego involves morals and values learned from the parent and society. The ego constitutes conscious human functioning in response to the demands of the id and the super-ego.
- Freud believed that anxiety stems from an individual's inability to appropriately manage the impulses of the id or the demands of the super-ego.
- Defense mechanisms are also a means by which people manage perceived and unconscious threats to the ego.
- Object relations theory places an emphasis on object-related behavior rather than id-related drives. The term 'object' refers to the mother, who is considered to be the primary love object.
- Winnicott coined the term 'good-enough mother', which refers to maternal behaviors which gradually teach the child how to self-regulate emotional and physical states.
- Fraiberg introduced the notion of 'ghosts in the nursery', which refers to the fact that difficult parenting behaviors often have their roots in parents' own problematic childhoods.
- Rogers believed that all individuals have a natural actualizing tendency to become mature, socially adjusted and independent individuals.
- Rogers believed that if therapists treat their clients with congruence, empathy and respect, positive therapeutic change will occur.
- Rogers introduced the notion of active listening, which requires therapists to listen deeply to their clients and reflect back key issues.
- Client-centered principles applied to parenting work include the use of I-messages. An I-message (e.g. I want, I think, I feel) is a direct statement that allows a parent to emphasize what he or she wants without assigning blame.
- Personal Construct Theory (PCT) is based on the premise that human thoughts, feelings and behaviors are informed by personal constructs, which individuals use to anticipate and explain everyday events.
- Constructs are informed by people's beliefs, as well as their experiences with the world.
- Some constructs are more permeable than others. Constructs linked to people's sense of self are often the most resistant to change.
- Practitioners should consider the extent to which their own personal constructs influence their perceptions of parents. Practitioners should also be aware that parents' constructions of therapeutic work may interfere with their ability to accept support.
- Cognitive Behavioral Therapy (CBT) is an umbrella term for a collection of therapeutic techniques aimed at improving people's thought processes.
- Behaviorism is the study of how behavior is learned and reinforced by external stimuli.
- Classical conditioning is the idea that natural, physiological responses can become associated with neutral stimuli.
- Thorndike's Law of Effect assumes that learning takes place through actions that are reinforced by satisfying consequences.

- Skinner's principles of operant conditioning consider the extent to which voluntary behaviors are reinforced by positive and negative consequences.
- Systematic desensitization uses operant-conditioning principles to treat phobic anxieties.
- Ellis's Rational Emotive Therapy (RET) assumes that emotional responses are determined by people's beliefs regarding the meaning of events. He explained this through his ABC model, with A standing for activating events, B standing for beliefs and C standing for emotional consequences.
- Beck identified a relationship between depression and what he identified as negative automatic thoughts.
- Beck asserted that depressive thinking is characterized by a dysfunctional belief system which he referred to as the negative cognitive triad that consists of feelings of inadequacy, a sense of failure and a sense of hopelessness.
- Rotter's social learning theory asserts that human behavior is influenced by one's subjective interpretation of his or her environment, expectations for success and the extent to which reinforcements are personally rewarding.
- Rotter believed that people have a tendency towards either an internal or an external locus of control. An internal locus of control is the belief that consequences are primarily determined by forces within one's personal control. An external locus of control is the belief that consequences are primarily externally driven by forces outside of one's control, such as luck, fate, etc.
- Bandura's model of social learning assumes that people learn vicariously by watching how others are reinforced for their behavior.
- Bandura also observed that behavior is reciprocally determined by the behavior of others, thus creating a behavioral environment.
- Bandura demonstrated how behaviors are determined by people's sense of self-efficacy, rather than their actual experiences in various activities.
- Bandura established that one's sense of self-efficacy is related to one's perceived capabilities.
- Family systems theory is the study of human behavior within the context of the family.
- Family systems theory asserts that families are homeostatic, self-regulating systems that achieve a sense of balance via corrective feedback loops.
- Family systems theory asserts that families are organized via subsystems and the quality of the boundaries between these subsystems. Dysfunction often occurs when the boundaries between subsystems are too rigid or too diffuse.
- Family therapists believe that the maladaptive behavior of one family member is a symptom of dysfunction within the entire family.
- Family therapists aim to improve the functionality within families by improving patterns of communication, maintaining a sense of connectedness and respecting personal boundaries.

Notes

1 Object relations theorists also include Freud's daughter, Anna (1895–1982), Melanie Klein (1882–1960) and her student John Bowlby (1907–1990) whose attachment theory is discussed in greater depth in Chapter 3.

2 Also known as person-centered, humanistic or Rogerian therapy.

3 Such as the use of suggestions, as used in process-experiential therapy.

4 Kurt Lewin's ideas are highly influential in the fields of social and organizational psychology. Aside from his 'behavioral equation' discussed in this section, Lewin is also credited with some of the systems theory concepts described in the next section, as well as the action research framework discussed in Chapter 6.

5 Lewin's behavioral equation, $B = f(P,E)$, simply means that behavior is a function, or result of both personality and environmental factors.

6 Minuchin described his ideas regarding structural family theory and structural family therapy in a series of books published in the 1970s and early 1980s. This section draws most heavily from *Families and Family Therapy* (1974), *Family Therapy Techniques* (1981) and *Family Therapy: An Overview* (Goldenberg and Goldenberg 1996).

5 Practitioner expertise

Understanding how to deliver evidence-based parenting support

Introduction

Practitioners must possess a unique combination of knowledge, skills and personal qualities to deliver parenting interventions effectively. The previous two chapters described the theoretical knowledge underpinning most parenting interventions. This chapter considers the practical knowledge involved in delivering parenting support, as well as the personal skills and qualities which enable practitioners to facilitate therapeutic change.

Understanding parents' needs and knowing how to meet them is an essential component of any evidence-based parenting intervention. This chapter begins with an overview of why parents attend parenting interventions and methods for assessing parents' needs. Program fidelity – delivering program content in a manner that is faithful to the program's original model – is also crucial for ensuring that parents gain the most from parenting intervention. This chapter therefore considers the issues involved in delivering parenting interventions with fidelity and the ways in which this can be supported through practitioner training and supervision. In order for parents to fully benefit from parenting interventions, parents must also feel psychologically safe. The chapter concludes with a discussion of how practitioner qualities (including their qualifications, knowledge and skills) facilitate the creation of a psychologically safe environment to support the process of therapeutic change.

Understanding the needs and values of parents

Why do parents seek help?

It is important to remember that the vast majority of parents do not need 'training' to raise their children successfully (Bhabra and Ghate 2004, Henricson 1999, Rutter and Smith 1995). Most parents are sensitive to their children's needs, know how to set standards, and provide discipline when appropriate. In the words of Donald Winnicott, most parents are 'good enough'.

When 'good-enough' parents seek help, they most often do so because they want particular information related to the care and/or management of their children (Ghate and Hazel 2004, Hebbeler and Gerlach-Downie 2002, Moran et al. 2005, Peterander 2004). As Miller and Sambell (2003) observed (see Chapter 2 for a complete discussion), parents want specific advice for improving or 'fixing' their children's behavior. Parents are also more likely to adhere to this advice if they know that it is coming from an expert.

Miller and Sambell also observed that parents value emotional support that is empathetic to their circumstances and validates their perspective as a parent. Sometimes parents want affirmation that they are doing a good job, or that they're 'not the only one' with a particular problem or challenge. Validating parents' feelings and experiences is often a good starting point for engaging parents in evidence-based parenting interventions.

Validating parents' experiences is rarely sufficient for improving parents' behavior, however (Hebbeler and Gerlach-Downie 2002, Scott 2002). While emotionally supportive services are often well liked, parenting interventions must also be able to provide parents with new skills in order to reliably improve child outcomes (Barnard 1998, Gomby 1999, Hutchings et al. 2007, Kazdin and Whitley 2006, McMahon and Forehand 2003). In addition, support that validates parents' negative feelings about their children runs the risk of reinforcing ineffective or destructive parenting attitudes and behaviors. Knowing when to validate a belief or challenge an assumption is an important part of parenting work that all practitioners must master (Davis et al. 2002).

Parents also often seek help because they are concerned about ongoing problems with their child. This may be a problem with the child's conduct, his or her learning at school or his or her emotional wellbeing. Parents in these situations frequently have many worries, including concerns about the causes of their child's problem, their role in contributing to it and the ways in which the problem can be treated. In these instances, parents often want a clear explanation of the child's problem and an understanding of how the child's treatment will impact on family life (Davis et al. 2002).

Parents also seek help when they are coping with personal issues which interfere with their ability to parent well. These issues may include psychological problems, such as depression or anxiety, or relationship problems between parents. In these cases, parents often want a combination of emotional and practical support which can help them to manage their own needs, along with the needs of their families.

In a minority of cases, parents do not want help but are forced into support because of very serious family problems and/or because their child has committed a crime. In these cases, it is not uncommon for parents to avoid support because they are in denial about their problems or preoccupied with other issues (McCurdy and Daro 2001). Parents may also feel estranged from statutory services because of a history of negative interactions which has resulted in their feeling hostile and persecuted (Day et al. in press). In these cases, it is not uncommon for parents to actively resist support, especially if they feel it is being forced upon them (Bentovim 2006, Biehal 2005, 2006, Patterson and Chamberlain 1994, Patterson and Forgatch 1985). In order to overcome this resistance, practitioners must have the right combination of qualities and skills which allow parents to feel that their needs are understood and that progress is possible (Day et al. in press).

Understanding parents' needs

Knowing why a parent is seeking help is just the starting point for understanding their needs. Practitioners must also gather knowledge of the characteristics of the parents attending their services and what their specific needs are. No two families are alike – with families varying in terms of their structure, income, location and challenges. For this reason, a 'one-size-fits-all' approach to parenting support is unlikely to be effective. Practitioners require methods for understanding the characteristics and needs of the parents attending their services, so that the support they provide is appropriate and relevant.

These methods should include systems for collecting information about parents' demographics, such as their age, gender, family structure, ethnicity and economic circumstances (if relevant), as well as child characteristics, such as age, gender, etc. Although most parents have more than one child, they often attend parenting interventions on behalf of a single, 'target' child. Parenting support must therefore be relevant to this child's age in order for it to be effective (Holmbeck et al. 2010, O'Connell et al. 2009). While many programs advertise themselves as suitable for parents with children of all ages, it is highly unlikely that such a broad focus will result in measurable and lasting changes for individual families. This is because parents require age-specific information that they can apply and rehearse with their children at the time of the parenting intervention. Otherwise, it is highly likely that they will forget what they have learned.

Parents and children also differ in terms of their needs. As noted previously, some parents seek occasional help because they want practical tips for dealing with normal parenting issues, such as toilet training, bedtime routines and negotiating teen privileges. Other parents require high levels of support to cope with ongoing and complex problems. Services should therefore be matched to each family's level of need. Figure 5.1 provides a spectrum of support for addressing a continuum of family mental health needs.

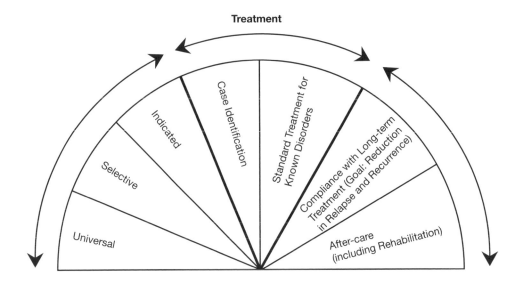

Figure 5.1 An intervention spectrum for mental health disorders (reprinted with permission from Mzarek et al. 1994)

At the left side of the spectrum are prevention services. Prevention services aim to prevent the occurrence of problems – not to treat them once they have occurred. Prevention services fall into one of three categories: universal, selective and indicated. **Universal prevention** services are available to all families within specific eligibility groups existing within the general population. Examples of universal prevention services include prenatal classes, health visiting services and courses delivered through schools at key transition stages. In many cases, universal prevention services are inexpensive to deliver and do not always require professional advice or assistance.

Selective prevention refers to services made available to specific groups of children or parents who may be at risk of having future difficulties. These groups include teenage parents, divorcing families or families living in poverty. Examples of selective prevention interventions include *Nurse–Family Partnership* (NFP, Box 1.2) and *New Beginnings* (see Box 5.1).

Box 5.1: The *New Beginnings* selective prevention parenting program for divorcing or separating families

New Beginnings is a selective prevention program for improving outcomes for children after a family break-up. *New Beginnings* involves ten weekly group sessions and two individual sessions delivered to divorcing parents and their children by fully trained and certified Master's-level psychologists. *New Beginnings'* content targets four factors that commonly place divorcing families at risk: 1) the quality of the residential parent's relationship with their children, 2) the maintenance of effective discipline post-divorce, 3) children's exposure to inter-parental conflict and 4) children's access to the non-resident parent. A six-year follow-up study demonstrated significant long-term program benefits, with 15 per cent of the child participants reporting mental health problems in comparison to 23 per cent of those in the control group (Wolchik et al. 2002).

Indicated prevention applies to services targeting individuals who have been screened as being at risk for a specific behavioral or emotional problem. An example of an indicated prevention service is the *Fast Track* program (see Box 1.6), which screens 5-year-olds to determine whether they are at risk of developing a conduct disorder.

In the middle of the spectrum are treatments. Treatments apply to identified and diagnosed mental health problems. Case identification refers to treatments which assess conditions that are relatively recent in onset. Standard treatment is applied to disorders that have been formally diagnosed. Standard treatment can be used to reduce and/or halt the problems associated with the disorder, as well as reduce the likelihood of other, co-occurring disorders. Co-occurring disorders are often referred to as **co-morbid** disorders. Examples of co-occurring disorders include ADHD and conduct disorders, conduct disorders and substance misuse, and low school achievement and mental health disorders. Standard treatments include time-limited therapies involving both children and parents. Weisz et al. (2005) have identified *Incredible Years* (see Box 1.7) as a time-limited, standard treatment for children diagnosed with a conduct disorder.

At the right of the spectrum are maintenance systems that might include drug treatments (as is often the case with ADHD or adolescent depression), aftercare services or follow-up booster sessions. The majority of parenting interventions fall into the prevention and treatment categories.

In order for interventions to be effective they must match the needs of the parents receiving them. In this respect, a universally available prevention program is unlikely to fully meet the needs of families experiencing complex problems. For example, a four-week parenting course providing parents with opportunities to socialize is unlikely to be sufficient for parents with a child who has recently been diagnosed with ADHD (Sonuga-Barke et al. 2006). Similarly, high-end, individualized services are not likely to improve outcomes for low-need families. For example, many of the home visiting programs initiated in the US in the 1990s targeted both affluent and economically deprived mothers. Evaluations of these programs suggested that more affluent mothers gained little from the interventions, which, in turn, significantly diminished their overall effectiveness (Gomby et al. 1999).

All interventions, including those that are universally available, should have **eligibility requirements** which include **inclusion** and **exclusion criteria**. Eligibility requirements should specify, at the very least, the family's level of need and the age range of the children. Examples of child age ranges include infants, toddlers, preschool, primary school, preadolescence and adolescence. Levels of need include low, moderate, complex and high needs:

- **Low need** refers to parents seeking support for stresses and difficulties experienced by most families at some point in their child's development.
- **Moderate need** refers to parents requiring support for issues that could potentially develop into serious problems, but are usually of recent onset and can be rectified with moderate levels of support.
- **Complex needs** refers to families with numerous needs that may have persisted over time. Examples of complex needs include ongoing conduct issues and antisocial behavior, an adolescent diagnosis of ADHD, multiple family problems and child protection concerns.
- **High needs** refers to families where a child may be coping with a serious mental illness, going into care or has committed a serious offense.

Eligibility criteria should also include exclusion criteria. For example, NFP specifies that mothers that already have a child, are in a committed couple relationship, or are over the age of 20 are not eligible for their program.

Individual needs assessments[1] are a good method for ensuring that a program or intervention is suitable for a family's needs. Needs assessments come in a variety of forms depending upon the intervention, the practitioner's qualifications and experience. An individual needs assessment may involve an interview with a skilled practitioner before the start of an intervention, or the use of a standardized instrument that has diagnostic capabilities. Needs assessments can be developed for use within specific agencies, or may be recommended as part of the parenting program model. For example, the *Incredible Years* program recommends an assessment tool developed by researchers at the Oregon Social Learning Center (see example at: http://www.incredibleyears.com/Measures/forms_GL.asp).

Needs assessments allow practitioners to determine the extent to which the intervention's content matches the family's needs. They can also be used to track parents' progress throughout the program and verify the extent to which the service continues to meet their needs. Needs assessments are essential when working with families with complex needs, but are also helpful for ensuring that the needs of families attending universally based services are met (Budd 2005, Taylor et al. 2009).

Recruiting and engaging parents

Barriers to recruitment

Recruiting parents to evidence-based parenting support can be a significant challenge (Whittaker and Cowley 2010, Winslow et al. 2009). This is especially true when it comes to universally available interventions, where parents are expected to self-refer and attend on a voluntary basis. Research suggests that, on average, only 17 per cent of eligible parents attend universal, community-based parenting interventions (Prinz et al. 2009, Spoth et al. 2007). While the recruitment rates for targeted interventions are somewhat higher (between 40 and 60 per cent), program attrition in these services is also often high (Haggerty et al. 2006, Redmond et al. 2002).

A variety of reasons have been cited for difficulties in recruiting and retaining parents in evidence-based programs (see Whittaker and Cowley 2010 for a recent review). These reasons include a lack of time, a perceived lack of relevance, parent characteristics (age, education, income, etc.), situational constraints (a lack of transportation and child care) and cultural barriers (Kazdin et al. 1997a and 1997b, Prinz and Miller 1996). Many of these barriers can be overcome, however, through additional services and strategic planning. Box 5.2 provides a summary of activities which can increase recruitment and retention rates in parenting programs. Further guidance can also be found in Forehand and Kotchick's (2002) *Behavioral Parent Training: Current Challenges and Potential Solutions*.

It should be noted that many of the practices described in Box 5.2 require additional financial resources and staff time. Financial resources include money for transportation, payment for staff working out of hours, payment for material translation (when necessary) and child-care provision (Nock and Ferriter 2005, Brookes et al. 2006). Activities involving high levels of staff time include the delivery of introductory sessions and telephone support (Nock and Ferriter 2005).

Box 5.2: Practices that can increase the take-up of parenting programs (Moran et al. 2005)

- Provide parents with an onsite crèche where children can stay while they attend parenting services
- Reimburse parents for transportation
- Locate services in convenient areas (close to transportation)
- Locate services in welcoming, non-stigmatizing venues
- Deliver parenting interventions when parents are available, including evenings and weekends
- Advertise the program through newspapers and leaflets
- Use other parents to promote the program through word of mouth
- Provide an introductory 'taster' session to acquaint parents with the goals of the program
- Involve parents in the selection and implementation of services
- Use trusted recruiters, including doctors and individuals whom children trust
- Treat parents in a respectful, non-patronizing or -condescending way
- Use interactive teaching methods
- Provide incentives, including money or gift vouchers
- Overcome cultural barriers by respecting cultural differences in parenting practices
- Use materials that reflect parents' culture and values
- Match the ethnicity of practitioners to parents' ethnicity
- Use recruitment calls to remind parents of the program and raise interest
- Pursue non-attenders in a friendly but persistent manner
- Provide one-to-one contact before, during and after services to make sure the program is meeting parents' needs
- Reward regular attendance (e.g. with certificates and qualifications)
- Incentivize attendance by providing access to useful or fun activities not necessarily related to parenting
- Warn parents that services may be withdrawn if they miss sessions
- Mandate high-risk parents to attend services.

The use of community recruitment teams provides an additional, cost-effective method of increasing recruitment rates (Spoth et al. 2007). Community recruitment teams involve the use of parent and practitioner volunteers (from health, education and the police) to recruit parents to evidence-based programs. Community recruitment team activities include sponsoring culturally relevant recruitment events, providing presentations at schools, phoning parents and determining incentives for program attendance. Haggerty and Spoth (2010) have observed that the most successful community recruitment teams use a three-pronged strategy which involves 1) saturating the local media with information about the program, 2) sponsoring a popular event and 3) telephoning interested parents after the event. Once community recruitment teams are established, they can remain self-sustaining by asking parents who have completed the evidence-based parenting program to join the team.

Inter-agency referral systems

Parent recruitment can also be enhanced through good inter-agency referral systems, particularly in situations where families have complex needs. Within England, the *Common Assessment Framework* (CAF) provides a common basis for local authorities to refer families across agencies (see Box 5.3).

Agencies delivering parenting support should also have systems in place to refer parents on to other services if it becomes apparent that a service is not meeting a family's needs. Good parenting programs include guidelines to help practitioners judge when a family requires additional services or to be referred on to another service. Agency-level systems must also be in place to allow practitioners to report child protection concerns. Given the nature of parenting work, it is not uncommon for parents to disclose information that could suggest child maltreatment. For this reason, practitioners must understand the appropriate procedures for reporting abuse within their local authority.

Establishing a therapeutic alliance

Once parents are recruited to a parenting intervention, regular attendance and active participation are necessary for it to have any impact. Unfortunately, approximately one-half of parents attending parenting programs stay for the duration and drop-out rates can be as high as 75 per cent for groups where attendance is mandatory (Harpaz-Rotem et al. 2004, Nock and Ferriter 2005, Orrell-Valente et al. 1999, Patterson and Chamberlain 1988). While parents drop out for a variety of reasons, the quality of the **therapeutic alliance** (established between the parent and practitioner) is frequently cited as a factor in determining whether a parent remains in a parenting intervention. A strong and positive therapeutic alliance consistently predicts higher retention rates and an improved likelihood of positive change (Kazdin et al. 2005, 2006, Kazdin and Whitley 2006, Orrell-Valente et al. 1999).

Edward Bordin (1913–92) identified the therapeutic alliance as the working relationship between a practitioner and client within the context of therapy (Bordin 1979). As a student of Carl Rogers (see Chapter 4), Bordin believed that the quality of the alliance – not the content of the therapy per se – enabled positive therapeutic change. From Bordin's perspective, a positive therapeutic alliance is a necessary prerequisite for the client 'to accept and follow treatment faithfully' (Bordin 1980, as cited in Horvath and Greenberg 1989: 224). Bordin also believed that the therapeutic alliance develops independently of any specific therapeutic model (Bordin 1979, Orlinsky and Ronnestad 2000). While the therapeutic alliance is clearly

Box 5.3: The *Common Assessment Framework*

The *Common Assessment Framework* (CAF) is a shared assessment and planning tool for use across all children's services in England. It aims to help identify children who may need more support than what is universally provided through their schools and health services. The CAF is intended to be introduced at the preventive level, before problems begin to interfere with children's wellbeing. It does this through the provision of personalized services that are provided universally to all children. Once needs become apparent within universal settings, a process begins whereby each child's strengths and weaknesses are assessed through a set of standardised measures. A key area of assessment is the parents' capacity to appropriately meet the needs of the identified child. Once the assessments are complete, a lead professional is assigned to the case and a Team Around the Child (TAC) is formed, which works with the parents to decide what additional support is required. The TAC then coordinates an integrated package of family support, which can include an evidence-based parenting intervention.It is important to emphasize that the CAF is not a tick-box exercise, but a strengths-based referral system that facilitates an ecological understanding of the risk and protective factors influencing the identified child's wellbeing. While the CAF involves the use of multiple assessment forms (depending upon each family's needs), CAF guidance stresses the need for sound professional judgment and skill when administering them. For this reason, training is necessary for practitioners to implement the CAF effectively.

While the CAF is frequently used as part of a child protection plan, the use of the CAF is not restricted to child protection cases. Children with a wide variety of needs (including mental health problems and learning disabilities) should be identified early within universal settings through CAF assessments, so that problems can be addressed before they become too serious. More information regarding the CAF and its implementation can be found at the *Every Child Matters* website at: http://www.dcsf.gov.uk/everychildmatters/strategy/deliveringservices1/caf/cafframework/ and the CWDC website at http://www.cwdcouncil.org.uk/caf.

a crucial part of client-centered therapy, it can also develop within the context of family therapy, CBT and evidence-based parenting interventions.

Bordin asserted that the quality of the therapeutic alliance is determined by three processes: 1) practitioner and client agreement on the therapeutic goals, 2) agreement on the tasks necessary for pursuing these goals and 3) the development of a bond between the practitioner and client. In describing these processes, Bordin believed that goals should be determined not by the practitioner, but by the client, through guidance and feedback from the practitioner. The tasks of the therapy must also be agreed by both client and practitioner and be recognized as relevant for achieving the therapeutic goals. Once the goals and tasks are established, a bond between the practitioner and client should form naturally through the shared experience of therapy. The practitioner–client bond is also facilitated through feelings of mutual respect, trust and positive regard that develop over time (Bordin 1994).

Research in adult psychotherapy repeatedly suggests that the strength of therapeutic alliance significantly predicts positive change throughout the course of individual therapy (Green 2006, Horvath and Bedi 2002, Lambert et al. 2004). Evidence also suggests that the therapeutic alliance predicts positive change in parents receiving evidence-based parenting support (Kazdin et al. 2005, 2006). While Horvath and Bedi (2002) have argued that the alliance itself is the mechanism of change (with stronger alliances resulting in greater changes), Kazdin and his colleagues believe that when it comes to parenting support, it is difficult to determine whether parent change is due to the therapeutic alliance or to program content (Kazdin et al. 2006). From Kazdin's perspective, the therapeutic alliance is likely to moderate parents' adherence to program principles which, in turn, improve parenting behaviors.

Findings from the evaluation of *Healthy Start America* (HSA), a home visiting parenting program for at-risk families, provide some evidence for Kazdin's argument. The collective findings from state-wide evaluations of HSA suggested that once families were recruited to the program, home visitors were generally able to establish a positive therapeutic relationship with them. However, the evaluations also found that there were consistent differences in program outcomes which varied by state, with some states showing greater family improvements than others. The evaluators believed that these differences were related to variations in the program content, rather than practitioners' relationships with the families. In addition, the evaluators found that some programs had better methods in place for improving the quality of the practitioner–parent relationship, which, in turn, increased retention rates (Gomby 2007). Considered together, these findings indicate that a positive therapeutic alliance is necessary for creating the context in which important program content can be learned, but that the quality of the content determines the extent to which positive parent and child outcomes can be achieved.

Practitioner and parent characteristics related to positive outcomes

It is worth noting that the quality of the practitioner–parent relationship is driven by both practitioner and parent characteristics. Practitioner characteristics include 1) the extent to which the therapist can empathize with the parent and express unconditional positive regard, 2) the therapist's previous experience with similar parents and 3) the therapist's skill in the use of specific therapeutic techniques, including the ability to implement intervention models with fidelity (Alexander et al. 1976, Forgatch et al. 2005, Horvath, 1994). The quality of the therapeutic alliance is also facilitated by similarities between the practitioner and client in terms of their personal attributes, such as their ethnic background and previous life experiences (e.g. the practitioner being a parent him- or herself – Orrell-Valente et al. 1999). The ways in which practitioner qualities and characteristics contribute to the efficacy of parenting interventions will be described in greater detail at the end of this chapter.

Parent characteristics also contribute to the quality of the therapeutic alliance (Rosenfeld 2008). Parents who are able to develop and maintain good relationships with others are more likely to form a positive therapeutic alliance with the practitioner, as well as achieve positive change from the parenting intervention (Kazdin and Whitley 2006). Alternatively, parents who have difficulty forming good relationships with others are less likely to benefit from parenting interventions, since they are less able to form a positive relationship with the parenting practitioner. High levels of parent stress are also known to interfere with parents' ability to form positive relationships with practitioners and benefit from evidence-based treatments (Kazdin 1990, Kazdin and Mazurick 1994, Kazdin et al. 1993).

Patterson and his colleagues (1985, 1988, 1994) observed that practitioners delivering evidence-based parenting interventions often experience particular challenges in establishing a positive therapeutic alliance with parents. This is related to the fact that the goals and the tasks of the program are predetermined and some parents will not perceive them as relevant to their situation. Indeed, as mentioned previously, approximately 50 per cent of all parents drop out of parenting programs and this number increases to 75 per cent if parental attendance is mandatory. Moreover, parental resistance and/or drop-out are likely to occur at the most critical phase of the treatment – when parents are learning new skills that will change their children's antisocial behavior (Patterson and Chamberlain 1988, 1994, Patterson and Forgatch 1985). Practitioners must therefore understand how to overcome these challenges.

Unfortunately, parental resistance often negatively influences the practitioner's behavior, which can, in turn, further reduce the treatment's overall efficacy. When parents resist, practitioners often respond by reducing their positive regard and spend less time covering key principles. In some instances, practitioners may even engage in confrontational behaviors. These negative practitioner behaviors, in turn, reinforce the parents' noncompliance and further reduce the efficacy of the treatment. In order to counteract this negative cycle, practitioners must learn how to resist confronting parents at the beginning of the therapy, so that a strong therapeutic alliance can be formed. Once a strong therapeutic relationship is established, practitioners are then in a better position to suggest changes to parenting behaviors and work through issues which may impede the therapeutic process (Forgatch and Patterson 2010).

Adopting a strengths-based perspective

When parents participate in parenting interventions, they often do so because of problems occurring with their child or family. This runs the risk of interventions becoming highly problem (or deficit) focused, placing a strong emphasis on what is wrong within the family, rather than what is right. A continual focus on family weaknesses runs the risk of demotivating parents and interfering with the efficacy of the treatment (Itzhaky and Bustin 2003).

In order to counteract this risk, evidence-based parenting interventions often begin with a focus on family strengths. Family strengths may include individual capabilities and talents, supportive relationships, economic and material resources (Allison et al. 2003, Naidu and Behari 2010). Once strengths have been identified, the practitioner and parent work collaboratively to generate strategies for how these strengths can be used to overcome difficulties identified during treatment. These strategies are then linked to a number of short-term goals which can be addressed within the context of the intervention (Davis et al. 2002).

When working properly, a strengths-based approach helps parents recognize areas of resilience within their family system which can improve their sense of efficacy and empower members towards change (Saleebey 1996, 2000). A strengths-based approach also supports the development of a strong therapeutic alliance (Allison et al. 2003). Evidence-based parenting programs which emphasize the use of a strengths-based approach include the NFP, FFT and FAST.

What makes a parenting intervention effective?

Core components

As discussed in Chapter 3, evidence-based parenting interventions are informed by evidence-based theories of parenting and child development. These theories should be evident in the intervention's design, content and activities. The program should also be underpinned by a clear and logical **theory of change** that links the intervention's theoretical basis to specific activities that should, in turn, achieve positive short- and long-term outcomes for the parent and child.

The reason evidence-based programs work is because they include a set of **core components** (sometimes referred to as mechanisms of change or active ingredients) that result in improved outcomes for parents and children. Examples of core components include the program's content (e.g. the use of praise incentive plans within a social learning theory perspective), activities (e.g. homework and role play) and processes (e.g. the quality of the relationship between the parent and practitioner). An intervention's theory of change should provide a framework for linking a program's core components to its theoretical basis and its short- and long-term outcomes.

Identifying a program's core components is more easily said than done, however. Weisz and Kazdin (2010) observe that while an RCT can demonstrate whether an intervention works, it cannot identify the specific mechanisms that make it work. The previous discussion regarding the importance of the therapeutic alliance illustrates this point. Is it the therapeutic alliance or the content of the intervention that facilitates change? As Kazdin et al. (2006) observe, both of these elements are likely to benefit parents and children, but the extent to which they each contribute to the program's effect size remains unknown. Indeed, evaluations of evidence-based programs suggest that positive child outcomes are generally best predicted by the combination of several core components, rather than any single one (Donaldson et al. 1994, 1995, Mihalic 2004, Sexton and Kelley 2010).

Content and activities

At the very least, the content of a parenting intervention should reinforce its primary short- and long-term goals. For example, an intervention which seeks to improve the attachment relationship should have specific activities which encourage parental sensitivity – not parent-and-child interaction more generally. Parenting interventions should also aim to change parents' behavior, as well as their knowledge and attitudes. This means providing parents with opportunities to digest information and practice new skills. In this respect, research suggests that active learning activities are preferable to didactic instruction (Arthur et al. 1998, Kaminski et al. 2008, Salas and Cannon-Bowers 2001, Swanson and Hoskyn 2001).

Ideally, learning activities should cater to a variety of learning styles (i.e. visual, auditory and kinesthetic) and include a mixture of methods. Examples of effective and engaging learning activities include group discussion, role play, homework assignments and reflective video-tape viewing. Parenting programs should also provide parents with opportunities to practice new behaviors and receive feedback. Kaminski et al. (2008) observe that some of the most effective programs provide parents with opportunities to interact with their children and receive direct feedback on their behaviors. Intervention materials (including books, workbooks, leaflets and videos) should also be engaging and easy to understand.

'Dosage'

Other factors that impact parenting intervention outcomes include the format of the intervention (e.g. one-to-one vs. group sessions), the number of sessions and the length of time between them. Collectively, these factors are referred to as the program's 'dosage', as they involve the amount and intensity of support parents receive (Berkel et al. 2010, Nation et al. 2003). Research consistently suggests that higher dosage is directly linked to greater program effectiveness (Mihalic 2004).

A program's dosage should be determined by the aims of the program and the needs of the target population. As a general rule, more complex problems require a higher dosage. As noted previously, a four-week parenting course involving didactic instruction is unlikely to be sufficient for parents learning how to manage the behavior of a child with ADHD.

Pre-service practitioner training

Practitioners require training which is sufficient for them to deliver the intervention to a high standard without continual support from the original developer. Effective training includes, at the very least, a detailed curriculum and specific learning objectives. The format, intensity and duration of the training should also be appropriate for the complexity of the program, the target population and practitioner qualifications. For example, a one-day training course is unlikely to be sufficient for a program model targeting families with complex needs.

Training materials should be clear and engaging and sufficient for practitioners to remember important information once the training is over. Many evidence-based parenting programs also include an accreditation or certification process to ensure that practitioners leave the training with a good understanding of the program's content. Many programs also offer a consultation or coaching service after the training is over, so that practitioners can understand how to apply the principles they learned during training to their specific practice (see following section on Supervision and Coaching for further discussion). As noted in Chapter 1, some of the most effective evidence-based program models provide technical assistance on program implementation after the training is completed.

In order for training to be effective, program developers should specify the qualifications, skills and qualities required to attend training. Most evidence-based parenting models are based on the assumption that their programs will be delivered by individuals with a Bachelor's qualification or higher in a helping profession. Those targeting more complex needs often require a Master's qualification in the fields of psychology, social work or nursing. This is because research suggests that parenting support is less likely to be effective if the practitioners delivering it are under-qualified (e.g. Korfmacher et al. 1999).

Appropriate qualifications and experience allow practitioners to understand a program's underpinning theories and principles, its content, the needs of its target population and methods for maintaining fidelity. Practitioners must also be able to understand what to do when the program is not meeting the needs of individual parents. This means knowing how to assess the needs of individual parents and understanding when and how to refer them on to other services.

Training manuals and materials

While a manual does not make an intervention evidence-based, it does help to ensure that practitioners learn the program content and deliver the intervention in a standardized manner (Kaminski et al. 2008, Moran et al. 2005, Westen et al. 2004). In this respect, the manual serves as a blueprint of the program's model and is considered a necessary component for ensuring program fidelity (see below). A good program manual (or manuals) should include a clear explanation of the theories underpinning the program, lesson plans for every session and guidance on how to respond to challenges and unexpected outcomes.

Fidelity

Program fidelity (also referred to as program integrity) is the extent to which the program is delivered as it is intended – i.e. as it is prescribed in the manual and pre-service training.

Program fidelity involves four primary components (Dane and Schneider 1998):

- **Adherence** refers to the extent to which the program is delivered in a manner that is faithful to its original model. Adherence assumes that 1) all staff have received appropriate training (including pre-training qualifications), 2) the program is delivered to its target population, 3) delivery involves the right protocols and techniques and 4) the program is delivered under the correct circumstances and setting.
- **Exposure** is similar to the idea of dose and refers to the extent to which all of the sessions are implemented, their length and whether or not the right techniques are taught.
- **Quality of program delivery** refers to the skill with which the practitioner delivers a program or intervention (see below).
- **Participant responsiveness** is the extent to which those participating in the intervention are engaged in the program's activities.

Research consistently suggests that program fidelity is essential for a parenting intervention to remain effective (Berkel et al. 2010, Blase et al. 2010, Durlak and DuPre 2008, Fixsen et al. 2005, Henggeler et al. 1997, Huey et al. 2000). This is because carefully adhering to the program's original model ensures that participants are exposed to all of the program's core components (O'Connor et al. 2007, Webster-Stratton 2004). In fact, research repeatedly demonstrates that there is a direct relationship between the degree to which a program is delivered with fidelity and its achieved effect size (Durlak and DuPre 2008, Mihalic 2004). In short, the greater the fidelity, the more effective the program will be. By contrast, failure to adhere to the program's model often significantly reduces the program's overall effectiveness and in some cases may create worse outcomes. For example, Aber et al. (1998) observed that children receiving the full dosage of the school-based *Resolving Conflict Creatively Program* (RCCP) were significantly less likely to engage in aggressive behaviors than those in the control group receiving no conflict-resolution training. However, children enrolled in the program with teachers who delivered fewer lessons exhibited significantly *more* aggressive behavior than the control group. While the reasons for these findings are unclear, the authors suggested that the teachers who reduced the program's dosage may have replaced it with activities that actually increased children's aggression.

Fidelity versus adaptation

Practitioners may have difficulty maintaining program fidelity for a variety of reasons. In some instances, practitioners may not understand the program model. In other cases, the training and supervision may be inadequate. This was the case with many of the US home visiting programs evaluated in the 1990s, which suffered from inconsistencies in training and supervision which, in turn, reduced practitioners' understanding of the program's core components (see Chapter 1 for further discussion). A second reason program fidelity may be lost is because of program 'drift'. This happens when practitioners gradually adjust the program's content to fit their facilitation style. Program drift is frequently related to low amounts of supervision and/or inadequate systems for monitoring fidelity (Backer 2001, Forgatch et al. 2005, Ogden et al. 2005). A third reason for fidelity loss is that service managers or practitioners feel that certain aspects of a program must be changed. This often occurs when a practitioner feels that the intervention is longer than parents can commit to, or that there is not a sufficient budget to hire appropriately qualified staff. Practitioners may also be tempted to remove or alter some of the program's content because they are uncomfortable with the material or believe that it is too difficult for parents.

Fidelity can also be lost when practitioners adapt program content to make it more cultur-ally relevant to program participants. Some researchers suggest that such changes should not be characterized as a loss of fidelity, but rather as program adaptation – especially when it involves adding program content, rather than omitting or changing program materials (Berkel et al. 2010, Castro et al. 2004). The extent to which program adaptation is helpful or detrimental remains unclear, however. Some argue that program adaptations are seldom necessary and usually reduce a program's effectiveness (Elliott and Mihalic 2004, Mihalic n.d.) whereas others believe that appropriate adaptations may enhance program effective-ness by increasing participant engagement (Blakely et al. 1987).

Adaptations to improve cultural acceptability often include changing the language and/or vocabulary to match that of the participating parents, replacing cultural references and adding relevant content (Box 5.4). SAMHSA has found that such adaptations may be appro-priate when the culture of the program differs from that of the parents (Emshoff et al. 2003).

Box 5.4: Types of program adaptations (from O'Connor et al. 2007)

Acceptable adaptations

- Changing language – translating or modifying vocabulary
- Replacing images to show parents and children that look like the target audience
- Replacing cultural references
- Modifying some aspects of activities such as physical contact
- Adding relevant, evidence-based content to make the program more appealing to participants.

Risky or unacceptable adaptations

- Reducing the number or length of sessions
- Lowering the level of participant engagement
- Eliminating key messages or skills learned
- Removing topics
- Changing the theoretical approach
- Using staff or volunteers who are not adequately trained to deliver the program
- Using fewer staff members than recommended.

Note that the acceptable adaptations involve changing the cultural context of the content, but not the actual content. In this respect, these are planned and purposeful changes. Mihalic (n.d.) observes that a majority of adaptations are unplanned and are often due to practitioners' lack of understanding of the program's model and/or a lack of resources to deliver the program in its entirety. When changes are unplanned, the risk of compromising a program's core components increases.

O'Connor et al. (2007) have identified a number of strategies for reducing the likelihood of unplanned or inappropriate changes in the delivery of evidence-based parenting programs:

- **Select a program that meets the target audience's needs**. Service providers should carefully consider who the target audience is and select an intervention that matches the needs of this population as closely as possible. It is almost always preferable to choose a program that does not need any adaptation.

- **Make sure that practitioners are committed to program fidelity**. Practitioners delivering the program need to understand its underpinning theories and principles, its content and how to best implement the material. They must also believe that it is important to maintain program fidelity.
- **Understand the program's core components**. Identifying the core components is sometimes referred to as a **core components analysis**. This information is usually provided by the program developers during training and will help practitioners to make sure that core components are not lost.
- **Contact the program developer before making changes**. Program developers often know whether adaptations have been successful or not. Practitioners should therefore contact program developers before making any changes to ensure that all adaptations are appropriate. Most program developers are interested in the ways in which their intervention can be enhanced and will carefully consider whether the adaptations are acceptable.
- **Assess whether there is a genuine need for cultural adaptation**. O'Connor et al. (2007) observe that the cultural aspects of an intervention are reflected at the surface level, in terms of the program's language and the visual images used, and at a deeper level, in terms of the risk and protective factors it addresses. Surface-level issues are unlikely to reduce the program's effectiveness if changed, whereas deeper cultural differences are likely to imply a mismatch between a program's content and its target audience.
- **Maintain the program's duration and intensity**. Changes to an intervention's length or dosage are frequent and are often due to budget or time constraints. However, these kinds of changes often interfere with an intervention's effectiveness because they reduce the time parents have to develop a relationship with the practitioner or learn a new skill. Agencies and practitioners should therefore make sure that they have sufficient resources for maintaining an intervention's dosage before they commission and implement it.
- **Have systems in place for avoiding program drift**. Systems for avoiding program drift include rigorous training and accreditation requirements, fidelity checklists, re-certification processes and sufficient supervision for practitioners (McGuigan et al. 2003, Webster-Stratton 2004). Supervision requirements are discussed in greater depth below.
- **Keep up to date with program changes and new materials**. Evidence-based programs are continually trying to improve their effectiveness. Service managers and practitioners should stay in touch with program developers to find out about any recent improvements or alterations.

Supervision and coaching

Good-quality supervision is an important part of ensuring program fidelity and quality assurance, which, in turn, contribute to a program's overall efficacy (Payne and Eckert 2010, Henggeler and Schaeffer 2010, Olds 2002, Stern et al. 2008). While pre-service training acquaints practitioners with the intervention's content, theories and principles, it is limited in its ability to help practitioners apply these concepts in real-life settings (Fixsen et al. 2005). Pre-service training also cannot teach practitioners skills that can be learned only on the job. Metz et al. (2007) refer to training without follow-up support as the 'train and hope' approach, which rarely results in positive program outcomes.

In the field of evidence-based parenting practice, the term 'supervision' can refer to two inter-related activities. Within the helping professions, clinical supervision (also referred to as case supervision) refers to ongoing meetings between practitioners and managers to discuss casework and professional issues in a structured way. This activity enables practitioners to reflect on their practice in a focused and purposeful manner, share their learning and improve the quality of support provided to parents and children. Through these discussions, practitioners are able to consider with others the extent to which their services are meeting the needs of parents or whether additional services may be required. Supervision also provides an important context in which issues pertaining to child maltreatment can be discussed. As noted previously, disclosures of child maltreatment are not uncommon in parenting work and ongoing supervision is necessary for ensuring that child maltreatment concerns are properly considered and acted upon.

In the field of evidence-based parenting work, the term 'supervision' can also refer to the coaching support provided to practitioners after their pre-service training. The purpose of coaching overlaps with supervision, but also involves teaching practitioners key program skills, giving them feedback on these skills and providing them with ongoing motivational and emotional support (Spouse 2001). Joyce and Showers (2002) suggest that coaching should be considered an extension of training in order to ensure that important behavioral skills are learned.

Most evidence-based parenting programs provide guidelines for supervision and coaching, which vary depending upon the program model. For example, *Triple P* facilitates supervision by helping practitioners establish peer-supervision networks (Sanders and Murphy-Brennan 2010). The *Incredible Years* program recommends a combination of peer support with direct supervision from the *Incredible Years* organization through the certification process (Webster-Stratton 2004). NFP provides supervision training to individuals who are employed as supervisory coaches in their host organization (Olds 2002). *Multisystemic Therapy* (MST) offers a combined approach to supervision which includes an on-site MST team supervisor and an off-site MST consultant (Henggeler and Schaeffer 2010). *Parent Management Training-Oregon* uses a four-tiered system of coaching and supervision to improve program fidelity and increase the expertise of practitioners involved in the delivery of the PMTO program (see Box 5.5).

What makes a good parenting practitioner?

Sexton observes that 'it is only through the person and actions of the [practitioner] that therapy works' (Sexton 2007: 374). By this, Sexton means that the practitioner is an additional core component in the success or failure of any parenting intervention. While most effective parenting interventions can successfully articulate and teach the theories and principles underpinning their intervention models, the skills and personal qualities required to deliver the program are often more difficult to understand and are likely to differ across parenting interventions (Sexton and Kelley 2010). This section considers what is known about the ways in which a practitioner's skills, knowledge and personal qualities contribute to the efficacy of evidence-based parenting interventions.

Practitioner skill

Although program fidelity is an essential part of an intervention's effectiveness, it is by no means a replacement for a practitioner's judgment and skill. Practitioner skill is crucial for

Box 5.5: Supervision and quality assurance in the implementation of *Parent Management Training–Oregon* (PMTO) in Norway (reprinted with permission from Ogden et al. 2005)

- **Supervision and quality assurance.** Four supervision levels guide practitioners in varying stages of PMTO expertise. Because supervision is based on observed therapy sessions, all levels of attendees are required to bring video-tapes to supervision groups.
- **National Implementation Team (NIT) supervision.** The NIT meets several times a year to discuss its own and its supervisees' therapy issues. Some of these meetings include video-conference consultation from senior clinicians at OSLC. To maintain PMTO fidelity throughout Norway, the NIT collects and views video-tapes of therapy sessions and rates competent PMTO adherence using the Fidelity of Implementation rating system (FIMP: Forgatch et al. 2005, Knutson et al. 2003), participates in regular reliability checks within Norway and with OSLC, and receives monthly one-hour retraining sessions from OSLC. The NIT also meets two or three days each month to plan and prepare implementation activities.
- **Maintenance supervision for certified PMTO practitioners.** Regional groups with up to eight practitioners meet one workday, eight times each year. Practitioners share experiences and challenges, and polish teaching and clinical skills. Supervisors record attendance, and PMTO candidates and practitioners must have 85 per cent attendance during a three-year period to attain or retain certification.
- **Training supervision for training candidates.** Regional groups of four candidates meet with a supervisor one workday every second week throughout the 18-month training period. Between-session telephone conferences are also available.
- **Colleague supervision.** Regional supervisors meet one workday, three or four times annually with their Regional Coordinator. They also attend a one-day maintenance seminar each semester arranged by the Behavior Center.

understanding the content of the program and knowing whether it is effectively meeting the needs of parents and children. While fidelity concerns *whether* a practitioner adheres to the program model, skill determines *how well* he or she does this (Alexander et al. 1976, Eames et al. 2009, Scott et al. under review, Waltz et al. 1993). Indeed, Forgatch et al. (2005) have observed that greater practitioner skill leads to more positive changes in parenting behavior. Practitioner skill in the delivery of parenting interventions involves:

1   Creating a safe and supportive environment for learning
2   Questioning parenting behaviors in a way that leads to openness and maintains an appropriate balance
3   Encouraging parents to develop and practice new skills
4   Relating the learning to each family's story line.

Studies considering the role of practitioner skill in delivering cognitive therapy have similarly observed that practitioner skill is as important, if not more so, as a strong therapeutic alliance in predicting positive outcomes in depressed adults (Davidson et al. 2004, Shaw et al. 1999, Trepka et al. 2004).

Research also suggests that practitioner skill affects the cost-effectiveness of evidence-based interventions. For example, a study considering the cost-effectiveness of FFT in the state of Washington found that the recidivism rates of antisocial youths were over twice as high amongst practitioners judged less competent by program developers than among those judged as highly competent (Figure 5.2). A cost analysis of the therapy revealed that highly competent practitioners saved the taxpayers $10.69, but that non-competent practitioners cost them $4.18 for every $1 invested in the FFT program (Barnoski 2002, 2004).

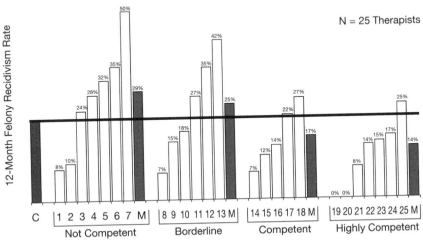

Figure 5.2 12-month felony recidivism rate for youth assigned to individual FFT Therapists (reprinted with permission from Barnoski 2002)

More worrying are findings that suggest that less competent practitioners actually make outcomes worse for parents and their children. For example, Scott et al. (under review) found that parent and child outcomes actually deteriorated after attendance at an *Incredible Years* program implemented by practitioners with relatively low levels of skill, as rated by a team of clinical coders (Figure 5.3). Practitioners who were rated as competent, however, measurably improved outcomes for the children of the parents attending their groups, with the most highly rated practitioners demonstrating the greatest improvements.

Professionals vs. paraprofessionals: what the evidence says

Paraprofessionals are generally defined as practitioners without graduate mental health training. Paraprofessional roles include caseworkers, family support workers, teachers, volunteers and other parents. The involvement of these individuals in the delivery of evidence-based parenting support is intuitively appealing, with some maintaining that parents are more likely to be responsive towards care providers who share similar characteristics to them – including their culture and life experiences (Ernst et al. 1999, Grant et al. 1996, 2003, Orrell-Valente et al. 1999). The use of paraprofessionals is also attractive to organizations, as it has the potential for increased service provision at less cost.

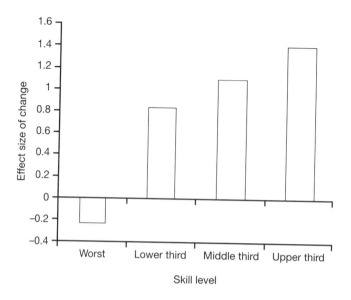

Figure 5.3   Impact of therapist skill on the outcomes of children whose parents are attending an *Incredible Years* program

The extent to which paraprofessionals can deliver therapeutic support to adults and children has long been debated in the research literature. There is now evidence to suggest, however, that paraprofessionals can deliver therapeutic services as effectively as professionals as long as two conditions are met: 1) the intervention is well-specified and 2) the practitioners receive high-quality training and supervision (Christensen and Jacobson 1994, Lambert et al. 2004). In two meta-reviews, Weisz et al. (1987, 1995) observed that when these two conditions were met, paraprofessionals were just as effective as professionals in treating children. Moreover, when it came to improving children's **externalizing** behavior, paraprofessionals appeared to be more effective than the professionals. However, when it came to treating **internalizing** problems (e.g. anxieties and phobias), professionally trained therapists were significantly more effective. When exploring the reasons for these findings, Weisz et al. observed that treatments targeting children's externalizing behavior were highly specified and training was most often delivered by the original program developers. The treatment of internalizing problems was less specified, however, requiring more professional judgment and skill.

When considering paraprofessional work with adults, Bright et al. (1999) found that individuals with a background in community outreach were just as effective as psychology professionals in alleviating symptoms of depression in adults attending group-based cognitive behavioral therapy (CBT) sessions. However, when the authors followed up the participants in the months following therapy, they observed that clients in the professionally treated group were less likely to report a recurrence of their depressive symptoms. The authors speculated that the professionals were better than the community-outreach workers in communicating CBT principles, so that their clients could better manage the recurrence of depressive symptoms on their own.

When it comes to the effectiveness of paraprofessionals delivering parenting support, the evidence is mixed. For example, Gordon and Arbuthnot (1988) observed that paraprofessionals can successfully implement FFT, as long as they are appropriately trained and supervised. However, evaluations comparing professionals and paraprofessionals in the delivery of home visiting support suggest that paraprofessionally delivered support is not as effective. In a study comparing the effectiveness of nurses and paraprofessionals delivering NFP, Korfmacher et al. (1999) found that while both groups of practitioners measurably improved parent and child outcomes, the nurse home visitors demonstrated greater improvements and lower drop-out rates. The authors attributed this difference to the fact that there was higher staff turnover amongst the paraprofessionals and that the nurses spent more time with the mothers on health- and child development-related issues. The authors concluded that while the training for both groups was identical, the nurses' background facilitated a more sophisticated understanding of the training content, which, in turn, enabled them to better cover key concepts during the home visits.

Collectively, the above findings suggest that paraprofessionals have the potential to provide effective parenting support, as long as other support systems are in place:

- **Trainee selection**. Processes should be in place for screening paraprofessionals for key characteristics, including the right qualities (including their attitude and beliefs, see below) and good interpersonal skills. Gordon and Arbuthnot (1988) note that cynicism regarding the treatment of families with delinquent children inevitably leads to treatment failure. Good interpersonal skills are also necessary to effectively engage parents and form a positive therapeutic relationship with them. Research repeatedly suggests that while parenting group leaders do not necessarily need to be graduate-level psychologists to effectively deliver a parenting intervention, a background in a helping profession, such as social work, nursing or teaching is often essential (Webster-Stratton 2004).

- **A rigorous accreditation process**. Appropriate accreditation processes work to ensure that practitioners fully understand the program content and know how to apply it to their work with families. For example, the *Triple P* program requires that practitioners pass a test before they are accredited. Accreditation in the *New Forest Parenting Program* model requires that practitioners deliver the program twice with complete fidelity.

- **A clearly specified intervention model**. Research suggests that paraprofessionals are capable of effectively delivering programs that are clearly specified. This means programs should have clear outcomes that are linked to specific activities. Paraprofessionals are less successful when treatment protocols are less specified and more reliant on professional judgment.

- **High-quality training**. Paraprofessionals, in particular, benefit from a systematic, step-by-step approach to training that makes clear links between their behavior and child and parent outcomes. Homework assignments and opportunities to practice skills during the training also improve learning (Gordon and Arbuthnot 1988, Webster-Stratton 2004).

- **Appropriate supervision**. Supervision is vital for ensuring that paraprofessionals grasp what was taught during their training and understand how to apply it to the implementation of the program (McGuigan et al. 2003). This supervision might include pairing practitioners with a more experienced professional, feedback on video-tapes of their work, staff support groups, on-site consultation from a trainer and regular telephone consultations with the trainer (see previous section).

- **Organizational support**. Agencies must also recognize the importance of evidence-based parenting support and endorse it appropriately. Agency endorsement includes salary enhancements for certification, appropriate budgetary allowances for staff supervision and support, sufficient time to implement parenting interventions, reasonable case loads and logistical support (e.g. provision of a venue, food, transportation and child care). Moreover, agencies should make explicit the expectation that practitioners will deliver evidence-based parenting programs with fidelity.

It is important to keep in mind that while paraprofessionals have the potential to effectively implement parenting programs, the extent to which they reduce costs remains debatable. For example, the evaluation of *Homestart* (a UK-based home visiting service delivered by trained volunteers) found that while the program resulted in measurable benefits for families, these were no greater than what they stood to gain through standard care, despite the increased cost of the *Homestart* program. Alexander (2009) has similarly observed that while paraprofessionals can effectively deliver FFT, they require considerably more supervision than do qualified psychologists and this supervision significantly increases program costs. Staff turnover amongst paraprofessionals also tends to be high, which additionally increases the costs to agencies. In short, these findings suggest that while paraprofessionals may improve outcomes for parents and children, there may be no savings in using them and they may ultimately reduce the overall cost-benefits of the evidence-based parenting intervention.

Practitioner qualities

As described in Chapter 4, parents must feel psychologically safe in order to learn new parenting skills. Rogers (1957) observed that a psychologically safe environment is created through congruence, empathy and respect expressed by the practitioner. Braun et al. (2006) observed that these qualities are difficult to learn through training, however, and are underpinned by a set of fundamental beliefs and attitudes involving parents and parenting interventions:

- **Respect**. Parenting practitioners should genuinely care about the parents they work with and believe that they are capable of positive change. Respect also involves valuing parents' expertise and a willingness to work alongside them (rather than taking over from them) throughout the therapeutic process. Practitioners must also be able to respect parents' opinions, even if they may differ from their own.
- **Empathy** involves the practitioner's being able to understand the parent's circumstances from the parent's own point of view and resist temptations to impose their own perspective on the parent's situation. This does not mean that the practitioner must assume that parents are always 'correct' in their assumptions, but the practitioner must be willing understand the parent's point of view before therapeutic change will take place.
- **Genuineness** involves being open to all experiences and not distorting them. In order to do this, practitioners should strive to be honest and non-defensive about their own weaknesses. Through genuineness, practitioners can build trust with parents and gain a deeper understanding of the parent's circumstances from the parent's point of view.
- **Humility** is necessary for one to be genuine. When the practitioner is able to understand and accept his or her own strengths and weaknesses, the practitioner is better able to accept parents' expertise and work alongside of them.
- **Quiet enthusiasm** refers to the drive required to overcome the challenges involved in parenting work. This involves the practitioner's commitment to the intervention, as well as an ongoing commitment to parents, no matter how distressing their circumstances may be. Enthusiasm should be maintained through an inner reserve of positive energy and expressed by a consistently calm and warm approach towards parents.

- **Personal integrity** refers to the practitioner's ability to remain self-aware and keep boundaries between his or her point of the view and that of the parent. While the practitioner must be able to empathize with the parent, he or she must also be able to maintain some objectivity and provide an alternative point of view when appropriate.

As stated previously, practitioner qualities are likely to differ across parenting interventions. For this reason, program models should consider first the kinds of qualities necessary to deliver their intervention and recruit and select practitioners on this basis (Sexton 2007, Sexton and Kelley 2010). Braun et al. (2006) also note that practitioner qualities can be supported through frequent supervision, which includes empathic support for the work of the practitioner.

The role of the practitioner: expert, partner or friend?

Over the past sixty years there has been an ongoing movement in the field of psychology to downplay the notion of the practitioner as expert (Darling 2000). This idea is central to Carl Rogers's client-centered perspective, which begins with the premise that each client is the world's best expert on him- or herself. This implies that clients are in the best position to interpret their feelings and experiences and this expertise should be acknowledged and respected by the practitioner.

Although Rogers recognized that clients themselves often seek the 'expert' advice of mental health providers, Rogers believed that practitioners should resist the temptation to provide their personal opinion and should encourage their clients to develop solutions on their own. Research suggests that parents similarly turn to practitioners for advice, and value it more if they believe that it is coming from an expert (Ghate and Hazel 2004, Hebbeler and Gerlach-Downie 2002, Miller and Sambell 2003, Moran et al. 2004, Peterander 2004). However, family problems often require much more than a 'quick fix' from an expert and parents often benefit more from collaborative interaction between themselves and their practitioner than they do from a simple piece of advice. For this reason, practitioners must often balance parents' desire for an easy answer against the need to help parents develop problem-solving skills of their own.

Davis et al. (2002) suggest that this tension is best resolved by practitioners' working in **partnership** with parents, by inviting parents to work collaboratively with them in resolving their child-management issues. The *Family Partnership Model* (FPM) acknowledges that while the expert judgment of practitioners is important, parents are experts when it comes to understanding their own circumstances, as well as their children's. FPM asserts that when practitioners genuinely acknowledge parents' expertise in their own lives, communication between both parties will improve and parents will feel more in control of the process.

As illustrated in Figure 5.4, FPM involves an explicit set of tasks that are negotiated between the practitioner and parent which include the formation of meaningful goals for the partnership. Once goals are established, the next task is for the parent and practitioner to mutually decide how best to achieve these goals through a sharing of their mutual expertise. Through this partnership approach, parents are more likely to develop enhanced problem-solving skills, a greater sense of empowerment and an improved sense of self-efficacy.

While the extent to which a partnership approach is more effective than expert or client-centered models remains to be tested, many believe that partnership working is better for engaging parents and motivating them to adhere to the program model (Appleton and Minchom 1991, Courtney et al. 1996, Davis et al. 2002).

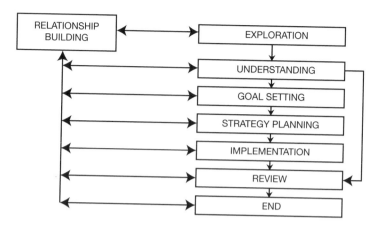

Figure 5.4 Tasks involved in family partnership work

It is important to note that working in partnership is not the same as becoming a parent's friend. While a partnership approach is often used in 'befriending' schemes, these programs nevertheless require carefully trained volunteers to maintain professional boundaries with the parents they work with (Cox et al. 1991, Cox 1993). Research suggests that becoming a parent's friend is not necessary, nor is it an effective way of improving outcomes for parents and children. This is because parents themselves say that they are not interested in practitioners becoming their friends (Hebbeler and Gerlach-Downie, 2002). Practitioners also report that personal relationships with their clients can be emotionally draining and inappropriate (Bignold et al. 1995, Hunter 2001).

Points to remember

This chapter provided an overview of the issues involved in working with parents. While many parents seek support on their own, others may resist it because they are not aware that there are problems with their child, or may have become estranged from services. Meeting the needs of parents can therefore be a challenging process, requiring a high degree of judgment and skill. Important practitioner skills include knowing how to engage and motivate parents and making sure that services are meeting their needs. Practitioners must also have the personal qualities and skills to develop a positive therapeutic alliance with families that can motivate learning and facilitate change. Adopting a strengths-based approach is a particularly fruitful method for developing and maintaining a productive therapeutic alliance with parents.

Practitioners must also be skilled in delivering parenting interventions with fidelity. Contrary to some beliefs, program fidelity is not a replacement for practitioner skill, but requires a high level of understanding for ensuring that the program's core components are not lost. While fidelity concerns *whether* a practitioner adheres to the program model, the practitioner's skill determines *how well* he or she does this. Parents are less likely to benefit from evidence-based programs if they are not implemented with fidelity *and* a high level of skill. While professionally trained psychologists and paraprofessionals are equally able to deliver effective parenting support, professionals are likely to do this with greater consistency and less supervision.

Box 5.6: Key points

- Most parents successfully manage their children without any additional help.
- When parents seek help, they most often want advice for improving their children's behavior. Parents are more likely to pay attention to this advice if they know that it is coming from an expert.
- Some parents are resistant to support because they are not fully aware of the problems with their children, or they feel estranged from services.
- Parents must attend and engage in parenting programs in order for them to be effective.
- Parents are more likely to engage in services if they have a positive therapeutic alliance with the parenting practitioner.
- The therapeutic alliance involves three processes: 1) agreement between the practitioner and parent regarding the goals of the intervention, 2) the activities necessary to meet the goals and 3) the bond that forms between the practitioner and the parent.
- A positive therapeutic alliance is a necessary but not sufficient component of evidence-based parenting programs. Actual improvements in parents' behavior are largely determined by the content of the program.
- There are multiple situational and motivational barriers to parent participation. Practitioners must be skilled in knowing how to overcome these.
- Practitioners must be careful before making adaptations to evidence-based parenting interventions, as these can significantly reduce the impact of the intervention.
- Maintaining program fidelity is necessary for parenting interventions to remain effective. Program fidelity involves processes which ensure that the intervention is reaching the right audience, that its full dosage is implemented and all core components are preserved.
- Ongoing supervision and coaching are necessary for ensuring that parenting programs are delivered with fidelity.
- The effectiveness of a parenting intervention is also determined by the characteristics of the practitioners, including their skill, knowledge and personal qualities.
- In some instances, parenting interventions delivered by less competent practitioners result in worse outcomes for parents and children.
- Paraprofessionals can effectively deliver parenting interventions if the program is well-specified and they are properly supported through supervision.
- Practitioners should have personal qualities which enable them to create a supportive therapeutic environment for parents. These qualities include empathy, respect, genuineness, humility, quiet enthusiasm and personal integrity.
- A partnership approach is considered to be an effective way of engaging parents in evidence-based support.
- Practitioners should maintain professional boundaries and not be tempted to become parents' friends.

Note

1   Individual needs assessment should be differentiated from community needs assessments, which are conducted to understand the need for family and children's services at the community level. See Chapter 7 for further discussion.

6 Developing and monitoring evidence-based parenting services

Introduction

Previous chapters of this book cover the methods used to understand and assess the quality of the evidence base. This knowledge is useful when commissioning services that already have an established track record. However, there are times when evidence-based parenting interventions are not practical or available for a specific problem or community. In these instances, it may be necessary to develop a new and unique intervention and this is when practitioners need to establish their own evidence base. As noted in Chapter 2, randomized controlled trials (RCTs) are the most rigorous way of understanding whether or not an intervention is effective. However, a full RCT requires a good deal of time and resources. Before practitioners and program developers invest large amounts of resources in conducting an RCT, it makes sense to carry out some preliminary research to determine whether an intervention has promise in the first place. This chapter provides an overview of the steps involved in exploring the potential of an intervention as it is being developed, as well as monitoring it after it has been developed.

Outcome-focused services

Outcomes vs. outputs

In order to understand the impact of a service or intervention, program developers must first ask themselves what the intervention hopes to achieve. In other words, what are the intervention's intended outcomes? Although the answer to this question may seem obvious, it is actually not that straightforward. The reality is that most programs have multiple objectives, as was the case with *Head Start*. Although this was a large-scale, community initiative, many smaller-scale services also have multiple goals, which can be difficult to define and measure.

Take, for example, a hypothetical prenatal course delivered by a team of maternity nurses to mothers expecting their first child. The primary objective of the service is to provide information to mothers about their pregnancy and what to expect during the initial weeks following birth. This service is made available to mothers who are in their third trimester and is delivered through six weekly sessions that take place in the evenings. If mothers attend, the service's primary objective is met, with mothers receiving information about the pre- and postnatal care of their infant. But is this primary objective (also known as an **output**) the same as the service's primary **outcome**?

Some of the nurses might answer yes to this question, but others would probably hope that the course would result in some longer-term benefits for both the mother and child. If asked, some of the nurses might also claim that the primary aim of the course was to boost immunization rates, whereas others might say that the course mainly aimed to increase breastfeeding. In this respect, the team's output of providing a prenatal course to mothers is expected to result in a specific **outcome** – improved immunization rates and increased breastfeeding. However, the maternity nurses have not given much thought to their course's outputs and outcomes at a practical level because they know the course is well liked (it is always oversubscribed) and are sure that it adds value to the lives of the mothers who attend it.

The nurses' assumptions are sufficient until they are pressed to find evidence of the course's effectiveness after their primary care trust's budget review. While it is clear to their manager that the prenatal course is popular, she now needs robust evidence of its effectiveness to justify its **inputs** – i.e. its financial resources and staff time. While the nurses could make some educated guesses about its effects on mothers and children, they know these will not be sufficient for their manager, who will need more substantial evidence in order to validate its expense.

SMART outcomes

The nurses therefore must come up with a quick and practical way to evaluate their course. This means that they will need to think 'SMARTly'. SMART is an acronym used by evaluators to identify outcomes for assessing service impacts when limited resources and timescales are available (see Box 6.1). To evaluate SMARTly, the nurses must consider their service's impact in terms of outcomes that are *specific, easy to measure, achievable*, and can *realistically* be assessed within a relatively short *time frame*.

When considering potential outcomes for their prenatal course, the nurses all agree that a primary aim is to educate mothers about the health of their infant and increase immunization and breastfeeding rates. They determine that immunization rates are a SMART outcome, since they are specific, measurable, achievable, realistic and measurable within a short time frame. In addition, information on immunization and breastfeeding rates is easy to find, since their practice routinely collects this information through their monitoring systems. This data allows the nurses to compare the immunization rates of mothers who attended their course and those who did not. This comparison suggests no differences in immunization rates between the groups, as immunization rates are generally quite high (over 98 per cent) throughout the community. The same is true for breastfeeding rates. The nurses therefore conclude that there are no outcomes that can easily be assessed through their trust's monitoring data.

The maternity nurses are now in a bind, as there is no readily available evidence to suggest that their service is needed or effective. As their search for measurable outcomes continues,

---

Box 6.1: Understanding SMART outcomes

SMART outcomes are:
   Specific and deal with discrete rather than broad dimensions
   Measurable so that they can be monitored
   Achievable and within the scope of the service provision
   Realistic in that they can be measured with limited resources
   Time-limited to provide quick answers.

one nurse finds an old newspaper article suggesting that mothers who attend prenatal services are more likely to have babies with higher IQs. Could it be that maternal participation in their prenatal course will actually help children become smarter? The nurses are intrigued by this claim, but when pressed to find the evidence to support it, they are disappointed to find that the original study is flawed, since it only considered mothers' self-reports and it did not compare their reports to mothers who did not attend a prenatal course. The nurses also realize that it is not possible to assess infants' IQs with their available resources.

Once again, the nurses find themselves hard pressed to identify an outcome unique to their service that would justify its expense. The nurses nevertheless continue to consider ways in which to evaluate their service. During their discussions, they recall that mothers who attend their groups often say that they feel more confident about what to expect when their baby arrives. One nurse also remembers hearing about a study that observed that maternal confidence improves the likelihood that a mother will respond sensitively to her infant. The nurses all know that maternal sensitivity has been linked to a number of improved outcomes for babies and children and feel that they may have identified an outcome that is both specific to their service and hopefully measurable.

Articulating a theory of change

With this new-found knowledge, the nurses feel that they have identified some outcomes relevant to their service. However, information on mothers' sense of self-confidence is not routinely collected by their primary care trust and they are still not quite sure how to link improved maternal self-confidence to increased child wellbeing. They find themselves needing a way to link their service to improved outcomes for mothers and children.

The nurses do some further research and find several studies which link increased maternal self-confidence to greater sensitivity. Within these studies is a **theory of change** which suggests that improved self-confidence increases maternal sensitivity, which, in turn, improves infants' developmental outcomes. They then link these short- and longer-term outcomes within the following theory of change involving their service: provision of prenatal course → attendance on the course → mothers' knowledge of the pregnancy and child care → improves mothers' confidence → enhances their maternal sensitivity → ultimately leads to improved outcomes for their children (Figure 6.1).

While the nurses are now confident that maternal confidence is an achievable goal of the course, the nurses are still unsure how to **operationalize** it so that it can be measured. Maternal confidence and improved infant wellbeing are indeed very broad concepts, so the nurses need to come up with a way to further specify them.

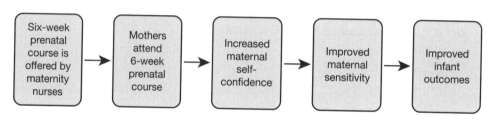

Figure 6.1   Initial theory of change underpinning a six-week prenatal course

Fortunately, one of the nurses has kept her textbooks from her nurse's qualification training. There she finds a standardized measure of maternal confidence – the Maternal Confidence Questionnaire (MCQ; Parker and Zahr 1985). The nurses also learn that some of their pediatric nurse colleagues have recently attended training in the Brazelton Neonatal Behavioral Assessment Scale (NBAS; Brazelton and Nugent 1995) and are looking for opportunities to refine their skills. These two discoveries provide the nurses with the information they need to better articulate their service's theory of change and design an evaluation to assess its impact. Their new, re-specified theory of change is shown in Figure 6.2.

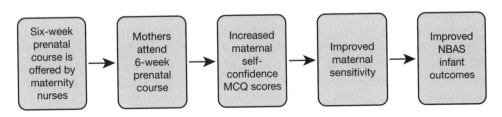

Figure 6.2   Revised theory of change for six-week prenatal course

Although the nurses do not have the resources to conduct an RCT, their course was over-subscribed anyway and they still have the details of the mothers who were turned away from their most recent group. This gives the nurses a natural treatment and comparison group from which to obtain a sample. Because the number of women attending their group is small (from an evaluation standpoint), the nurses invite everyone from both the treatment and comparison groups to participate in their study. After gaining ethical clearance from their local health service's ethics committee,[1] the nurses offer each of the participants a gift voucher from a local pharmacy as a 'thank you' for agreeing to participate in their study. Their participation will require the completion of a short questionnaire and a health assessment of their baby within one month of their baby's birth. The nurses are pleased when they find that they have easily recruited 90 per cent of the mothers to participate in their treatment and comparison groups. This results in 21 participants in total (11 treatment and 10 comparison) and while the nurses know that this is not a very big sample, they hope it will be sufficient to detect differences between the two groups.

It takes three months to complete the study and the results are better than the nurses had expected. Not only did the mothers who attended the prenatal group report greater confidence in caring for their infants, they also had infants who were easier to calm and responded more appropriately to adverse stimuli during their NBAS assessments. Moreover, the confidence scores of the mothers who attended the antenatal course were significantly higher than those of the mothers who did not attend the course. Although the differences between the treatment and comparison group infants' NBAS scores were not significant (probably due to the small sample size), they were nevertheless in the predicted direction. And while these findings were not sufficient for publication in an academic journal,[2] they were enough to justify the continuation of the course. In fact, they were sufficiently robust to gain the attention of their head of children's services, who decided to provide their service with more funds to further evaluate the prenatal group, so that it could be developed further and offered across the community.

Steps for developing a parenting intervention

It should be noted that the hypothetical findings from the maternity nurses' evaluation are extraordinary for a number of reasons. First, the nurses were lucky to have retained the details of the mothers who were turned away from their course, as well as to have recruited so many participants to their study. The nurses were also fortunate to have the support of the pediatric nurses, who were trained in the administration of the NBAS. Third, it is unusual that their findings regarding maternal confidence were significant – partially because of the small sample size, but also because they used outcome measures that were identified on a **post-hoc** basis. In other words, the nurses developed their theory of change to fit what they were already doing. In an ideal world, a theory of change would be developed before the service was implemented – not after. Jackson and Dickinson (2009) observe that a good theory of change should be the first of eight steps in developing an effective and professional service.

Step 1: Produce a logic model of the intervention

The terms **logic model** and 'theory of change' are often used interchangeably to describe how an intervention's activities are linked to its short- and long-term goals. Strictly speaking, a theory of change links the intervention's theoretical basis and underlying assumptions to short- and long-term goals for the target population. An intervention's logic model takes this one step further by differentiating between the intervention's inputs (resources), activities, outputs (immediate effect of the intervention – such as attendance) and outcomes (e.g. increased breastfeeding, improved sensitivity, better child wellbeing, etc.). Figure 6.4 (below) provides an example of the logic model underpinning the maternity nurses' prenatal course. While the nurses developed their theory of change and logic model after their course had been running for some time, Jackson and Dickinson recommend that these activities take place before the intervention is offered.

Step 2: Specify precise, unambiguous intervention objectives

As stated previously, an intervention's objectives should include SMART, short-term outcomes. Jackson and Dickinson (2009) suggest that these outcomes should also be relevant in terms of the research literature. These outcomes will, in turn, provide the basis for monitoring the extent to which the intervention is effective in meeting its short- and long-term goals.

The maternity nurses identified their outcomes through the research literature, which linked greater confidence to increases in maternal sensitivity. The research literature also established a link between maternal sensitivity and improved child outcomes. The standardized measure of maternal self-confidence provided them with a precise, unambiguous intervention objective. Ideally, they should have also identified a way of measuring maternal sensitivity. This way, they could establish the extent to which maternal self-confidence and sensitivity were related, as well as the extent to which sensitivity predicted the babies' NBAS scores.

Step 3: Build an intervention blueprint

This step involves identifying specific activities to support the intervention's primary objectives. For example, knowledge of what to expect during childbirth and how to care for a baby is likely to give first-time mothers greater confidence. The ability to discuss these ideas with others in a group format is also likely to help them explore their feelings and validate their concerns, which could also provide them with greater confidence. Specific information about responding sensitively to a baby's cues and soothing a baby is also likely to increase mothers' sensitivity.

Once an intervention's activities have been identified, developers can then define specific objectives, which are directly linked to the program's short- and long-term outcomes. These objectives become the intervention's blueprint. Table 6.1 provides an example of potential blueprint objectives for the maternity nurses' prenatal course.

Table 6.1 Sample objectives for the maternity nurses' prenatal course

Week 1	Mothers will understand their nutritional requirements during their last trimester through didactic teaching and interactive discussion.
Week 2	Mothers will understand their childbirth options. This will be supported through a video of real women discussing their births. A group discussion involving pain management, birthing options and the likelihood of a c-section will follow.
Week 2	Mothers will learn breathing techniques to help with pain management. Learning will take place through demonstration and opportunities to practice and receive feedback.
Week 3	Mothers will understand their infants' nutritional requirements.
Week 3	Mothers will understand the benefits of breastfeeding. Mothers will receive a presentation on the value of breastfeeding. Mothers will also be given information about how to deal with issues arising from breastfeeding. Mothers will then practice various breastfeeding methods with a doll.
Week 4	Mothers will understand how to meet their child's basic health needs. This will be taught via demonstrations and mothers will have opportunities to practice cleaning and changing a baby with a doll.
Week 5	Mothers will understand how to balance their needs with the baby's. Mothers will watch a video of young mothers discussing how they learned to develop a routine with their baby in the weeks following its birth. This will be followed by a group discussion where each mother will be helped to develop her own individualized postnatal support plan, identifying friends, family members and services that will help her to manage her new responsibilities as a mother.
Week 6	Mothers will understand the community resources available to them and their baby after their birth, including the importance of immunization. A local pediatrician will be available to answer questions.
Weeks 1–6	Mothers will understand the benefits of social networks. Mothers will have the opportunity to form social networks between themselves during a group meal that takes place during each of the six sessions.

It is important to note that the maternity nurses never had the opportunity to develop a blueprint for their course linked to its outcomes before it was already running. Had they done so, they might have considered adding information about how to respond sensitively to the new infant. This step might have further increased the efficacy of their course.

Step 4: Obtain participant input before developing intervention materials

Once the intervention's activities have been identified, developers can consider how these activities will be supported through intervention materials and resources. Materials cost money, however, so it is important to consider the extent to which the activities will be engaging and relevant for program participants. If the intervention is still in its planning stages, focus groups with parents who are representative of the service's target population can be used to understand the acceptability of the proposed activities. Had the maternity nurses had the opportunity to do this, they might have explored whether first-time mothers would be interested in having a weekly meal, what their concerns were about breastfeeding and immunization, the information they wanted regarding the postnatal period, etc. If the intervention is already up and running, practitioners can still get this information from user-satisfaction surveys and focus groups following the intervention. For example, the nurses could have easily used the last group meal to discuss with the mothers what they did and did not like about the course so that they could develop it further.

Steps 5 and 6: Develop and field-test prototypes of intervention activities

Before investing in final materials, it is a good idea to test them to make sure that they are clear. This can be done by developing draft copies of materials (Step 5) and then asking parents about their clarity (Step 6). This can be done informally, but Jackson and Dickinson (2009) suggest that it be done formally, through the use of semi-structured interviews which ask parents representing the target population their views about the intervention's activities and materials. Key questions should include asking parents what they think about the quality and clarity of the materials, what they understand from them and how they think they can be improved.

Step 7: Add professional illustrations and graphic designs

After the intervention's developers are 100 per cent happy with their activities and their materials, it is a good idea to make them look professional by sending them out to a graphic designer who can add illustrations, develop an intervention logo, etc. This is an important step for ensuring that participants perceive the program as legitimate.

Step 8: Produce intervention activity guides and supplemental materials

Once the intervention's developers are happy with the materials and the intervention, they are in a position to 'standardize' the activities through lesson plans, a manual and a training program. It is advisable that the intervention should undergo a number of pilot evaluations before this takes place, however, as findings from the evaluations can be used to better understand the needs of the target population, improve the materials, alter activities, etc. – so that these are completely clear in the manual. These evaluations will also allow developers to understand how to further refine and develop their program.

It is advised that pilot evaluations also measure whether any change has taken place during the course of the intervention. Recall that the maternity nurses initially evaluated their program by making cross-sectional comparisons between the mothers who attended their course and those who did not, at one point in time after the baby was born. When they evaluate the program again, it would be ideal if they measured the mothers' confidence before taking the course and then again right after it is completed. This way they will have an initial understanding of whether the mothers' confidence actually changed during the six weeks of the course. Ideally, the evaluation would also include pre/post measures of mothers not attending the service.

Service planning and evaluation

Evaluation as part of service planning

The purpose of evaluation is generally threefold: 1) to provide accountability, 2) to inform development and 3) to produce new knowledge (Fetterman and Wandersman 2005). The maternity nurses' evaluation was conducted for accountability purposes – i.e. they did it because they had to justify the expense of their activities. Fortunately, they were able to come up with a way of efficiently measuring the prenatal course's effectiveness after it had been in operation for a period of time. They would not have felt caught out by their primary care trust's budget review, however, if they had built evaluation processes into the delivery of their service during its planning stages. This would have allowed them to monitor the effectiveness of the service as they were implementing it, so that they could develop it to best suit the needs of its participants, as well as of the wider community.

The additional funding from their children's services director gave the maternity nurses the opportunity to do this. A second evaluation would enable them to further specify their course's outcomes and also consider the extent to which variations of their course (e.g. a prenatal course for fathers) might additionally improve outcomes for mothers and infants. When used to develop services, the goal of evaluation is thus not to prove, but to *improve*. These developmental aspects of evaluation are sometimes referred to as the **cycle of evaluation**, or **action research**[3] (Figure 6.3).

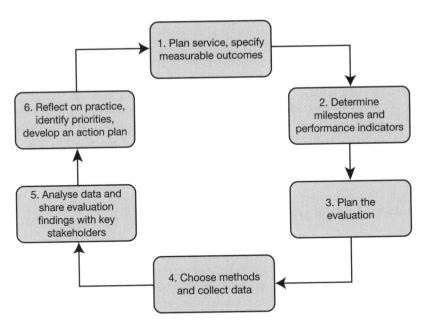

Figure 6.3 Cycle of evaluation

As the above figure illustrates, well-planned services have a focus on outcomes right from the start, when evaluation processes are automatically built into the service's delivery. For this reason, it is considered good practice for an intervention's developers to meet with evaluators during the planning stages of their service to determine:

- What the service is trying to achieve
- Short- and long-term outcomes that include milestones that will help evaluators and service providers to assess whether they are on their way to achieving these outcomes
- Methods for collecting the evidence necessary to determine whether the milestones and short- and long-term outcomes have been achieved
- Systems to assess outputs as well as outcomes
- The resources required for the service to achieve its outputs and short- and long-term outcomes.

Figure 6.4 provides an illustration of the prenatal course's logic model which identifies elements that can be measured as part of its ongoing evaluation.

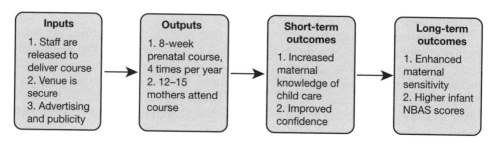

Figure 6.4   Inputs, outputs and short- and long-term outcomes

This model suggests that at the service-planning stage, processes should be put in place to collect information regarding the service's inputs, outputs and short- and long-term outcomes. For example, an evaluation (or good monitoring system) can consider whether the appropriate resources are available (venue, transportation, etc.), whether key activities took place and whether parents attended the course, when evaluating the extent to which the course achieved its intended short- and long-term outcomes. This information can also be used in drafting a **service level agreement** or contract as part of commissioning arrangements (see next chapter for a more in-depth discussion).

Identifying stakeholders and use

When planning service evaluations, it is considered good practice to specify who the primary user(s) and stakeholders are. If, for example, the main purpose of the evaluation is to demonstrate accountability to funding agencies (including the government and/or the children and young people's service directorate), then evaluations should be designed in a manner that will provide information that is useful for these stakeholders. This information might include costs, the service's **reach** or throughput, service user demographics and a consideration of how the users may be similar or different to families who do not use the service.

Michael Quinn Patton (1997) refers to this emphasis on the needs of evaluation stakeholders as 'utilization-focused' evaluation. Utilization-focused evaluation begins with the premise that evaluations should be judged by their actual use – not just by their findings. For this reason, evaluations must also carefully consider how the design will affect its use by its intended users – i.e. those individuals who have the responsibility to apply the evaluation findings and implement the recommendations. Since no evaluation can be value free, its primary stakeholders should be identified at the outset of the evaluation and it should be designed according to their specific needs. When considering the evaluation's use and stakeholders during its planning stages, the following questions should be asked:

- How will the evaluation contribute to service development?
- How will the evaluation inform major decisions about the service?
- Will the evaluation generate new knowledge, and if so, who might be interested in this knowledge?
- What might be the **process use** of the evaluation components?

By process use, Patton is referring to the potential benefits of the actual evaluation process. While many senior managers and frontline workers frequently resent participating in evaluations, the process itself often results in direct benefits for the organization. For example, a group-based theory of change exercise is often a positive experience for everyone who participates in it. If done correctly, it can double as a useful team-building exercise that helps managers and frontline workers articulate the purpose of their service within the broader aims and objectives of the organization. Another example of a process use benefit is that program developers and service providers develop new skills when contributing to the evaluation process (e.g. defining outcomes, assessing monitoring data, etc.).

Despite these potential benefits, the evaluation process often puts service providers on the defensive because it can be viewed as judgmental or critical. There is no question that there are judgmental aspects to the evaluation process. Evaluations have the unfortunate habit of bringing out the 'white elephants' that most managers and frontline workers try to avoid. However, most people working with parents and children want confirmation that what they are doing is effective – so, while aspects of the evaluation process may be judgmental or time consuming, they often also provide a sense of accomplishment when they are completed. While a well-designed evaluation will definitely uncover inefficiencies in service delivery (that is what they are intended to do!), it will also confirm what is working well, and occasionally will reveal some pleasant surprises, as was the case with the maternity nurses' prenatal course.

This last point highlights a further advantage of the evaluation process: the generation of new knowledge. It is highly likely that other nursing teams would benefit from the knowledge generated from the maternity nurses' evaluation. This is a core part of evidence-based working – finding out what works and sharing this knowledge with others, so they can improve outcomes for children and parents.

Commissioning and conducting evaluations

Hiring an external evaluator

The maternity nurses in the above example were fortunate in that they had sufficient resources within their team to evaluate their own service. Self-evaluation is not always practical, however, as practitioners do not usually have the time, the expertise or the objectivity to evaluate what they do. In these cases, it may be necessary to hire an external evaluator. Although external evaluations cost money, their expense is usually returned in the more efficient running of services. For this reason, it is generally recommended that 5–10 per cent of a service budget be allocated to evaluation. This budget should ideally include some funding for external evaluation consultancy.

Hiring an external evaluator has many clear benefits. A chief advantage is that a reputable academic institution or evaluation agency can add a degree of credibility or 'weight' to findings that will ensure that all stakeholders take them seriously. Another benefit is that external consultants have areas of expertise that go beyond the scope of most agencies. Thirdly, external evaluators often have access to resources, such as standardized measures, that may be difficult for individual organizations to obtain. Finally, external evaluators provide a degree of objectivity which makes the evaluation more credible.

There are nevertheless some drawbacks to hiring an external evaluator. First, most external evaluators work to their contract. This means that there is less flexibility if changes are required and the contract may need to be renegotiated if the agency finds that it needs to go beyond what was originally agreed. If evaluators are busy, this may also result in delays in the work being completed, and this can be a serious disadvantage if the service needs some quick answers.

A second problem is that the evaluation may be designed around assumptions that are not necessarily true. Take, for example, an external evaluator who is hired to assess the impact of a home visiting service implemented by family support workers. This is done with the assumption that home visits are taking place on a regular basis. However, when the evaluator begins her job she finds that no home visits have occurred, because no families have met the eligibility criteria. The evaluation must thus be scrapped – but the agency must still pay the evaluator for her time, and perhaps a penalty. Other assumptions that should be considered are whether participants are willing and available to partake in the evaluation and whether it will be possible to obtain ethics approval, if it is required.

A third caveat is that an external evaluator is not always easy to monitor, and misunderstandings occasionally occur because there are fewer opportunities to communicate. This means that key issues should be clarified right from the start and communication systems should be built into the evaluation process accordingly.

A fourth point to consider is who actually 'owns' the evaluation. While commissioners generally 'own' the evaluation findings, the evaluators (especially if they are academicians) may want permission to publish the findings and/or the methodologies. The issue of ownership also comes up when there are stakeholders who go beyond the commissioning agency. These situations often occur when agencies commission an evaluation for accountability purposes. While the agency technically 'owns' the evaluation, it is nevertheless accountable to its parent agency to report the findings and in these instances the evaluator can find herself playing 'piggy in the middle'. Take, for example, a parenting program offered by a team of youth workers. The children's services director is concerned that it is not reaching its target population, so she asks that it be evaluated. The team hires an external evaluator to do the work and the findings are not positive. The team decides not to share them with anyone – but a few months later, the evaluator receives a call from the children's services director, wondering where her evaluation report is. The evaluator cannot give it to her, because the youth offending team actually 'owns' the findings. This nevertheless creates ill-will between the evaluator and the children's services director, which may ultimately affect the evaluator's ability to work in the local authority again.

The above example illustrates a fifth caveat regarding external evaluators: evaluators may not always be as objective as they should be, for the simple reason that they may want repeat business, or a good referral. In this respect, evaluation findings may appear more positive than they really are. This may result in short-term gains for the agency commissioning the evaluation and the external evaluator, but is likely to undermine both parties in the long run, if it is determined later on that the findings are not, in fact, valid.

Despite these shortcomings, hiring an external evaluator to establish an evidence base for parenting support is more often than not a worthwhile investment, especially when it involves an intervention with particular promise. Many of the above drawbacks can be overcome if the following issues are specified in the evaluation contract at the time the work is undertaken:

1   The scope of work is carefully defined, including its key deliverables, their contingencies and assumptions and who is responsible for them.
2   The contract identifies pre-agreed deadlines when key aspects of the work must be completed.
3   The assumptions underpinning the evaluation's design have been carefully considered. For example, is the service being delivered as it should be? Is there an adequate pool of eligible participants? If the evaluation involves service providers, are they willing to participate and do they have sufficient time? Is ethics approval required and will this be a lengthy process?
4   The primary stakeholders are identified, as are the reporting procedures.
5   Ownership of the evaluation has been specified. This includes agreement involving who will be able to disseminate the evaluation findings. For example, will the evaluator have opportunities to share the findings with stakeholders who go beyond the commissioning agency? If the findings are published, who will be the authors?
6   All plans for disseminating the findings should be pre-specified. These plans should include the extent to which the evaluator will participate in this process.

Data collection methods

A number of data collection methods have been mentioned throughout this book. These include structured questionnaires, observational methods, structured, semi-structured and in-depth interviews, focus groups and standardized measures (see Chapter 2 for a more in-depth discussion). Other methods not mentioned previously include **video diaries**, **time diaries** and **reflective diaries**. Depending upon resources and the outcomes being measured, any one of these methods may provide good information about a service's effectiveness and the experiences of its users, although a mix of methods is generally preferable.

It should be emphasized that the data collection methods described in this book should be used for evaluation and research purposes *only*. For example, many of the standardized questionnaires described in Chapter 2 can also be used to make clinical judgments about an individual child or parent to determine their course of treatment. Clinical training is often required to make these judgments, however, and for this reason data collected as part of an evaluation study should *never* be used to make a clinical diagnosis, unless the evaluation is being conducted by a trained clinician and it is within his or her authority to do this. It is unethical to use evaluation data for any purpose other than to evaluate the qualities of a service.

Hoagwood and Cavaleri (2010) observe, however, that it is not uncommon for researchers to become aware of co-occurring mental problems during the course an intervention's evaluation, which may suggest the need for additional services and which may confound the evaluation's findings. In these instances, it could be considered unethical not to refer an individual to additional services if it becomes apparent during the course of the evaluation that the individual could benefit from them. For this reason, it is wise is to consider ahead of time the potential of the study in identifying co-morbid problems and to determine procedures for referring participants on to other services if participants may benefit from them. In some instances, it may be wise for the study team to include a clinician who can make referrals if the need arises. However, the potential need for referrals should be explained to the participants at the time they are recruited to the study and referrals should never be made without a participant's informed consent. If the participant is a child, the consent of the parent is also required (see below).

Ethical considerations

All evaluations should be conducted in a manner that is ethical. This means:

- There should be a clear purpose for the study and its benefits must outweigh any risks or inconveniences potentially affecting the individuals involved in the study
- Study participants must consent to the study and have full knowledge of what they are consenting to
- All of the details of participants should be kept confidentially, unless they give their consent that they can be shared or there is a life-threatening reason as to why they must be shared.

   Most health and educational bodies provide detailed guidelines describing how the above principles apply to the research conducted within their organizations. Academic bodies also have requirements for how their staff can carry out research. Researchers must consult these guidelines and gain ethical clearance from their organization's ethics committee before they begin a study or evaluation. If ethics approval is required (and it most often is for studies involving parents and children),[4] this could cause delays to the project. For this reason, evaluators and program developers should consider whether ethics approval is necessary during the planning stages of their study. While it is not possible to provide the details of specific requirements of individual ethics committees, the key issues underpinning most committees' decisions are summarized briefly below.

Risk or harm

While non-pharmaceutical research involving social interventions generally does not pose many physical risks, psychological risks are always present when asking someone personal questions. Examples of psychological harm include embarrassment, discomfort or stressful memories. Although it is not always possible to anticipate all of the potential risks of a study, evaluators need to carefully consider what the potential psychological risks are and to identify processes for reducing these risks before they start their work. Measures for reducing risks include systems for debriefing individuals after the study is complete and providing them with resources for finding help or further information if they require it. An additional risk is not wasting the participants' time. This means that there must be a clear and beneficial reason for the research or evaluation to take place and that the evaluation does not unduly waste service providers' or participants' time.

Informed consent

It is important that all evaluation participants know what they are consenting to. This means that they understand the purpose of the study, what will happen to the findings and what will happen with the information they provide. This also means that participants know about the study's potential risks and benefits. Participant consent should be voluntary, not coerced or forced. In order to ensure that participants know what they are consenting to, it is necessary to seek their informed consent at the beginning of the study. This is done by giving participants an information sheet explaining the purpose of the study, including how their information will be used and stored and asking them to provide their signed consent for participating in the study. When investigating children, consent must be received from the parent and child. In cases where a child does not want to participate in a study, a parent cannot override this decision by giving consent (Hoagwood and Cavaleri 2010).

Confidentiality

The information that participants provide should be kept completely confidential. This means that any information collected about participants, including standardized scores, interview data or observations, should be kept anonymously, unless participants give explicit permission for it to be shared, or if the researcher learns something that suggests that the participant or someone close to them is in danger. This also means that information gained through the evaluation process should never be shared with other professionals in other contexts, unless 1) the participant knows and agrees that it can be shared or 2) there are child protection concerns.

Incentives

Recall that the maternity nurses offered their participants a gift voucher from a local pharmacy as an incentive for participating in their evaluation. Gift vouchers often help the recruitment process by providing an incentive. They are also a good way of thanking participants by acknowledging their time and trouble. Most stores offer gift voucher options and it is sometimes nice to allow participants to choose where their vouchers come from. Vouchers should not be too expensive or elaborate, however, as this may influence the representativeness of the sample and could be viewed as a form of coercion. It is therefore good practice for gift vouchers be modest (no more than $20 or £15), unless the study requires a great deal of time, which is unusual for most service evaluations.

Analyzing data

As mentioned in Chapter 2, evaluation methods tend to fall within one of two categories: quantitative and qualitative. When establishing an evidence base for parenting services, quantitative analyses are advantageous in that they can directly quantify impacts and determine if they are significant. In many instances, **descriptive statistics** are sufficient for understanding an intervention's outputs. They can answer the questions of *who, how many* and *what is the average*. Going back to the maternity nurses' evaluation, a descriptive analysis of the data could determine the following:

- Who attended the service – i.e. what were the characteristics of the mothers who attended the group?
- How many mothers attended the group?
- What was the range of the confidence scores and what was their average?
- What was the range of NBAS scores and what was their average?

Descriptive statistics are generally easy to calculate, do not require sophisticated software (in most cases, a spreadsheet will do) and do not require training in statistical analyses. Descriptive statistics cannot, however, answer the more complex questions that will help to determine the impact of the maternity nurses' service. These questions include:

*   Is the difference between the 'treatment' and 'control' mothers significant – i.e. is the size of the difference more than what might have occurred by chance?
*   Do the mothers' confidence scores predict the infants' NBAS scores – i.e. is a more confident mother more likely to have a baby who is easier to calm?

These questions require **inferential statistics** and these generally entail some specific training. While the first question could be answered by a **t-test** (which is relatively easy to calculate) the second question involves a **simple regression** or correlation, and this requires special software, such as SPSS or STATA. Had the maternity nurses used pre- and post-treatment measures of maternal confidence for the mothers attending their course and a comparison group, they would have had to conduct an **analysis of variance**, which also requires some familiarity with more complicated, multivariate analyses.

Qualitative data can also be challenging to analyze. It is often extremely time consuming and generally requires the knowledge and skills of a specialist who knows how to sift through lengthy interviews, identify key themes and interpret their implications in a way that is valid and easily understood. It is therefore considered best practice for qualitative studies to be undertaken by an individual external to the service. It should also be remembered that qualitative studies cannot definitively determine whether a service has had any impact. They can, however, provide information as to why a service is (or is not) effective, and this is often important to know.

Returning to the example of the maternity nurses' antenatal service, the data they collected indicated that the mothers who attended their group were more confident than the control group. However, they did not know why they were more confident. While the nurses assumed that participation in their service had led to greater confidence, they still did not know what aspects of their service had contributed to it. Had they been able to interview the mothers, it would have been possible to directly ask them what they had liked best about the group, what knowledge they had gained, and the extent to which this had improved their confidence. While a short questionnaire might have shed light on some of these issues, it would not have allowed the nurses to explore possibilities that they had not already considered.

Another advantage of qualitative studies is that they often provide rich and descriptive quotes, which are effective when disseminating findings to diverse audiences and stakeholders. While people find statistical data difficult to understand and interpret, most people can understand and relate to a personal quote. Although statistical analyses are necessary for providing evidence of an intervention's impact, they do not always generate much enthusiasm. When enthusiasm is necessary (and this is often the case when funding is sought) a descriptive quote often goes a long way in creating interest in an intervention.

Outcome evaluation versus user satisfaction surveys

In the field of evaluation and research, the terms 'impact' and 'effectiveness' have a specific meaning. If a service has been proved to be effective or have an impact, it means that a statistically significant change in the treatment group has been observed (see Chapter 2 for a more in-depth discussion). The meanings of impact and effectiveness are less precise outside of research and evaluation communities, however, and occasionally findings from user-satisfaction surveys are used as evidence of a service's effectiveness.

While using satisfaction surveys as evidence of impact is often well intentioned, it is, in fact, bad practice. The only information user-satisfaction surveys can provide about a service is whether or not it is well liked. This is why user-satisfaction surveys are sometimes referred to as 'happy sheets'. Although it is *often* true that well-liked services are effective, it is certainly not *always* true. Take the example of a parenting program that uses a trip to the seaside to 'hook' parents into a parenting group. The program developers' theory of change assumes that: parents come to the service because they want to go to the seaside → parents have fun and make new friends → parents come to their service again to have more fun and meet friends → parents receive information about good child rearing practices → parents put information to use and improve their parenting skills à child behavior improves. The program developers are excited because the program is over-subscribed and their user-satisfaction surveys suggest that it is very well liked. According to their theory of change, this satisfaction should lead to longer-term benefits for parents and children.

The second half of their theory has not yet been proved, however. While there is no question that their service is popular, the service providers do not really know what effect it has had on parenting or child behaviors. *Unless methods are in place to specifically measure change in parenting and child outcomes, the service providers have no way of knowing whether these outcomes have been achieved.* Program developers must always remember that a service's popularity is *never* a guarantee of its effectiveness. While it is good practice to routinely collect user-satisfaction data as part of a service's monitoring and quality assurance processes, they should not be used as a measure of impact, nor as the sole form of evaluation.

Disseminating findings

All too often, evaluation findings are never reported or used (Patton 1997). The most frequent reason why evaluation findings are not reported is because adequate time and resources were not allocated to the dissemination process. A second reason why evaluation findings are not used is because they are not 'owned' by the evaluation stakeholders. This is often the case for evaluations that take place because services are told they have to conduct an evaluation – not because they want to. A third reason that evaluation findings are not used is because they are disseminated in long-winded technical reports. A fourth, more sinister reason why evaluation findings are not reported is because they are not positive, and hence get 'buried'.

These pitfalls can be avoided if plans for disseminating evaluation findings are made during the planning stages. This ensures that the correct stakeholder groups are identified and sufficient resources are allocated to the dissemination process ahead of time. During this time, it is also helpful to inform all key stakeholders that the evaluation is taking place and that meetings are tentatively scheduled to discuss the findings. This step in the planning stages of the evaluation will help to ensure that unfavorable findings do not become buried or 'lost.'

In instances where evaluations are used to develop services, it is often helpful to build in evaluation processes to ensure that service development actually takes place. Aubel (1999) advocates the use of a five-phase evaluation process that ensures that the evaluation findings inform service development and are shared with the right stakeholders:

- **Planning**: This takes place at the beginning of the evaluation, when stakeholders are asked to come together and define the evaluation's focus, processes and methods.

- **Data-gathering**: This is the data collection phase of the study, when interviews are conducted and observations are made.
- **Consensus-building**: This process is also known as a 'validation' workshop. This takes place when the data has been collected and analyzed, but before the final report has been written. During this phase, the primary stakeholders reconvene at a workshop designed to discuss the findings and agree on their implications.
- **Action planning**: This often takes place during a second workshop where all of the stakeholders meet to develop an action plan for taking the evaluation findings forward.
- **Dissemination**: This is the final stage of an evaluation, where the findings will be disseminated through reports and presentations to a wider group of stakeholders. Evaluation stakeholders can include other practitioners, service managers, commissioners, policy makers and academicians.

Reports are not always necessary if the primary purpose of the evaluation is to develop a service. However, in instances where there is a wider stakeholder audience, a report is often necessary. Reports that include the decisions made during the consensus-building and action-planning phases of the evaluation are more likely to get disseminated even when the findings are unfavorable, because they describe the positive steps the organization will take to address the negative issues raised.

In order to ensure that evaluation reports are read and used, the following points should be observed:

- They should include an executive summary
- They should include visual information, such as tables and graphs
- They should break up long slabs of text with bullet points
- Quotes, if used, should be highlighted and italicized
- Technical details should be separated from the main body of the text and be included in the appendices
- They should report the findings confidently and definitively
- They should include recommendations.

Understanding costs

Documenting costs

In order to ensure that parenting programs are providing value for money, it is good practice to carefully document all of their costs. This involves knowing the start-up costs of the service, as well as its running costs. All service inputs, including staff time (e.g. calculating the proportion of their time spent on their service against their salary, including all related taxes and pension costs), supervision time, support staff, site costs, venue hire, crèche services, food or refreshments, transportation and publicity should all be included as part of a service's overall cost. An example of how this was calculated for the *Incredible Years* program in Wales is provided in Edwards et al. (2007). Once all of the program costs have been accounted for, it is possible to calculate the costs for running the program (or service), as well as the cost per each participating parent or child. Table 6.2 provides a summary of how Edwards et al. did this (2007).

Table 6.2 Total costs and cost per child of running parenting group over 12-session *Incredible Years* program (reprinted with permission from Edwards et al. 2007)

	Mean (SD) unit cost (£)	Mean (SD) units	Total cost (£)
Non-recurrent initial training and group setup costs:			
Materials (programme kit)	735.00	1	735.00
Initial group leader training			
Training course fee	350.00 per leader	2 leaders/group	700.00
Time at training course for two leaders	22.94 (5.27)/hour	45 hours	1032.10
Travel time to training course	22.94 (5.27)/hour	8 hours	183.52
Mileage to attend course for two leaders	0.34/mile	160 miles	54.24
Subtotal			2704.86
Recurrent group running costs			
Supervision of group leaders before start of programme:			
Time for two group leaders with trainer	22.94 (5.27)/hour	6 hours	137.61
Travel time for two group leaders to supervision	22.94 (5.27)/hour	4 hours	91.70
Mileage	0.34/mile	640 miles	217.60
Trainer† costs‡	62.50/hour	1 hour	62.50
Recruitment of parents:			
Time for two group leaders spent in visits to recruit parents	22.94 (5.27)/hour	24 hours	550.56
Group leader travel time to recruit parents	22.94 (5.27)/hour	12 hours	275.28
Cost of telephone calls to recruit parents	0.03 per min	210 mins	6.30

Continued overleaf

	Mean (SD) unit cost (£)	Mean (SD) units	Total cost (£)
Group costs:			
Group materials pack			611.45
Time for two group leaders running sessions	22.94 (5.27)/hour	51.81 (2.94) hours	1188.35
Time for two group leaders outside sessions (preparation, administration, follow-up with parents)	22.94 (5.27)/hour	139.11 (13.73) hours	3190.51
Time for two group leaders in three hour weekly supervision with trainer	22.94 (5.27)/hour	72 hours	1651.36
Travel time for two group leaders to attend weekly supervision with trainer	22.94 (5.27)/hour	48 hours	1100.91
Mileage	0.34/mile	1920 miles	650.88
IY trainer† costs for weekly supervision	62.50/hour	12 hours	750.00
Costs of clerical support to group	9.70/hour	8 hours	77.60
Telephone calls to parents	0.03/min	1129.8 (688.8) mins	33.98
Transport and crèche facilities			1057.57
Venue rental and refreshments			1109.63
Subtotal			12763.65
Cost of establishing and running parenting group over 12 week programme:			
Total			15468.51
Cost/child based on 8/group			1933.56
Cost/child based on 12/group			1289.04
Costs of running parenting group excluding non-recurrent costs:			
Total			12763.65
Cost/child based on 8/group			1595.46
Cost/child based on 12/group			1063.64

Note: In some cases, total costs do not equal product of mean unit costs and mean units because of rounding.
†Consultant clinical psychologist.
‡Supervision delivered to three sets of group leaders at a time

Understanding cost-effectiveness

A service's starting and running costs are generally sufficient for service developers and providers, but there may be times when managers want to compare the effectiveness of their provision to other services. This is when a cost-effectiveness analysis is helpful. It is beyond the scope of this book to provide all of the details of conducting a cost-effectiveness exercise, but it is worth reviewing some basic principles so that program developers can consider the extent to which their service is providing value for money.

A cost-effectiveness exercise essentially asks four questions (Meadows 2001):

1   How much did the program or service cost?
2   What did that use of resources really achieve?
3   Did the benefits from that use of resources exceed the costs?
4   Would an alternative use of the resources have achieved either a larger number or a higher quality of outcomes?

The first question is relatively straightforward to answer. The last three are more difficult, particularly if the service's outcomes are not clearly defined and there is not a clear understanding of how these outcomes contribute to the broader targets of the organization or local authority. This is why it is important to consider how the resources allocated to the service contribute to its impact during the service-planning stages.

Take the example of 'Families Together', a Children's Centre drop-in developed to increase parents' participation in their community. The drop-in runs twice weekly throughout the year with the exception of the school holidays. Each session lasts three hours and provides opportunities for parents to socialize, children to play, and parents to receive advice from psychologists, speech and language therapists, health visitors and nutritionists. It is offered by a team of speech and language therapists and is well attended. The staff members are convinced that it effectively creates a sense of community and empowerment.

Their primary care manager is not convinced that this is the most cost-effective use of her staff members' time, however. She is concerned that the expense of her professional staff's time is not justified and feels that less-qualified staff would be able to run the group just as efficiently. She cites other locally available services that facilitate community involvement that run at less than half the cost. These comparisons suggest that the resources required to run 'Families Together' are more than what was required to achieve its intended outcomes – i.e. the drop-in is not providing value for money. This means that 'Families Together' has to carefully reconsider its inputs, outputs and outcomes to ensure that the resources allocated to it are appropriate for what it is trying to achieve.

Monitoring the impact of parenting services

Establishing monitoring processes to assess impact

A well-designed monitoring system is not only useful for keeping track of an agency's activities, but can also be used to understand whether parenting interventions are achieving their intended outcomes. Returning to the hypothetical example of the maternity nurses' prenatal course, let us assume that the maternity nurses take advantage of the funds provided by the director of children's services and use them to conduct a second evaluation of their course to further test its effectiveness and establish a monitoring system. This time, they have the resources to do a more robust 'experiment' that randomly assigns mothers into their course by providing a cut-off date by when mothers can express their interest. All interested mothers are then randomly assigned to the group or no service (as the course is still oversubscribed). This measure will address a potential confound created by the 'first come – first served' basis of the group. This policy may have inadvertently biased the findings of the first study towards the group attendees, as these mothers may have been more organized and confident to begin with.

At this time, the maternity nurses ask both groups to fill out a standardized questionnaire querying their general confidence (as the MCQ is for mothers who have babies already) and both groups are asked to complete the confidence questionnaire again at the end of the service. The mothers then complete this same pre-/post-group confidence questionnaire a third time, along with MCQ one month after their infants' birth.

Once again, the maternity nurses discover that the mothers who attended their group demonstrated a greater increase in personal confidence when compared to those who were not able to attend. In addition, their post-test scores were positively correlated with the MCQ scores, as well as their babies' NBAS scores, taken within one month of the babies' birth. These are *extremely* positive findings, but keep in mind that this is just a hypothetical example.

With these findings, the nurses are more confident that their service is effective and their manager decides to roll out more groups so that it is no longer necessary to turn away expectant mothers. The nurses also decide that a new standardized measure of maternal confidence will be used pre- and post-service for all future groups, since the MCQ can be used only with mothers who have a baby. This will allow the nurses to monitor whether their service continues to achieve its primary intended outcome (increased maternal confidence) for all future services without having to do follow-up assessments with the MCQ and NBAS measures. Although the midwives and health visitors may decide to continue to use these measures as a part of other screening and monitoring processes within their primary care trust, they will no longer be required to assess the impact of the antenatal group, once systems for routinely monitoring its effect on maternal confidence are in place.

Tracking service use

Pre- and post-service measures are a good way of understanding the potential effectiveness of all parenting services. Many evidence-based interventions recommend pre and post measures that are compatible with their intervention model. However, there are many instances when practitioners may want to consider whether their service is achieving additional outcomes that go beyond the intervention's original goals. Take, for example, a team of youth workers that is offering *Strengthening Families 10–14* as a way of reducing youth offending in its community. A comparison of parents' self-reports, the Strengths and Difficulties Questionnaire (SDQ) pre- and-post program participation, suggests that the intervention appears to be effective in improving children's behavior immediately after the course. The youth workers now also want to know if the program has any impact in their community in the years after parents have completed the course.

A good way to answer this question is to track what happens to the parents and children after the parents have completed the course, and the youth workers should be able to do this if their local authority has a good interagency monitoring system in place. Such a system should allow the youth workers to track the children whose parents attended their program through schools, health services and other community programs. If the system routinely collects information on important community outcomes, the youth workers should be able to determine whether the children whose parents attended their program went on to commit a crime, truant from school, and complete their secondary education.

Good monitoring systems are also extremely useful for determining the extent to which an intervention may result in any sleeper effects. Recall from the example of *Head Start* that it was the unmeasured outcomes which ultimately resulted in longer-term benefits for participating children. Returning to the example of the maternity nurses' prenatal group, the nurses suspected that mothers who attended their groups were also more likely to access other health services as their children matured. If their local authority has systems in place for data sharing, the nurses will be able to track the mothers and babies across all statutory services. This can be done anonymously by giving each parent and child a unique identifying number which is shared across agencies. Thus, in a year's time the maternity nurses can track the mothers who used their services against those who did not and make comparisons regarding their service use. Positive findings from such an exercise would not be absolute proof that participation in their prenatal group had led to greater access to health services (the mothers who accessed the prenatal course might have been more likely to access them in the first place), but it can provide meaningful information regarding patterns of service use that can inform the planning of new services.

Monitoring reach

Robust monitoring systems are also essential if a service wishes to understand its impact in terms of its **reach**. The term 'reach' (or throughput) refers to the proportion of the population exposed to an intervention. Returning to the example of the youth offending team's *Strengthening Families 10–14* service, the team's manager asks it to demonstrate whether it is reaching the most vulnerable families in the community. It knows from the housing and census data, as well as its own records, where the most deprived families live. Through the use of geographic information systems (GIS) software, it can map the reach of its service by plotting the addresses of its participants against the population densities within its communities.

Figure 6.5 provides an example of how this was done to monitor the extent to which a children's center in north London was reaching all of the children aged 4 and younger living in its area. The map on the right shows the proportion of children living within postal code

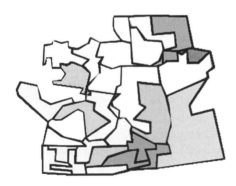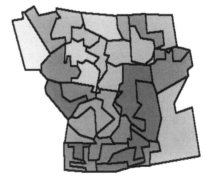

Figure 6.5 A comparison of a children's center's reach to the actual number of children under four living in a north London borough

areas attending the children's center's services. The map on the left shows the actual number of children living in these areas, using information collected from the area's birth records.

Data management systems

None of the monitoring activities described above is possible if service providers do not have access to good data management systems. While a robust data management system involves a considerable amount of time and expense, it can result in significant benefits for the organ-ization as a whole and should be considered an *essential* part of evidence-based practice. For this reason, those working with parents and children should make a concerted effort to ensure that they have sound systems for collecting and storing information. At the very least, these systems should include:

- The demographic details of all parents and children using their services
- Attendance records
- Systems for comparing outputs and outcomes
- Systems for sharing anonymized data.

All of this information is best managed through the use of a relational database. Microsoft Access is one example of a relational database, but when very large amounts of data are involved, bespoke systems are usually required. These systems need to be user friendly, built around effective software packages (that can interact with statistical and geographical mapping software systems) and to be adaptable to accommodate ongoing changes. As practi-tioners get into the habit of evaluating their services, it is likely that they may want to collect new or different data on parents and children as their service develops. It is also good practice to have a dedicated post or specified person(s) to oversee the data management and moni-toring process.

Developing an evaluation strategy

A framework for assessing area-wide impact

The above sections provide examples of how evaluations can be used to develop an evidence base for individual services. It is also often beneficial for organizations and local authori-ties to develop an overarching evaluation strategy so that they can achieve a fairly robust understanding of how their services are collectively meeting local need. Figure 6.6 provides a framework for understanding how evaluation and monitoring systems can be integrated to inform area-wide planning and service integration.

The above framework illustrates how robust monitoring systems and community data (described in more detail in Chapter 7) lay the foundation for assessing local need and targeting services. This information, in turn, informs the development of services and cross-agency target setting. Individual service evaluations then provide specific information regarding service impacts that can then be considered collectively across agencies in order to assess area-wide impact, within the context of locally defined targets and national objectives. A good evaluation strategy will also include systems for assessing cross-cutting issues, such as the quality of inter-agency working and the extent to which services are collectively reaching vulnerable populations.

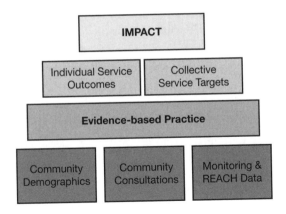

Figure 6.6   Building blocks of a community-wide evaluation strategy

The elements of a good evaluation strategy

When specifying how all of this information will be integrated, a good evaluation strategy should include the following:

- The ways in which evaluation will support the agency's and/or community's overarching aims and objectives
- Methods for assessing and understanding community needs (see Chapter 7)
- Methods for matching community needs to tiered support (see Chapter 7)
- Monitoring systems and the extent to which these will link to evaluation processes
- Methods for tracking service use across authorities and agencies
- Plans for evaluating individual services
- The extent to which services will be evaluated via internal systems, or external consultants
- Systems for ensuring that evaluation findings will inform the development of practice
- Structures for managing the evaluation (including steering groups and advisory committees)
- Staffing arrangements to support evaluation processes
- A designated evaluation lead
- Processes for disseminating evaluation findings
- A timetable for planned evaluation work
- Processes for dealing with ethical issues.

Points to remember

Most organizations have built-in systems to help them automatically monitor their quality and effectiveness. This is because they have clear targets and outcomes by which they can assess progress. For example, a store knows if it is effective if it makes money. Educational bodies monitor their effectiveness through grades and standardized testing. A health organization monitors its effectiveness by tracking whether its patients get better or worse.

Monitoring the effectiveness of social interventions is not as straightforward, however. This is because their outcomes are often difficult to identify and measure. Just because it is difficult is not an excuse for not doing it, however. Hopefully this chapter has provided some examples of how family-based interventions can identify key outcomes and monitor their progress in achieving them.

There is no question that monitoring and evaluation processes require resources and time. However, when used properly, these processes should greatly improve services and ultimately improve job satisfaction. This is not to suggest that all services must be undergo an RCT, but it is important that services aimed at children and parents are closely monitored to ensure that they are doing what they were intended to do. At the very least, agencies should routinely monitor their outputs so that they know who is using their services and what happens to them after they leave. With the proper resources, good monitoring systems can also allow a local authority to assess the collective impact of multiple services in meeting the needs of its communities. The ways in which this can be done are discussed in greater depth in Chapter 7.

Box 6.2: Key points

- There are times when it is necessary for practitioners to develop the evidence base for their own services.
- Program development should always start with the intended outcomes in mind and include methods for specifying and measuring them.
- It is good practice to build evaluation into service development at the very beginning, by pre-specifying the service's inputs, outputs and short- and long-term outcomes.
- The purpose of evaluation is threefold: accountability, development and the generation of new knowledge.
- Evaluations should consider how the findings will be used at the beginning of their design, as well as who will use them.
- When managed properly, evaluation work conducted by an external agency can help a service establish its evidence base.
- Evaluations should always be conducted in a manner that is ethical.
- User-satisfaction surveys cannot provide evidence of a service's effectiveness.
- Program developers should keep close track of costs to verify whether their service provides value for money.
- Services should consider the routine use of pre- and post-service measures to monitor their impact.
- Tracking systems enable practitioners to understand what happens to intervention participants after the intervention is over. They are also effective for understanding whether a service is reaching its target population.
- Robust monitoring systems can help practitioners to assess how their services contribute to local and national targets.
- An area-wide evaluation strategy is a helpful way to integrate services and monitor their collective impact.

Notes

1 Following ethical guidelines is described in the following sections.
2 Although it might be possible to publish this study in a practitioner-based newsletter, the study is not sufficiently robust for academic audiences, as the participants were not randomly assigned to a treatment and a control group and the sample was drawn from individuals who were actively seeking to join an antenatal group. For this reason, the findings cannot be generalized to other service populations, particularly those who might be more isolated and less likely to participate in group-based antenatal services.
3 The concept of action research was first introduced by Kurt Lewin, whose ideas have also influenced the work of Uri Bronfenbrenner (Chapter 3), Julian Rotter (Chapter 4) and Ludwig von Bertanlanffy (Chapter 4).
4 Unless it qualifies as part of a service's audit or monitoring system. In these cases, the need for ethical clearance is sometimes waived. Researchers should verify that ethical clearance does not apply, however, before starting an evaluation, even if they are pretty sure it does not qualify as research.

7 Evidence-based commissioning and implementation of parenting support for community change

From the clinic to the community: disseminating evidence-based parenting support

While the previous chapters highlighted methods for developing and delivering individual evidence-based parenting interventions, this chapter describes strategies for maximizing their impact at the community level. As mentioned in Chapter 2, the evidence base for most parenting programs is established within research organizations where a variety of factors are within the program developers' control. These factors include sufficient financial resources, access to the right client group and strict adherence to the program's model. These ideal conditions ensure that the model's core components are not lost and the program has the best chance of achieving its intended outcomes.

Once programs are disseminated across a variety of settings, it becomes more difficult to maintain the ideal implementation conditions, however. This frequently results in a substantial amount of program drift, which inevitably interferes with a program's impact. As noted in Chapter 5, factors that reduce a program's effectiveness include poor referral routes, practitioners who do not understand or respect the program's model, a workforce lacking the necessary qualifications to deliver the program and insufficient systems for their ongoing supervision. This chapter covers what commissioners, service managers and parenting practitioners need to do to make sure that the right conditions are in place so that evidence-based parenting interventions have the best chance of achieving their outcomes at the community level.

Developing a 'portfolio' of evidence-based parenting support

Evidence from the US and UK

As noted in Chapter 1, a growing body of research suggests that the implementation of a 'portfolio' of evidence-based parenting services contributes to community-wide improvements in key areas of child development. These improvements include measurable reductions in antisocial behavior, reduced child maltreatment rates, higher levels of academic achievement and reductions in child mental health problems. These improvements are seldom realized through the implementation of just one or two evidence-based programs, however. Rather, a constellation or 'portfolio' of universal and targeted evidence-based interventions matched to a population's needs is required for community-wide benefits to be achieved (Aos 2009).

In Chapter 5, family needs were discussed in terms of low, moderate, complex and high needs. A spectrum of prevention and intervention services linked to level of need and access was also provided (see Figure 5.1). Figure 7.1 provides a framework for considering how to proportionately distribute services based on a mix of needs within a given population (adapted from Hardiker et al. 1991).

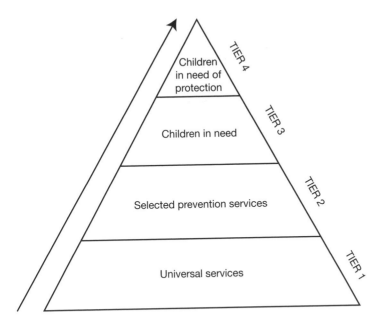

Figure 7.1   Tiers of need in child and family support

The bottom of the pyramid begins with universal needs. This implies that universal services are made available to everyone with the aim of preventing the need for services at the higher tiers. Tier 2 refers to services for smaller, selected groups within a larger population that may be at risk for developing problems. As noted in Chapter 5, these groups may include young parents, impoverished families or families confronting specific kinds of problems, such as parental separation and divorce. Tier 3 applies to an even smaller proportion of the population who are coping with problems that have been diagnosed, including problematic child behavior, learning difficulties, emotional problems or physical disabilities. Tier 4 refers to an even smaller proportion of the population who are confronting very serious problems, including youth offending and child maltreatment.

The tiered triangle presented in Figure 7.1 also assumes that the family support that is available is matched to the level of need across communities. Aos (2009) suggests that positive community change can be achieved if evidence-based services are proportionally available at each tier of need. When implemented properly, these services can collectively save communities money, since evidence-based services offered at the universal level should prevent the need for more costly services at Tiers 3 and 4.

As described in Chapter 1, communities within the US, the UK and several other countries are starting to witness community-level change through the implementation of a portfolio of evidence-based parenting interventions. For example, the US state of Washington expects to save the cost of a new prison by the proportionate implementation of evidence-based interventions at each tier of need. Table 7.1 provides a list of these interventions, many of which include parents within their delivery models.

Table 7.1 A portfolio of evidence-based programs to reduce the need for future prison construction in the US state of Washington (Aos 2006)

Selective prevention

Nurse–Family Partnership (NFP)

Pre-K education for low-income three- and four-year-olds

High needs for children already in the juvenile justice system

Functional Family Therapy (FFT)

Aggression Replacement Therapy

Multi-systemic Therapy (MST)

Multidimensional Treatment Foster Care (MTFC)

Interagency coordination in juvenile courts

Family Integrated Transitions

Juvenile drug courts

Restorative justice programs in juvenile courts

Washington State's portfolio includes only programs that are evidence-based and cost-effective (Aos 2006). Thus, all of the programs listed in Table 7.1 have high benefit–cost ratios, with those including parents resulting in some of the highest savings. These ratios were calculated with the Washington State Institute for Public Policy's (WSIPP) economic models that conservatively estimated NFP's benefit–costs at $6 to $1, FFT's and MST's at $28 to $1 and *Multidimensional Treatment Foster Care*'s (MTFC – see Box 7.1) at $43 to $1 (Aos et al. 2001). While it is too soon to determine whether Washington's strategy has resulted in any actual cost savings, monitoring data suggests that recidivism rates are dropping in the predicted direction (Aos 2010).

The US state of Pennsylvania provides a second example of a successful portfolio approach informed by the *Communities That Care* (CTC) prevention model. CTC (see Box 7.2) involves the formation of collaborative community partnerships to identify and implement evidence-based social programs targeting a constellation of risk and protection factors unique to each community (Feinberg et al. 2010). The partnerships then select a 'menu' of evidence-based programs from the CTC Prevention Strategies Guide to match the specific needs of their communities. Each community menu includes a combination of school-based, community-based and family-based support. Examples of evidence-based parenting support implemented through CTC in Pennsylvania include *Strengthening Families 10–14*, *Incredible Years*, FFT, MST and MTFC. Findings from the ongoing evaluation of Pennsylvania's initiative indicate significant reductions in youth reports of antisocial behavior and higher levels of school achievement in CTC communities (Feinberg et al. 2010).

Once the plan is implemented, CTC becomes an ongoing community process. The process of monitoring implementation progress and community-level changes in risk, protection and youth outcomes is repeated every two years by re-conducting the CTC survey. Based on a review of survey results, CTC boards revise their action plans as needed.

Findings from cross-sectional evaluations of CTC in the state of Pennsylvania have observed significant reductions in adolescents' reports of risks associated with antisocial behavior and increases in school achievement (Feinberg et al. 2010). An RCT of the initiative also suggests a significantly decreased risk of antisocial behavior among students attending CTC schools in comparison to those in control communities (Hawkins et al. 2008). CTC is endorsed by the Center for Substance Abuse Prevention (CSAP) in the office of the United States Government's Substance Abuse and Mental Health Services Administration (SAMHSA).

Box 7.1: *Multidimensional Treatment Foster Care*

Multidimensional Treatment Foster Care (MTFC) is an alternative to residential treatment, prison, or hospitalization for children who have serious emotional and behavioral problems, including delinquency. Children are removed from their parents and placed with a 'treatment foster family' that has been trained to implement parenting strategies based upon the principles of social learning theory (see Chapter 3). Within these positive and structured family environments, children receive consistent positive reinforcement for appropriate behavior and negative consequences for inappropriate behavior. MTFC foster parents receive support on a weekly basis through weekly meetings with other foster parents and MTFC supervisors. In addition, foster parents are contacted daily by telephone so that MTFC staff can provide individual support for the foster child's problems. MTFC supervisors are also available 24 hours a day for consultation and crisis intervention.

While the young person is in placement, family therapy is also provided to the biological (or adoptive) family, with the goal of the child returning home once the treatment is completed. During this time, parents are taught the same parenting strategies which are endorsed in the MTFC foster home. MTFC children are encouraged to have frequent contact with their parents during supervised visits. Biological parents are also provided with high levels of MTFC supervision and support.

Multiple randomized controlled trials (RCTs) suggest that children placed in MTFC homes are significantly less likely to be rearrested, run away from home and misuse hard drugs in comparison to adolescents not assigned to the program. MTFC children also demonstrate better school performance 24 months following their original foster care placement. Girls participating in the program are also significantly less likely to become pregnant and engage in risky health behavior during their teenage years (Chamberlain et al. 2007, Smith and Chamberlain 2010). The cost savings of the program have been calculated at $43 for every $1 invested (Aos et al. 2001).

CTC has also been used by more than 30 authorities in the UK and in communities in Australia and the Netherlands.

The US state of South Carolina provides a third example of how a 'spectrum' of evidence-based interventions can result in positive community change. This was achieved through the implementation of the full range of universal and targeted *Triple P* interventions (see Box 1.3). Counties that were randomly assigned to *Triple P* interventions demonstrated significant reductions in child maltreatment in comparison to counties not implementing *Triple P* interventions (Prinz et al. 2009).

As mentioned in Chapter 1, Norway has also implemented a 'suite' of evidence-based programs that have begun to demonstrate positive change at the agency level (Hellend 2009). Norway's suite of programs includes evidence-based interventions at every level of need, including *Incredible Years*, PMTO and FFT. Findings from the initiative's ongoing RCT suggest significant improvements in parent and child behaviors, as well as improved job satisfaction reported by those delivering the interventions (Ogden and Hagen 2008).

Within the UK, eleven *Sure Start* Children's Centres across North Wales have been running a continuum of *Incredible Years* (Box 1.7) interventions since 2001 (Hutchings et al. 2007). This continuum includes the standard twelve week BASIC *Incredible Years* program (for parents of children aged 3 to 6), the *Incredible Years Dinosaur* program aimed at reception-aged children, the *Incredible Years* Teacher Classroom Management Program and, most recently, the newly

> **Box 7.2: *Communities That Care***
>
> *Communities That Care* advocates a five-phase process to the planning and implementa-
> tion of integrated prevention efforts:
>
> - **Get started**: Community leaders interested in beginning the CTC process define
>   the scope of the prevention effort, assess their community readiness, address barriers
>   to community readiness and engage key community stakeholders.
> - **Get organized:** CTC leaders form a community board to oversee and implement
>   the CTC process.
> - **Develop a profile:** CTC leaders are trained to conduct a community needs assess-
>   ment of risk and proctective factors through the use of a standardized questionnaire.
>   Risk and protective factors are assessed within four ecological domains: 1) the family,
>   2) school, 3) community and 4) individuals, friends and peers. Data from this exercise
>   are then analyzed to prioritize risk and protective factors unique to the community.
> - **Create a plan**: CTC leaders develop a plan to select and implement evidence-
>   based programs that are likely to reduce the risk and protective factors identified in
>   the CTC profile.
> - **Implement and evaluate**: The plan is implemented with the aim of supporting
>   fidelity so that programs can achieve their maximum effectiveness.

developed *Incredible Years Toddler* program. Ongoing evaluations of the program consistently demonstrate significant benefits for parents and children. For example, in a recent RCT of the BASIC program, *Incredible Years* participants reported significant increases in their perceived level of parenting competence, significant decreases in their levels of stress and depression and significant improvements in their children's behavior (Hutchings et al. 2007). Similar positive results have been observed in the pilot of the school-based *Dinosaur* program, demon-strating significant improvements in children's social competence and academic achievement (Hutchings et al. 2004). The pilot additionally observed that the greatest improvements were among children whose parents participated in the BASIC program while they simultane-ously attended the *Dinosaur* program. Webster-Stratton and her team in Seattle, Washington have similarly observed that program impacts are the strongest in cases where children's parents and teachers both receive *Incredible Years* training (Reid et al. 2003).

Creating a portfolio of evidence-based services for parents and children

As noted in Box 1.7, the *Incredible Years* program has achieved positive outcomes for parents and children when delivered universally to families through preschools, as well as to families confronting more complex child behavioral problems, including ADHD. Not all evidence-based programs are suitable for all levels of need, however. In order for evidence-based programs to achieve their maximum effectiveness within communities, they must be care-fully matched to the needs of the community, as well as the needs of individual families.

As discussed in Chapter 5, no one evidence-based program is likely to be suitable for all parents. This is because the needs of families change as children mature. For this reason, the most effective programs target specific risks at each developmental stage (O'Connell et al. 2009). Table 7.2 provides an overview of the kinds of interventions targeting risks at each stage of a child's development.

Table 7.2 Examples of needed evidence-based interventions by children's developmental stage (reprinted with permission from O'Connell et al. 2009)

Developmental stage	In the absence of interventions	Examples of intervention opportunities
Conception, pregnancy and postpartum	• High risk of postpartum depression	• Pregnant women screened routinely for risk factors and provided with needed interventions, such as mood management training, home visitation and nutritional counseling to prevent maternal depression during children's critical developmental stages
	• Baby at risk for problems of attachment, later preschool or school problems, or later depression if mother is depressed	• Well-baby visits to screen and intervene for developmental problems, abnormal feeding patterns, interactions with mother or other caregiver
Infancy	• Infant at risk for abnormal development	• Screening is offered for age-appropriate behaviors and evidence of normal brain development
	• Early behavioral difficulties increase risk for later bonding problems, negative patterns of parent–child interaction	• Remedial interventions are offered, such as parent training and referral to a developmental specialist
Preschool years	• Child does not receive early cognitive stimulation	• Caregivers are encouraged to read to their children
	• Child does not learn self-efficacy, pro-social skills or appropriate school behaviors	• In-home and out-of-home enrichment experiences such as early childhood education are offered for the child to build skills needed for school and social success
Primary school	• Child has difficulty establishing positive relationships with peers, caregivers or teachers	• Families and schools increase nurturance and decrease punitive experiences
	• Child does not experience early successes	• Children learn skills to enhance school performance and manage problem behaviors
Early adolescence (10–13)	• Early adolescent engages in risky behaviors, such as smoking, using alcohol or other drugs, delinquency or risky sexual behavior	• Families and schools provide high-level reinforcement for pro-social behavior
	• Early adolescent experiences few academic successes and bonds with deviant peers	• Young people at risk due to academic or peer-interaction problems are identified and provided with individual or family intervention options
Adolescence (14–18)	• Adolescent lacks self-esteem, has limited academic success, engages in antisocial behaviors, and does not develop positive health habits	• Family- and school-focused programs shape attitudes and behaviors around substance abuse, delinquency and sexual behaviors and provide self-identity and coping skills
	• Depression, conduct disorder and substance abuse increase	• Adolescents are routinely screened for early signs of depression and other disorders, with appropriate interventions provided

Continued overleaf

Developmental stage	In the absence of interventions	Examples of intervention opportunities
Young adulthood (18 and older)	• Young adult flounders in transition to independence, including continued education, employment, marriage and childrearing	• Community programs support decisions about education, work and relationship, and model parenting skills, including constructive parent–child communication
	• Young adults struggle with readiness to have and to parent children	• Interventions are available in university, training, the workplace and community settings as needed to reduce obstacles to raising a family, including academic, job-related and marital difficulties

As noted in the previous chapters, a number of evidence-based programs are now available that address specific developmental milestones based upon a family's level of need. Table 7.3 provides an overview of evidence-based[1] parenting programs currently available with respect to the developmental stage and level of need they address.

As Table 7.3 suggests, a range of evidence-based parenting programs are now available at the universal, selected prevention, complex and high needs levels for all age groups. Before commissioning an intervention, however, it is important to consider its costs in relation to what it is expected to achieve, as this will ultimately determine the intervention's cost-benefits. For example, while all families are likely to benefit from individualized one-to-one parenting support, not all families require this level of intervention. Recall from Chapter 1 that more affluent mothers receiving home visiting support reported fewer benefits, which reduced the home visiting programs' overall effectiveness. In this respect, home visiting support is likely to cost more than it can achieve if it is offered universally. Conversely, sending parents with extremely high needs to universally provided services is not likely to meet their needs and could waste time if a child's circumstances are getting worse. The need to match parenting support to the needs of families cannot be overemphasized. Methods for assessing community needs (as opposed to individual needs, which were discussed in Chapter 5) are described in further detail in the following sections.

Outcome-focused commissioning

Just as Chapter 6 highlighted the need for outcome-focused evaluations, this chapter emphasizes the need for outcome-focused commissioning. As the previous section illustrates, a portfolio of evidence-based parenting support has the potential to improve parent and child outcomes in a way that also benefits communities. Communities differ, however, in terms of their needs. In order for parenting interventions to have their biggest impact, they must be well matched to the needs of individual families *and* the needs of communities. Once a community's needs are understood, areas for change can be identified, outcomes can be prioritized and a plan for achieving these outcomes can be developed.

The Commissioning Support Program (CSP) defines commissioning as:

> the process for deciding how to use the total resource available for families in order to improve outcomes in the most efficient, effective, equitable and sustainable way
>
> (CSP 2009:7)

By definition, strategic commissioning involves the use of logic models that assign inputs (community resources) to outputs (e.g. services, including evidence-based interventions) to

Table 7.3 Evidence-based parenting programs by family needs and children's age group

	Universal low needs	Selected prevention	Complex needs	High needs
Prenatal to infancy (pre-birth to 2 years)				
Family Foundations	✓			
Infant Parent Psychotherapy			✓	✓
Nurse–Family Partnership		✓		
VIPP		✓	✓	✓
Preschool (age 2–5)				
Incredible Years Toddler	✓	✓	✓	✓
Incredible Years BASIC	✓	✓	✓	✓
New Forest Parenting Program			✓	
Parent Management Training-Oregon			✓	✓
Multidimensional Treatment Foster Care-P				✓
Middle childhood (age 5–12)				
Dads for Life		✓		
Incredible Years School Age	✓	✓	✓	✓
Families and Schools Together	✓			
New Beginnings		✓		
New Forest Parenting Program			✓	
Parent Management Training-Oregon			✓	✓
Triple P	✓	✓	✓	✓
Multidimensional Treatment Foster Care-C				✓
Adolescence (age 10–18)				
Strengthening Families 10–14	✓			
Functional Family Therapy			✓	✓
Multi-systemic Therapy			✓	✓
Multidimensional Treatment Foster Care-A			✓	✓

outcomes, which can include community-level improvements in children's and parents' well-being. Within this framework, communities must first identify the outcomes they need to achieve and then assign resources and commission services accordingly (Chinman et al. 2004).

The CTC model provides one example of outcome-focused commissioning, which considers outcomes in terms of a constellation of risk and protective factors identified through a community-wide survey conducted with young people between the ages of 11 and 14. The *Common Language* approach (Box 7.3) offers a second method of outcome-focused commissioning through the use of inter-disciplinary training to help those involved in the delivery of children's services to identify community-specific outcomes, which can be addressed through evidence-based interventions. *Outcome-based Accountability* (OBA, see Box 7.4) provides a third method for bringing together children's services stakeholders to identify positive and negative trends within their community data. These trends then provide the baseline which should be reversed through the strategic commissioning of services (Friedman 2005).

Box 7.3: *Common Language*

The *Common Language* approach underpins the selection of evidence-based parenting interventions implemented through the city of Birmingham's *Brighter Futures* investment-to-save scheme described in Chapter 1 and Box 7.6. *Common Language* helps strategic partners involved in the delivery of children's services to identify priorities and outcomes through three integrated processes: 1) the implementation of practice tools, 2) methods for planning and implementing effective services and 3) training to enable practitioners to understand scientific concepts core to the delivery of children's services. This training includes an introduction to common risk and protective factors within a developmental framework. *Common Language* practice tools include methods for helping commissioning stakeholders to audit their services and assess community needs. Once a community's needs have been assessed, *Common Language* methods assist practitioners in developing a logic model that prioritizes community-wide outcomes and identifies resources and activities to achieve these outcomes. Throughout this process, practitioners also receive training that enables them to select evidence-based interventions for children and parents (Axford et al. 2006).

Box 7.4: *Outcome-based Accountability*

Outcome-based Accountability (OBA) provides a framework for helping multiple agencies involved in the delivery of children's services to identify and prioritize outcomes that their services can collectively achieve (Friedman 2005). First developed in the US, OBA has been used in over 20 English authorities to develop their Children and Young People's Plans and is endorsed by the *Center for Excellence and Outcomes* (C4EO) as a best method for commissioning children's services. As with the CTC and *Common Language* approaches, a well-conducted needs assessment is critical for identifying relevant outcomes. While OBA advocates a mixed-methods approach to needs assessment, it places an emphasis on understanding population trends to identify current and future community needs.

The OBA process begins by bringing commissioning stakeholders together to identify priority populations in need of improved services. These populations may involve a relatively small number of families (for example, parents who misuse drugs and alcohol) or a large group of children living in a particular geographic location. Planners identify the outcomes relevant for these populations and determine the extent to which these outcomes will add value to the entire community.

Once these outcomes have been agreed, strategic partners establish the community's baseline by considering time trends within community data to forecast what might happen if current services and budgets remain the same. Planners must then explain the 'story' (i.e. theory of change) underpinning the trends. After the stories are understood and agreed, strategic partners develop plans for reversing or 'turning the curve' of these trends. Each plan must include specific targets and outcomes, as well as identify agency partners who will work together to achieve the targeted outcomes. The partners then agree the activities necessary to achieve the outcomes and allocate community resources accordingly.

While these three models differ from each other in terms of the order in which commissioning activities take place, they all include similar processes (Figure 7.2).

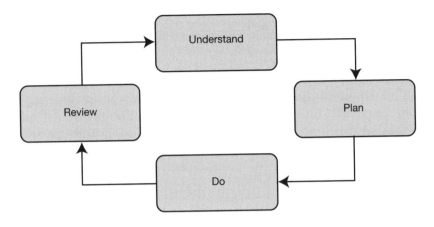

Figure 7.2 The commissioning cycle

1   **Understand** the needs of the community and the outcomes the services aim to achieve. Understanding involves having good information on population-level outcomes and the needs and wants of families living in the community.
2   **Plan** services that address the needs, priorities and outcomes identified through the needs assessments. These plans should draw from all of the resources available within the community, including funding, workforce and facilities. There should also be a good match between the plans and the needs of the community (Chinman et al. 2004).
3   **Do** through the implementation of evidence-based services that are matched to the needs of parents and children identified in the needs assessment.
4   **Review** through the use of robust monitoring systems that enable service providers to understand whether their plans and activities have achieved community-wide change.

The processes underpinning the four phases of the commissioning cycle are described in greater detail below.

Understanding community needs

Using population data to conduct a needs assessment

In order to understand the needs of a community, stakeholders involved in the delivery of children's services must have a thorough and accurate understanding of their community. This understanding is facilitated by a well-designed and -conducted needs assessment that should fulfill the following three objectives:

• Profile the community in terms of its strengths and weaknesses, so that priority outcomes can be identified

- Provide an objective point of view to reduce the tension that can occur between strategic partners competing for resources
- Provide a baseline from which progress can be measured.

A well-designed needs assessment should include data from multiple sources – including population-level data and data collected through the monitoring and evaluation of services (Chinman et al. 2004). Box 7.5 provides a list of the kinds of information communities collect about their population. Cox and Hughes (2007) suggest that population-level data can be conceptualized as a community's 'outcomes'.

When starting a community needs assessment, it is good to consider first the most recent data a community has on itself. For example, a school may have just published a five-year report on educational outcomes, or a hospital may have completed a study on the use of its accident and emergency services. Health services also keep statistics on births, immunization rates, breastfeeding and smoking.

Census data also contains ward-level or community-level demographics, including employ-ment rates, birth rates, a population's age, housing mobility, housing structure, family struc-ture and ethnic minority representation. In the US, the Census Bureau provides information about population trends, as well as maps that link population characteristics to geographical areas. In the UK, census data can be accessed at National Statistics Online, which includes ward-level data, as well as GIS mapping software that allows users to observe population trends on a geographic basis. The CTC, *Common Language* and OBA approaches also include methods for consulting various sources of population data to profile a community's outcomes.

Once community-level data has been collected, it is helpful to compare it to national and international trends regarding children's wellbeing. This exercise further enables commis-sioning stakeholders to consider the community's strengths and weaknesses within the context of its country's and international standards for children's wellbeing.

Box 7.5: Examples of community-level 'outcomes'

- Overall level of deprivation
- Unemployment rates
- Child population
- Low birth rates
- Teenage pregnancies
- Accident and emergency rates
- Child protection statistics
- Rates of antisocial behavior
- School exclusions
- Educational achievement and attainment
- Single-parent households
- Percentage of families from black and minority ethnic communities
- Mobility
- Availability of housing

Understand the views of parents and children

A community needs assessment is never complete without the views of its resident parents and children. Such exercises are particularly important for understanding how the 'felt' and 'expressed' needs of residents may differ from the needs identified in population data (Petersen and Alexander 2001). For example, comparisons between local data and national data may suggest that a community's crime rate is relatively low. However, community members may still perceive community crime as a problem. For this reason, it is good practice for authorities to routinely consider the views of its residents through community consultation exercises. Examples of consultation exercises include information road shows (that promote services while gathering the views of parents and children), community consultation events, surveys conducted with children in schools and door-to-door surveys conducted with parents and children.

Door-to-door surveys are arguably the best way of obtaining an understanding of parents' felt needs in a way that is representative of all families living within a community. Surveys conducted in schools are also an excellent way of obtaining representative information from children. Surveys have the additional advantage of yielding information that can be quantitatively analyzed and used as a baseline from which to monitor change. Both the CTC and *Common Language* approaches include methods for conducting community-wide and school-based surveys with children and parents.

Focus groups and consultation events are best used when the needs of smaller priority groups (e.g. fathers, parents with disabilities or parents from ethnic minorities) must be assessed (Utting 2009). This is because door-to-door surveys are designed to capture the views of the majority of parents, and thus smaller groups will be less well represented. Focus groups and consultation events should never be used as a substitute for conducting a door-to-door survey, however. Parents who attend consultation events rarely represent the views of the entire community, but rather those who are the least vulnerable and most vocal.

Understand the views of service providers and community organizations

When assessing a community's need, it is also considered good practice to routinely solicit the views of service providers and frontline staff. These individuals are in a good position to know who is and is not accessing their services and where further provision is needed. A good way of systematically collecting the views of service providers is through a service audit that 'maps' local services through the use of a survey that asks providers where their service is located, what they offer, who their target audience is, how much it costs, its demand (e.g. how often does it run, who attends and is there a waiting list) and where further provision is needed.

A well-conducted service audit can provide valuable information about community resources, as well as an understanding of the strengths and weaknesses in service provision. This information is vital for making decisions regarding where additional resources might be needed and where services should be decommissioned.

Identify groups of parents and children with specific needs

Once the sources of data have been identified, it is possible to identify specific areas of need. The *Common Language* method accomplishes this through an exercise entitled 'matching needs to services' whereby stakeholders involved in the delivery of children's services audit their case files and then meet to analyze the data. Although need groups will vary across communities, Tunnard (2002) has identified 12 'need groups' commonly identified through the *Common Language* matching exercise (Table 7.4).

Table 7.4 Typical 'need groups' of parents (adapted from Tunnard 2002)

Primary need	Description of need
Practical support	Parents seeking practical advice regarding their children or personal matters, including housing, day care, finance, etc.
Confident parenting	Parents wanting more confidence in dealing with temporary and common parenting issues, such as caring for an infant, dealing with temper tantrums, establishing household routines or coping with the common challenges of adolescence or young adulthood.
Adult conflict	Parents seeking relationship advice, especially in the area of conflict resolution and/or issues pertaining to children's living arrangements in situations involving divorce or separation.
Much improved care	Parents who are at risk of neglecting their children by not attending to their physical needs, including their hygiene and/or physical health. Parents may require an understanding of how to adequately care for their child and may need intensive support for a long period of time.
Parent–child relationships	Families need support in how to resolve conflicts between parents and children. Parents and children require improved communication and listening skills and strategies for resolving conflict in a non-violent and -abusive manner.
Emotional/ mental health issues	Parents struggling with their own mental health problems require support in attending to the emotional needs of their children. Mental health problems may range from depression or coping with life crises, to severe and enduring mental difficulties. This category also includes parents seeking help for dealing with a child who has emotional difficulties.
Physical health/ disability	Parents in this category may be coping with a physical illness or disability. Physical problems can range from physical and learning disabilities to a long-term health condition, such as asthma, or a terminal illness. Support may range from needing equipment to increase mobility, to help managing in the home and support in managing their illness.
Improve child's behavior	Parents require help to improve a child's behavior. Child behavioral issues may or may not be related to a difficult parent–child relationship. The primary focus is to control a child's antisocial behavior, reduce conflict at home and/ or improve attendance at school and academic performance. Parents may also need support for dealing with the police and juvenile justice system.
Loss or trauma	Parents falling into this category need support in coping with current or past traumatic events, including sexual or physical abuse, the bereavement of a close family member, managing a difficult separation or divorce, adoption breakdown, racial conflict or war.
Immediate protection	This category involves parents who are abusing or neglecting their child and his or her protection is an immediate concern. Once the child has been removed from harm, other family needs can be addressed.
Alcohol and drug misuse	Parents require support in reducing and/or stopping their drug and/or alcohol use, as well as in caring for their children.
Asylum seekers	Parents require specific support for managing problems related to their asylum status, including social isolation, poverty, housing and language difficulties. Parents within this category may also require support in coming to terms with traumatic events such as war or separation from loved ones.

O'Connell et al. (2009) stress that children's needs must also be considered in terms of developmental risks described in Table 7.2. Both CTC and *Common Language* make use of a developmental framework for capturing information about community-level risk and protective factors, which can then be used to identify developmentally appropriate interventions for reducing these risks.

Plan

Develop a strategy that identifies priorities and resources

Once a community's needs have been assessed and need groups have been identified, it is possible to establish baseline indicators from which to measure change. The CTC model advocates using findings from the standardized CTC youth survey to establish a baseline. The OBA approach recommends that, to the extent possible, baselines should be understood in terms of trends over time, rather than time-specific data points. Box 7.6 provides an example of how the UK city of Birmingham used the *Common Language* approach to identify needs and establish a baseline.

Box 7.6: Birmingham's *Brighter Futures* strategy

Birmingham is the UK's second-largest city and the largest local authority in Europe, consisting of over one million residents. Ethnic minority groups represent one-third of the total population and one-half of the quarter million child population. Unemployment is twice the national average and single parent households are four times the national average. In order to improve the wellbeing of Birmingham's children, the council used the *Common Language* approach (Box 7.3) to develop a five-year strategy to improve outcomes specific to the city's unique needs. The *Common Language* process begins by helping community planners to assess their community's needs and identify priorities for change.

Understand
Birmingham council brought together 35 stakeholders representing over 200 practitioners involved in the delivery of children's services to work together over nine days to develop a five-year strategy for children's services. In order to understand the needs of the city's children and parents, the team consulted information from the following sources:

- Community-level data
- Findings from a wellbeing survey conducted with a representative sample of 500 parents of children under the age of 6
- Findings from an online survey with over 6,000 children aged 7 to 18
- Focus groups
- A review of national policy
- An audit of staff capacity
- Research evidence of what works.

Plan

Through this exercise, the Birmingham team identified six priority areas:

- *Physical health:* Population data suggested that children's physical health was generally consistent with the majority of children living in England, but there were a number of areas of concern, including high infant mortality rates and high levels of teenage pregnancy and obesity.
- *Behavior:* Parents had concerns about the behavior and anxiety of just under one-fifth of all 5-year-olds. Seventeen per cent of 7- to 18-year-olds had an increased likelihood of a conduct disorder. Community data also revealed that rates of conduct problems were higher than the national average.
- *Emotional health:* Eight per cent of 7- to 18-year-olds had an increased likelihood of problems with anxiety and depression.
- *Literacy and numeracy:* The strategy team identified a link between children's behavioral problems and problems at school. By improving children's literacy and numeracy, the team assumed that there might be an additional pay-off in terms of children's behavior and emotional health.
- *Social literacy:* Findings from the survey with children also suggested that there were more peer problems than elsewhere in the country.
- *Job skills:* The strategy team identified a link between children's literacy and numeracy skills and their social literacy in improving their ability to successfully find a job in early adulthood.

The strategy team then considered the priorities within the context of children's development to identify where services could be enhanced through the implementation of evidence-based interventions. The team was also keen to provide a mix of services at each level of need – starting with universally available support through schools to specialist services provided by mental health professionals.

Through this exercise, the team matched the following interventions to the following priorities:

Priority	Intervention
All six priorities	*Family–Nurse Partnership* (FNP)
Social literacy	PATHS
Behavior	*Incredible Years / Teen Triple P*
Emotional wellbeing	*Triple P / Teen Triple P*

The team also identified the need for evidence-based services for families with complex or high needs, as well as universal interventions for all families. The team is therefore now investigating the feasibility of offering FFT to families with high needs. Plans are also being considered to offer the media-based version of *Triple P* so that all parents can receive advice regarding common parenting issues.

Do

In order to improve the commissioning process, Birmingham's Children and Young People's Board established a joint commissioning framework to decide which services would be jointly supported by funding agencies across the city. The framework aims to ensure that all providers have the same opportunity to offer services that have evidence of working in the priority areas. In doing so, the commissioning framework has set standards for how each service will be evaluated as part of its commissioning arrangements. Services that cannot provide evidence of adding value within one of the six priority areas will be decommissioned.

Birmingham has also improved its project management routines to ensure that services are delivered on time and to a high standard. To this end, services must provide information on their costs. Systems have also been put into place to ensure that evidence-based programs are properly supervised and delivered with fidelity.

The City of Birmingham has also developed an audit tool to assess the skills and qualifications of its parenting workforce, in order to ensure that they are adequately prepared to deliver evidence-based parenting interventions. The information gained through this exercise is then used to plot the training needs of the entire local workforce. Practitioners with a Bachelor's qualification or higher in a helping profession are identified for training in specific evidence-based programs, such as *Triple P* or the *Incredible Years*. Practitioners with less than a Bachelor's qualification in a helping profession are nominated for core skills training in working with parents. Birmingham council also provides training in the implementation of the *Common Assessment Framework* (see Box 5.3) to everyone involved in parenting work.

Review

The City of Birmingham has also introduced a robust monitoring system to capture outcome data on all of its children. The impact of its strategy will additionally be assessed through the wellbeing survey that will be conducted after the strategy has been in place for five years. To this end, the city has funded several studies involving a comparison group on the implementation of the *Triple P* and *Incredible Years* programs. Evidence-based services will also undergo **cost–benefit analyses** based on the WSIPP model and **benefit realization** processes will be used to monitor the progress of the five-year strategy and make real-time adjustments when necessary.

Once a baseline has been established, priorities can be identified and broken down into achievable milestones and targets. Priorities should also be **operationalized** into specific activities and behaviors. For example, a priority of 'improving parents' confidence' might be defined in terms of specific behaviors, such as their confidence in accessing community services or by measuring change through the use of a standardized assessment of parental self-esteem. No matter how this is done, there should be a clear and logical link between parents' behaviors and the community's identified priorities and outcomes.

Once priorities have been agreed and operationalized, strategies for meeting these priorities can be identified and targets set. A good commissioning strategy should also specify which partners will deliver against the targets and how they will be measured.

These planning principles can be applied to the case example provided in Box 7.7. In this instance, a community's needs assessment observed that rates of acquisitive crime were going up in the area, especially among youths between the ages of 13 and 16. Statistics from local schools also indicated an increase in truancy rates. The parents' consultation further identified youth crime as an issue.

When analyzing these trends, the commissioning team observed that the crime rates increased shortly after a new housing estate was built. The estate consisted mostly of one- and two-bedroom units that were occupied predominantly by single-parent families. The commissioning team believed that some of the parents living within these units might be struggling to parent their adolescent children effectively. This assumption is supported by police records that indicate that many of the recent arrests involve youth living in the new units. The local authority has thus developed a 'story' that has linked the housing estate to the crime rates (Figure 7.3).

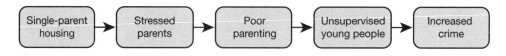

Figure 7.3   Story explaining crime rates

Through this exercise the commissioners identify the housing estate as contributing to the recent increase in crime and are in a position to consider how to reverse this trend through its local service strategy. As it develops its strategy, the commissioning team first considers the resources and services currently available within its community. In doing so, it observes that resources are available through a housing improvement strategy. It also sees that a local leisure center exists several blocks away from the housing estate. The center currently offers a wide range of activities, but all of them charge money and very few of them target young people specifically.

The commissioners agree that while both of these resources are likely to benefit the community more generally, neither one specifically addresses the needs of parents, which they believe are at the heart of the negative trend in youth crime. The commissioning team believes that it has thus identified a gap in its service provision that can be filled by applying funds to a parenting intervention with evidence of reducing youth crime. The commissioners then develop a plan that links the parenting support group to its local priority of crime reduction. Table 7.5 provides an example of how this can be done, linking the parenting group to the local priority, national indicators (within the UK), specific outputs and longer-term outcomes.

Plan services

Cox and Hughes (2007) identify a number of areas of good practice when planning services:

- Services should be commissioned by need – not by the availability of resources
- The planning of services should be mapped to specific, area-wide outcomes
- Commissioning should include preventive services
- Service plans should also include the specifics of how the service should be delivered, including an implementation action plan
- Service plans should include their intended outcomes and how they will be measured
- Planning should allow for risk and innovation.

Chinman et al. (2004) also note that services 'fit' within communities. A good fit implies that services reflect the values and practices of the community, as well as the community's needs. In addition, a community must be 'ready' for the intervention. Community readiness is discussed in greater depth at the end of this chapter.

In the case example provided in Box 7.7, the commissioning team has wisely adhered to all of these guidelines. Its strategy is driven by the needs of the local community and not its available resources. In addition, it has carefully mapped service activities to specific and measurable area-wide outcomes that have been agreed at the strategic level. Its strategy includes a mixture of preventive and remedial services and it is noteworthy that not all of them are evidence-based. Table 7.5 provides an abbreviated overview of the parenting support offered within the community, including only those services that involve parents in their delivery models. Table 7.6 demonstrates how these combined services constitute a portfolio of universal and targeted support.

Box 7.7: Developing an evidence-based commissioning strategy

'Trenton' is a hypothetical urban community with a child population of approximately 14,000 representing 5,700 households. A commissioning team has been brought together to determine how resources can best be used to improve outcomes for the children and families living in the community. The team includes representatives from education, health, youth justice and social work. With support from an external consultant, the team conducts a needs assessment that combines data on population-wide trends with findings from a door-to-door survey conducted with parents, as well as a survey conducted with children in schools. This exercise identifies a number of strengths and weaknesses within the community. Areas of economic stability and afflu-ence characterize the west side, whereas on the east side there are several areas of economic deprivation. In particular, social work data have identified several child maltreatment 'hotspots' within several housing estates on the east border of the community. The hospital admissions due to unintentional and deliberate injuries are particularly high within this population. Most troubling are the recent deaths of two toddlers who fell out of the windows of their housing units.

Educational data also reveal an uneven profile across the schools. There are six preschools. Two of these schools are located in the more affluent neighborhoods. The heads of these schools are particularly good at accessing various funding streams to improve the schools' curriculum and facilities. The children leaving these preschools tend to do well once they enter primary school. While the educational attainment across the community is average to above average, there are several primary schools where standardized test scores are well below the national mean. The language and literacy scores are particularly low in two primary schools, where they are below the national average, even for deprived communities. School officials believe that these rates are low because they are located in areas with a high concentration of ethnic minority families who speak English as a second language.

While community crime rates are only slightly higher than the national average, police records have identified a number of districts where there are high levels of acquisitive crimes committed by young people between the ages of 13 and 17. Many of these individuals are first-time offenders. There are also higher-than-average truancy rates in two secondary schools.

This community profile has led the commissioning team to identify the following priorities:

- Reduce the number of children suspected of child maltreatment living within designated hotspots
- Improve the educational attainment in the primary schools where it is particularly low
- Reduce the truancy rates in the designated schools
- Reduce the number of first-time offenders.

Findings from the door-to-door survey suggest that breastfeeding rates are higher than the national average, but so are smoking rates – and these rates are particularly high in the most deprived areas. In addition, parents responding to the survey have identified the reduction of youth crime as a top priority, along with a lack of opportunities for their children to play outdoors. This survey has confirmed some of the priorities identified through the needs assessment conducted with the population and has also identified two further priorities:

- Reduce smoking rates amongst parents
- Create opportunities for children to play outside.

In order to better understand the available resources, the commissioning team maps the family support already available in the community. From this exercise, the team sees that there are a number of parenting groups already running. While most of these services are morning drop-ins, the team observes that *Strengthening Families 10–14* is being offered within one of the schools in a more affluent part of the community. It also sees that there is a non-evidence-based parenting support group being provided by a voluntary organization. Although this organization is not faith based, the program is delivered twice annually out of a church. The team additionally discovers that *Incredible Years* BASIC used to run out of a preschool, but is no longer being offered because one of the practitioners has changed posts (*Incredible Years* requires two practitioners to co-facilitate the program). The commissioning team is also disappointed to discover that there are no evidence-based programs for the parents of young people linked to the youth offending team, although MTFC is being offered as part of pilot scheme for children who would otherwise be put in out-of-home placement.

The commissioning team discovers that there are no outreach activities available for vulnerable families living within the community, although the council pays for a local voluntary agency to run a baby massage course out of a community center. The team also discovers that the preschools have good monitoring systems in place which allow them to track children's progress after leaving their services.

With all of this information, the commissioning team is now in a position to identify priorities and strategically plan its services. By working closely with representatives from health, education, social work, youth offending teams, voluntary organizations and adult education, a portfolio of services are identified, as described below.

Priority 1: Reduce child maltreatment and injuries. Nursing teams will conduct three 'welcome' home visits with parents of children under the age of two living within the child maltreatment hotspots. During these visits, parents will be told about community services, be provided with child safety advice and be invited to participate in a smoking reduction program. During these visits, the nurses will use a standardized assessment to determine whether parents may be at risk of maltreating their children. Families identified as at risk for child maltreatment will be referred to an *Incredible Years Toddler* program that will be delivered by four of the nurses. Health records are used to estimate that there will be 30 new births within these estates each year, which will enable the nurses to estimate their caseloads. The commissioning team has also procured funding to pilot the VIPP program with families with infants living in the hotspot areas.

The commissioning team also asks the voluntary agency sponsoring the baby massage group if it would be interested in evaluating its service to determine whether it might also improve parents' sensitivity in a way that could reduce child maltreatment. The agency refuses, saying it is sufficiently evaluated because all of the parents attending it like it. The commissioner decides not to include this service in her strategy, as it does not contribute to the area's priorities and the agency has refused to evaluate its efficacy.

Priority 2: Improve language and literacy scores in schools where they are assessed to be lower than the national average. In order to address the low language and literacy scores in two primary schools, the commissioning team asks two teacher trainees to conduct a literature review to determine whether they can identify an evidence-based program which aims to improve children's literacy skills. The team identifies a pre-literacy program that uses picture books to teach parents how to do 'dialogical' reading with their children. Although its research evidence is not conclusive, there is fairly consistent evidence to suggest that the program improves children's pre-literacy skills within ethnic minority populations (Whitehurst et al. 1988, 1994a, 1994b, 1999, Zevenbergen and Whitehurst 2003). The team is also pleased to learn that the program is easy to implement, as training can be achieved via videotapes that are easily purchased over the internet. The commissioning team therefore agrees that it is worth implementing on a trial basis with careful monitoring. In making arrangements to implement the reading program, the commissioning team is pleased to learn that it can access free books via a library funding scheme. It also identifies workers from an adult learning center to provide teachers who can implement the program during mornings at preschools in the areas with high ethnic minority concentrations. The teachers are then paired with two speech and language therapists who are released half a day a week to help deliver the program. Children are referred into the program through a standardized language assessment delivered by the speech and language therapists. Because there are more children than there are resources available to deliver the program, 3-year-olds are randomly assigned into a treatment and non-treatment group. The progress of the children participating in the program is then assessed at the end with the same standardized language measure.

Priority 3: Reduce youth crime. To address the rising rates of youth crime in the community, the commissioning team decides to get the previous *Incredible Years* BASIC program up and running in preschools in the areas with the highest crime rates. A teacher from the preschool agrees to go on *Incredible Years* BASIC training so she can deliver the groups with the other practitioner who was previously trained. The commissioning team also tries to convince the teacher delivering the *Strengthening Families 10–14* training in the affluent school to offer two further courses in one of the schools with high exclusion rates. The affluent school's head refuses to release the practitioner for this, however. The commissioning team does, nevertheless, get the practitioner and the school head to agree to collect pre and post measures on *Strengthening Families 10–14* so that they can monitor progress. The commissioning team also secures funding so that *Triple P* can be implemented in schools in the neighborhoods where the youth crime rates are the highest. Practitioners will receive training in *Triple P Teen* and *Triple P Group*, so that families with teens who have truanted or committed a crime can receive one-to-one support.

The commissioning team also works with the voluntary agency to determine how the non-evidence-based parenting group could support its community. It works out a deal with the voluntary organization whereby the local authority will support the implementation of the parenting groups under the condition that the organization properly evaluates it using standardized pre- and post-treatment measures. A local school also agrees to refer parents with pupils who have identified conduct problems into the program. In addition, the voluntary agency agrees to send its practitioner for *Triple P* training, so that she can better understand the similarities and differences between her program and the *Triple P* model.

Priority 4: Improve physical fitness through increased opportunities for outdoor play. In order to address community concerns about the lack of opportunities to play, the commissioning team has made arrangements to run a sports scheme out of the leisure center on Saturday mornings. Information on children's physical fitness will be gathered, with the aim of assessing the feasibility of the program for combating childhood obesity. Should the program indicate promise, it will be offered in schools across the community.

In order to monitor its strategy, the commissioning team looks into the possibility of expanding the preschools' database. The commissioning team convinces the head of children's services to invest further in this system and establishes methods for collecting data on the parents participating in her parenting services and monitoring their progress through standardized measures. It also initiates talks with service managers working out of local mental health agencies to consider ways in which evidence-based services can be commissioned for young people who are already in the youth offending system.

A key priority identified in the strategy is the reduction of child maltreatment. The commissioning team has therefore identified a mixture of preventive and targeted services to reduce the number of maltreatment-related hospital admissions and entries onto the child protection register. FNP is not available in the area, so the team, in partnership with stakeholders from health and social services, designs its own home visiting service that aims to reduce the abuse and neglect of very young children living in the area's most deprived housing estates. The service will be carefully monitored to observe the extent to which it can improve short-term outcomes that could be associated with decreases in child maltreatment rates. The commissioning team will also investigate the possibility of offering FNP in the future.

Table 7.5 Priorities, indicator, baseline and improvement targets

Targets	Baseline (2007)	Improvement targets in 2000			Activities / Outputs	Outcomes	Partners	Referral routes	Delivery dates
		08/09	09/10	10/11					
Priority 1: Reduce number of children on the child protection register									
Hospital admissions caused by unintentional and deliberate injuries to children and young people.	112	<90	<70	<50	Provide an extended package of home visiting during the first year after a birth of a new baby living within designated housing estates, providing home safety, child care and smoking cessation advice, with a target of reaching 50 new families annually.	Home safety advice provided to all visited families. Measurable improvements in mothers' knowledge of child care, maternal sensitivity and disciplinary strategies as measured via standardized measures. Increased access to health care and community services.	Health Social work	Families will be identified at birth via address	Sep. 07–indefinite
					Offer *Incredible Years Toddler* program to mothers with children aged 1–3 screened as 'at risk' in designated neighborhoods. Three courses will be run three times annually in three communities, totaling nine courses reaching 110 parents.	Measurable improvements of parents' wellbeing, disciplinary strategies and sensitivity. Measurable improvements of parents' self-reports of their children's behavior.	Health Social work	GPs Home visiting nurses Self-referral	Sep. 07–indefinite
Children becoming the subject of a Child Protection Plan for a second or subsequent time.	92	<80	<70	<60	Offer VIPP to parents with an infant where there is a child protection concern.	Measurable improvements of parents' wellbeing, and sensitivity. Improvements in children's attachment status.	Nursing Social work	CAF Child protection plans	Ongoing

Continued overleaf

Targets	Baseline (2007)	Improvement targets in 2000			Activities		Partners	Referral routes	Delivery dates
		08/09	09/10	10/11	Outputs	Outcomes			
Timeliness of placements of looked after children adopted following an agency decision that the child should be placed for adoption. Stability of placements of looked after children: number of moves. Stability of placements of looked after children: length of placement.					Continue with MTFC pilots.				
Priority 2: Improve health									
16+ current smoking rate prevalence.	45% of parent population	<43%	<40%	<35%	Provide an extended package of home visiting during the first year after a birth of a new baby living within designated housing estates, providing home safety, child care and smoking cessation advice, with a target of reaching 50 new families annually.	A target of 10 mothers per year will stop smoking and this information will be compared against area-wide statistics. Progress towards smoking cessation will be recorded via smoking diaries, and peak flow assessments that will measure lung capacity at various points throughout the home visits.	Health Social work	Families will be identified at birth via address.	Sep. 07– indefinite

Priority 3: Improve educational attainment

Targets	Baseline (2007)	Improvement targets in 2000			Activities / Outputs	Outcomes	Partners	Referral routes	Delivery dates
		08/09	09/10	10/11					
Achievement of at least 78 points across the Early Years Foundation Stage with at least 6 in each of the scales in Personal Social and Emotional Development and Communication, Language and Literacy.	31% demonstrating proficiency in CLL	35%	40%	45%	Implement pilot study of dialogical reading program in schools where literacy attainment is low. Children aged 3 assessed to have low English vocabulary will be randomly assigned to a dialogical reading program aimed at the children and their parents that meets once a week for 6 weeks. The pilot will take place with 20 families and be repeated if successful.	Significantly improved vocabulary and phonological awareness skills as measured via standardized pre- and post-program measures.	Education Adult learning	3-year-olds at designated preschools will be assessed and randomly assigned into the program	Jan. 08–Apr. 08 and then repeated if program is effective
Secondary school persistent absence rate.	45	<40	<35	<30	Provide standard *Triple P* individualized sessions to parents whose children have high absence rates – reaching 20 parents in each school.	Significant improvements in school attendance and behavior, as reported via standardized behavioral measures given to the children's teachers.	Education YOT	The parents of children with high truancy rates will be asked to participate in the program.	Jan. 08 and ongoing

Continued overleaf

Targets	Baseline (2007)	Improvement targets in 2000			Activities	Outcomes	Partners	Referral routes	Delivery dates
		08/09	09/10	10/11	Outputs				
Priority 4: Reduce area crime									
First-time entrants into the youth justice system.	1,143	<1,150	<1,050	<950	Deliver eight sessions of *Group Triple P* to parents of children aged 8–13 in two target schools annually – four sessions per school, reaching 48 parents in each school.	A significant increase in parents' positive reports of their children's behavior, as measured by pre- and post-treatment comparisons of the SDQ is achieved.	Police Education YOTs		
					Deliver two sessions of *Incredible Years* BASIC annually via preschools in neighborhoods experiencing the highest crime rates.	A significant increase in parents' positive reports of their children's behavior, as measured by pre- and post-treatment comparisons of the SDQ is achieved.	Health Education	Preschool referrals	Jan. 08
					Deliver two sessions of *Strengthening Families 10–14* annually via extended school where it is currently implemented.	A significant increase in parents' positive reports of their children's behavior, as measured by pre- and post-treatment comparisons of the SDQ is achieved.	Education YOTs	Referral via school	Ongoing
					Deliver two sessions of voluntary sector parenting skills course to parents of children entering secondary school, reaching 30 parents per year.	Significant improvements in parents' disciplinary strategies and self-confidence; improvements in their perceptions of their children's behavior.	Education Voluntary sector	Self-referral	Jan. 08– ongoing if effective

Priority 5: Improve outdoor opportunities for play

Targets	Baseline (2007)	Improvement targets in 2000			Activities / Outputs	Outcomes	Partners	Referral routes	Delivery dates
		08/09	09/10	10/11					
Obesity among primary school age children in Year 6.	33%	30%	29%	28%	Use lottery funds to run a weekend sports scheme to operate on Saturday mornings out of all primary schools. There will be activities for parents and children. The program will be open to all children, but there will be a referral process for children who are obese.	Collect health information on children participating in the scheme, as well as physical fitness skills via standardized measures at the beginning of each school term.	Education Health	Self-referral Referral by school nurse	Jun. 08– ongoing

Table 7.6 Portfolio of parenting support

Service/Program	Evidence-based	Non-evidence-based
Tier 1: Universal		
Saturday morning sports scheme		✓
Parenting course for children entering secondary school		✓
Tier 2: Selected prevention		
Apartment estate home visiting scheme		✓
Incredible Years Toddler program	✓	
Incredible Years BASIC program	✓	
Dialogical parent–child reading program		✓
Strengthening Families 10–14	✓	
Group Triple P	✓	
Tier 3: Children in need/targeted early intervention		
Standard *Triple P*	✓	
Smoking cessation delivered via home visitors	✓	
VIPP	✓	
Tier 4: Children in need of protection		
Multidimensional Treatment Foster Care	✓	

Additional preventive services include the wider implementation of a parenting group aimed at parents of teenagers. The commissioning team has agreed to support this activity upon two conditions: 1) the facilitator works closely with local schools to target families with children entering middle school, 2) the voluntary agency will evaluate the program's effectiveness via pre and post measures with a comparison group. Funding for this evaluation is included in the voluntary agency's service budget.

Program innovation is supported in the strategy through the dialogical reading program that will be piloted for the first time within the UK. The service portfolio also includes a number of evidence-based programs, including VIPP, *Incredible Years Toddler* and BASIC, *Standard* and *Group Triple P*, and *Strengthening Families 10–14*.

Although not all of the services included in the commissioner's strategy are evidence-based they are performance-based. They all include a well-articulated delivery plan (including arrangements for appropriate training and supervision), specific referral routes and systems for measuring outcomes and tracking progress. The strategy also has an implementation action plan which includes delivery dates. These plans are included in the contractual agreements (also referred to as **service level agreements**) with the agencies delivering the services. Data collected via predetermined outcome measures will allow the commissioner to assess each service's efficacy and make comparisons across services. These comparisons will then inform the commissioning team's future commissioning and decommissioning decisions. It is noteworthy that the team has not included local drop-ins and adult services in its current strategy because these services do not contribute to any local priorities or national indicators, nor do they provide any outcome-based performance data.

It is also noteworthy that the commissioning team has included a number of short- and long-term goals in its strategy. Short-term goals include the close monitoring of the services that the commissioning team believes will contribute to short-term area-wide priorities. Longer-term goals include systems for understanding how all services contribute to the ongoing needs of the community, as well as methods for making them all evidence-based. The strategy also includes long-term goals for evidence-based provision targeting families with children already within the youth offending system. A good commissioning strategy should include an explanation of how short- and long- term goals will be addressed through the available resources.

Do

Determine commissioning arrangements

The commissioning process can begin once a strategy has been agreed and specific interventions have been identified. Commissioning processes are facilitated by effective governance structures which ensure that processes are fair and transparent. Effective governing bodies include representation from a wide variety of agencies, including voluntary organizations.

Trust within governing bodies is established through a shared understanding of community need and the extent to which the strategy is meeting these needs. Trust is additionally achieved through a history of positive partnership working (Audit Commission 2008). It is also considered good practice for commissioning teams to establish a set of working principles before the commissioning process begins. Box 7.8 provides an overview of commissioning principles advocated by the CSP (2009).

Additional examples of good commissioning principles include a commitment to joint commissioning, being inclusive in the tendering process, involving parents and children in the commissioning process and using outcome-based performance management frameworks. In

---

Box 7.8: Principles to guide the commissioning process (reprinted with permission from CSP 2009)

Commissioning decisions should be based on:

- Evidence of a favorable impact on outcomes and value for money
- Adherence to changing policy and government guidance
- Providing early intervention services at the earliest appropriate moment
- Agreeing to close the gap between those falling behind and the rest
- Sustaining stable relationships between key practitioners and vulnerable families
- Using open and transparent processes that build confident partnerships
- Using commissioning not just to retain existing services or commission new ones, but, where necessary, to decommission services which are inefficient, ineffective, inequitable or unsustainable
- Making all processes lean and aiming for continuous improvement
- Using contestability and packaging of work for small providers
- Providing challenge for all practitioners
- Taking account of value for money in all decisions
- Making use of shared processes.

the case example provided in Box 7.7 it is evident that services would only be included in the strategy if they had input from multiple agencies and were monitored against key outcomes.

Pooling budgets

If services are procured through a joint commissioning process, a system for pooling or aligning budgets should be established. This process begins by agencies involved in the commissioning process identifying all available funding streams. In some cases, the budgets are completely pooled and managed separately by a host agency. A less formal method of pooling budgets is by having all contributing agencies align their budgets. This takes place by partner agencies identifying all available funding streams, but keeping them separate in their individual agency budgets. Money is then aligned towards agreed joint outcomes, with agencies individually contributing to separate services. In the case example, the organizations aligned their budget and then separate agencies paid for separate services. Funding for the group for parents of teenagers came out of the participating schools' budget and the dialogical parenting group was to be paid for by the participating preschools.

Whatever the budgetary arrangements are, it is important that they are predetermined and completely transparent. Cox and Hughes (2007) observe that while a great deal of work is involved in setting up and managing pooled budgets, they tend to be more efficient in the long run. This is because pooled budgets provide greater fluidity in the commissioning of services, as each service contract does not require the separate negotiation of each contributing agency. They also facilitate spending on capital improvements, the co-location of staff and the joint delivery of services. Legal agreements are often required when establishing a pooled budget and the joint agencies will need to agree a host to manage it. The staff members involved in managing the budget are also likely to need training in budget administration. Because these processes take time to establish, many bodies start the commissioning process with aligned budgets, with the aim of pooling them once their partnership work is fully established (Audit Commission 2008).

Understand and develop the workforce

As noted in Chapter 5, evidence-based parenting interventions are more likely to be effective if they are delivered by appropriately trained and qualified practitioners. For this reason, commissioning stakeholders must ensure that the practitioners delivering evidence-based parenting support have the knowledge, experience and skills to deliver services effectively. Fixsen et al. (2010) observe that four factors are important for ensuring the competent delivery of evidence-based services: 1) staff selection, 2) staff training, 3) ongoing, on-the-job supervision and coaching and 4) regular assessments of staff performance. As described in Chapter 5, evidence-based program developers often specify the necessary skills, training, supervision and performance assessments necessary for the successful delivery of their programs. However, it is often up to the commissioning body to recruit practitioners with the right skill mix to deliver parenting interventions and assess their performance on a regular basis.

Research conducted within the US and UK suggests that it is often difficult to recruit appropriately trained and qualified practitioners because of shortfalls within the mental health workforce (IOM 2003, PwC 2006). In particular, findings from the ongoing evaluations of the National Academy for Parenting Practitioners evidence-based training offer (see Chapter 1 for an overview) observed that less than half of those attending training had a Bachelor's qualification and less than a third had a Bachelor's qualification or higher in a helping profession (PwC 2010, Asmussen et al. 2010). The lack of qualified practitioners attending training is attributed to shortfalls in the number of individuals trained to work with families more generally (PwC 2006).

Collectively, the above findings suggest that commissioning bodies need to assess the qualifications of their workforce before commissioning parenting services. The Birmingham Council has developed its own workforce audit tool to determine who might be suitable to deliver evidence-based parenting interventions, as described in Box 7.6.

The above research also suggests a role for governments and educational institutions in developing the workforce (Fixsen et al. 2009, O'Connell et al. 2004). A community on its own is unlikely to have the resources to create a fully qualified workforce and therefore national qualification and training efforts are necessary to ensure that sufficient numbers of qualified individuals are available to deliver effective mental health services. The Institute of Medicine (Annapolis Coalition on the Behavioral Health Workforce 2007, IOM 2003, 2006) has identified five 'levers for change' necessary for developing a fully qualified workforce:

- **Core competencies**: A set of core competencies and language should be identified and provided in training across all sectors involved in the delivery of services for parents and children. There should also be consistent methods to assess these competencies (IOM 2003).
- **National licensing and credentialing** standards should exist which make use of common examination procedures.
- **Accreditation standards** are also required to ensure consistency in the training and workforce practices. Training programs must be able to demonstrate that they are teaching a core set of competencies in order to receive accreditation.
- **Financing** is also necessary to pay for the necessary training for staff. This should be provided at both the national and local level.
- **Faculty development** should be an ongoing process to ensure that those teaching the practitioners understand the latest developments in the competencies and skills necessary to support parents and children. Faculty development requires both training and financial incentives to encourage ongoing professional development.

Commission services

Once the availability of the workforce has been assessed and accounted for, commissioning teams are in a position to commission services. Commissioning bodies vary in terms of their commissioning strategies – with some preferring a competitive tendering process and others favoring the preferred-supplier approach. Both of these strategies have advantages and disadvantages, depending upon the services being commissioned. Competitive tendering has the advantage of being inclusive and transparent, although it can also take up unnecessary time when it is clear that only a few providers have the capacity to deliver evidence-based parenting services. The preferred-supplier approach has the advantage of immediately engaging providers with the expertise for delivering specific kinds of services. The commissioning team in the case study relied on a preferred-supplier tendering process that enabled it to commission services by practitioners with the proper skill mix.

Before services are commissioned, a set of transparent rules should be established for the monitoring and evaluation of performance standards. Cox and Hughes (2007) advocate the use of highly specified contracts which include systems in place for describing the service and specifying how it will be delivered, as well as methods for determining outcome-based performance targets and measuring progress towards them. Evidence-based parenting serv-ices lend themselves well to such contracts, as they frequently have their own built-in systems for measuring parent and child outcomes. Highly specified contracts should also include forms for recording data and gathering user-satisfaction information. However, as noted in Chapter 6, user satisfaction data should not be used as a service outcome, nor should they be used as evidence of a service's efficacy. While user satisfaction can be used for quality assur-ance purposes, it does not verify whether the service has achieved its intended outcomes.

When negotiating a service contract or service level agreement, it is important to estab-lish methods for developing and monitoring services. In the example described in Box 7.7, systems were identified for referring families into the program and monitoring their progress. Each agreement also included pre-established targets and milestones for measuring progress. However, it should be noted that it is unlikely that all services will meet their performance targets even when they have been carefully pre-specified. For this reason, commissioning bodies need to have processes in place for determining how funding will be used to develop services that are underperforming and when decommissioning will be considered. Service providers should be willing to evaluate their own services and commissioner bodies may want to make extra funding available to enable them to do this. As noted in Chapter 6, it is considered good practice for providers to allocate between 5 and 10 per cent of their budget to the ongoing evaluation of their service.

Review

Monitor progress and evaluate success

Much has already been said about the monitoring of parenting interventions. Chapter 6 provides an example of how an area-wide evaluation strategy can be used to help strategic partners monitor their progress towards pre-specified targets and goals. Birmingham's *Brighter Futures* strategy (Box 7.5) is also underpinned by a centralized monitoring system which collects performance-related information on all agencies delivering evidence-based parenting programs. This information is then compared to key information routinely collected on all of the parents and children participating in the parenting groups. Parent-level information includes the reason for referral, family demographics and pre- and post-training measures of the key outcomes related to the program. Agency-level data includes the qualifications of the practitioners implementing parenting groups and the amount of supervision they receive. Parents are asked for their informed consent and are each assigned a unique identifica-tion number that ensures that their information is anonymized. The data is then held and managed in a central database that is configured to report against area-wide milestones and targets.

Birmingham's data management system is currently tracking only its evidence-based parenting support. However, Cox and Hughes (2007) believe similar systems can be used to assess the collective performance of all children's services. Effective data management is best accomplished through high-powered IT systems that are purpose-built in line with each local authority's reporting needs. As noted in Chapter 6, it is considered good practice to have a dedicated post or team to coordinate and oversee a community's data management and monitoring processes.

Making it happen

In the hypothetical case example provided in Box 7.7, the implementation of a coordinated strategy that addresses local priorities appears relatively easy. In real life, commissioning and implementing good-quality services is extremely hard work. Although the example in Box 7.7 is hypothetical, all of the services described were based upon real-life cases that were implemented through various agencies within a real council in north London. Some of these services were successful, whereas others failed well before the implementation stage. For example, the home visiting service failed because of a shortage in the health-visiting nurse workforce. The dialogical reading program also failed – not because of a shortage of suitably trained staff, but because of a lack of commitment from the head of the preschool, who ultimately refused to refer families into the program even though all the materials had been bought and the staff had been trained. The end result of the failed program was that some parents received free books, but no methods were used to ensure that they were given to the families that needed them the most. The parenting program run by the voluntary agency was also not implemented, because of a breakdown in the service level agreement negotiations.

The sports program was successful, however, and was subsequently expanded through schools across the council. However, no one knows the extent to which it has improved the health of children because the practitioners stopped collecting data, despite the fact that outcome measures were originally developed for the program. The council has also successfully implemented a number of evidence-based parenting programs, including *Strengthening Families 10–14*, which has been expanded to run in three schools. Funding has also been procured to implement FNP, which will be piloted in the areas identified as child maltreatment hotspots.

The council also abandoned its plans to expand its data management and monitoring systems. This means that the council cannot monitor the extent to which its children's services are contributing to community-wide outcomes, although data continues to be collected in conjunction with the evidence-based parenting programs, including *Triple P* and *Strengthening Families 10–14*. With the exception of FNP, the council also does not know whether its services are reaching the families who need them the most, because adequate referral systems have not been established and most of the participating families are self-referred.

The above example illustrates how a lack of commitment and good multi-agency relations frequently interferes with the delivery of good-quality services. Cox and Hughes (2007) observe that these problems can be overcome, however, if the following factors are in place:

- **A strong performance management culture**. This means having a robust performance management framework in place that is integrated into the authority's long-term strategies for children and families.
- **A skilled commissioning function**. This means that all individuals involved in the commissioning process know how to commission services and are supported by the relevant training and experience.
- **Excellent data and information management systems**. This includes good information management protocols and a commitment between agencies to share information.
- A commitment to conducting **a full and valid community needs assessment**, which includes the consultation of children and parents who are representative of the entire community.
- **Flexibility** within the system to shift resources when necessary to meet new priorities as they arise.

- **A common language** and understanding of commissioning that is shared by all commissioning partners.
- **Strong and effective leadership** that is capable of convincing others of the importance of the strategy.
- **A commitment towards new ways of working** shared by all agencies involved in the delivery of services for parents and children.
- **A clear vision for commissioning** that has buy-in from all partners.
- **Good working relationships and trust** between all partner agencies, which are developed through complete transparency throughout the commissioning process.

Implementing evidence-based parenting interventions

Intervention effectiveness versus implementation effectiveness

Once an evidence-based intervention has been commissioned, there is still no guarantee that it will be effective. As mentioned in previous chapters, evidence-based interventions must be implemented in a way that ensures that they are delivered to a high standard and with fidelity. Fixsen et al. (2005) characterize the distinction between the intervention and its implementation effectiveness as the 'what' and the 'how' of improved outcomes for parents and children. As Table 7.7 suggests, improved parent and child outcomes are achieved only when an effective program is implemented effectively. While program developers most often assume the responsibility for the 'what' of the intervention, communities and agencies must be responsible for the 'how' of its implementation.

Developing structures and infrastructures

Once an evidence-based intervention has been commissioned, it needs to be 'installed' within the agency that will implement it. Recall from Chapter 5 that evidence-based interventions are rarely effective if they have been adapted to fit the needs of the host agency. Instead, evidence-based interventions work best when agencies have altered their infrastructures to meet the intervention's delivery requirements. The National Implementation Research Network (NIRN 2008) has identified the following infrastructure changes common across most evidence-based interventions:

Table 7.7 The interaction of intervention effectiveness and implementation effectiveness (adapted from Fixsen et al. 2005)

| | | *Effectiveness of implementation practices* | |
		Effective	*Ineffective*
Effectiveness of intervention practices	*Effective*	Good implementation outcomes Positive outcomes for parents and children	Poor implementation outcomes Poor outcomes for parents and children
	Ineffective	Good implementation outcomes Poor outcomes for parents and children	Poor implementation outcomes Poor outcomes for parents and children

- Securing new funding streams to ensure the sustainability of the intervention
- Realigning current staff and recruiting new staff to ensure that practitioners have the appropriate qualifications to deliver evidence-based services
- Support in the form of time to attend pre-service training and receive on-the-job training through supervision
- Securing the space to deliver the intervention
- Purchasing and implementing the necessary technology to monitor the outcomes of evidence-based interventions
- Establishing appropriate interagency relationships to maximize resources and reduce redundancies between agencies
- Developing good referral routes between agencies to ensure that interventions are reaching the families who need them the most.

Core implementation components

Once an evidence-based intervention has been installed, ongoing implementation processes must also be in place to optimize its efficacy. Fixsen et al. (2009) have identified seven integrated processes (also referred to as core implementation components) necessary for the successful implementation of evidence-based interventions (Figure 7.4).

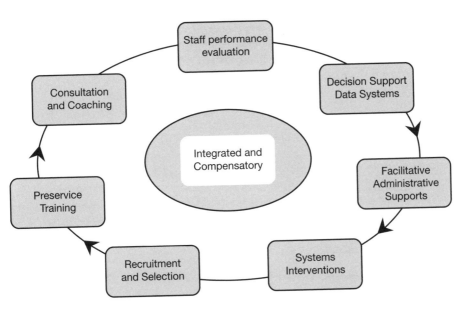

Figure 7.4 Core implementation components (reprinted with permission from Fixsen et al. 2009)

Fixsen et al. observe that these seven components are integrated and not consecutive. In addition, it is likely that stronger components may potentially compensate for relatively weaker ones. For example, weak recruitment and selection processes (due to inadequacies in the workforce) can potentially be compensated for by strong coaching and supervision processes.

Blase et al. (2010) further observe that staff selection, training and coaching are all **competency drivers** which contribute to high performance evaluations linked to an intervention's fidelity and effectiveness. Decision support data systems, facilitative administrative supports and systems interventions are all examples of **organization drivers** which also contribute to the effective delivery of evidence-based interventions.

Competency drivers and the use of purpose-built data management systems have all been discussed in depth in previous sections of this chapter and Chapters 5 and 6. 'Facilitative administrative supports' refers to leadership in the organization of staff and the development of policies and procedures to support the implementation process. 'Systems interventions' refers to strategies for working with external systems to ensure that funding, organizational and human resources remain available to support the ongoing implementation of the intervention. More information about how these components support the implementation process can be found at http://www.fpg.unc.edu/~nirn/implementation/01_implementationdefined.cfm.

NIRN (2008) notes that host agencies implementing evidence-based interventions assume the responsibility for coordinating and managing the quality of the core implementation components. For example, the host agency must oversee the selection of personnel to deliver the program and negotiate funding from external systems. However, many evidence-based interventions also provide support for the implementation process through **purveyor** arms which work with agencies to facilitate the implementation process (Fixsen et al. 2009, 2010). For example, MST, MTFC and NFP all offer implementation support through national centers which offer training, consultation and advice.

Fixsen et al. (2005) note that intervention implementation is a multi-stage process, sometimes requiring up to four years before evidence-based services are fully effective. Figure 7.5 provides an overview of the six stages of program implementation.

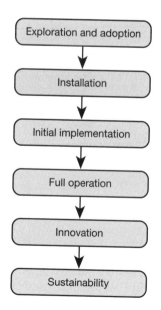

Figure 7.5 Six stages of program implementation

The first stage, **exploration**, occurs when communities and host agencies consider what is needed by conducting a needs assessment and analyzing the findings. Methods for conducting a community needs assessment have been described previously in this chapter. **Installation** involves the structural changes required to adopt and install an evidence-based intervention, which have also been discussed previously. **Initial implementation** refers to the first stage of a program's implementation, where the host agency and practitioners are learning how to implement the intervention as they implement it for the first time. **Full implementation** occurs when the intervention is fully operational, delivered by competent staff who are delivering services to families from the appropriate target population. **Innovation** occurs when the program has been in operation for some time and new challenges occur because of the program has expanded to new settings, or there have been changes in the staffing and funding streams. In this respect, innovation should not be confused with adaptation or a loss of fidelity, but should instead be viewed as small changes that reflect larger organizational changes. **Sustainability** refers to the systems developed to help services maintain efficacy in the event of large organizational and staff changes. Such systems include access to diversified funding streams, ongoing staff training and development of robust monitoring systems. More information about the stages of implementation can be found at the NIRN website at: http://www.fpg.unc.edu/~nirn/default.cfm.

Readiness

Evidence-based interventions are unlikely to be adopted by communities and agencies unless there is a shared understanding that such services are needed (NIRN 2008). In other words, communities and agencies must be 'ready' for the changes described in the previous sections. Blase et al. (2010) observe that 'readiness' is not something that can be created through incentives (e.g. government funding) or sanctions. Rather, communities must be aware that there is a need for common practices and services to change. Edwards et al. (2000) have observed that community 'readiness' can be conceptualized in terms of nine stages of awareness. These stages, and strategies for moving forward through these stages, are summarized in Table 7.8.

Community readiness must be determined at the community level by community stakeholders. Community readiness can sometimes be facilitated by a highly publicized event, such as a tragic death. More often than not, however, community readiness is achieved through the hard work of a local champion or an implementation team that is dedicated to improving community outcomes through the use of evidence-based programs (Blase et al. 2010). This individual or team must work hard throughout the implementation process to prepare communities and organizations for the new intervention and facilitate the processes necessary to implement it effectively.

Points to remember

The beginning of this chapter outlined the advantages of implementing a portfolio of evidence-based parenting interventions at multiple tiers of need. A growing body of research now suggests that when evidence-based programs are implemented in this manner, multiple community benefits can be achieved. However, transporting an evidence-based intervention into a new community is not a straightforward process. The commissioning of evidence-based parenting interventions imposes numerous challenges, requiring a significant amount of knowledge and skill to overcome. In order for commissioning to be effective, the

Table 7.8 Stages of community readiness (adapted from Edwards et al. 2000)

Stage	Level of awareness	Goals and strategies for improving awareness
No awareness	There is no awareness that a problem or need for change exists.	Raise awareness of the issue by: One-to-one visits with community leaders Visits with small community groups Phone calls with potential supporters.
Denial	There is some recognition of the problem but it is confined to a small group. There may also be a feeling that the problem is not owned by the community, but by the government or society as a whole. There may also be a belief that nothing can be done to solve the problem.	Raise awareness that the problem exists by: Highlighting local incidents related to the issue through media articles and newsletters Working with local education or health programs One-to-one visits with community leaders, asking for assistance.
Vague awareness	There is some recognition that things can change or that something must be done, but no clear understanding of what can be accomplished. There may also be a lack of leadership or motivation for addressing the problem.	Raise awareness that the community can do something by: Presenting information about the issue at local community events Sponsoring specific events to raise awareness about the issue Posting flyers and media announcements Conducting door-to-door surveys and visits.
Preplanning	There is a clear recognition of a problem and a belief that something can be done. Leaders may be identified and a committee may be in place, but there are no specific plans or focus.	Raise awareness with specific ideas for dealing with the problem by: Introducing information about the issue through the media and presentations Developing support from community leaders Reviewing existing efforts in the community for dealing with the problem to determine what needs to change Conducting local focus groups to discuss issues and develop strategies.
Preparation	Plans are articulated which provide detail as to what will be done and who will implement it. This stage also involves the identification of resources and partnerships are formed.	Gather existing information to help form a plan: Conduct school and community surveys Consider and publish local statistics regarding the problem Assess the costs of the problem for the community Sponsor an initiation event Hold public meetings to consider strategies for dealing with the problem Engage community leaders and influential leaders to raise awareness about the issue.

Stage	Level of awareness	Goals and strategies for improving awareness
Initiation	Policies and actions are underway. Enthusiasm for the new services is high and problems at this point are few.	Provide community-specific information by: Offering in-service training for practitioners Publicizing the start-up of the program Attending strategic meetings to provide updates on the progress of the initiative Identifying service gaps to improve existing services Identifying longer-term funding streams.
Stabilization	Programs are up and running with support from administrators and community leaders, staff have been trained and are experienced, limitations have been encountered and resistance overcome.	Stabilize the program by: Sponsoring community events to maintain support for the issue Offering training for community professionals Introducing program evaluation Conducting quarterly meetings to review the progress of the program and modify strategies Publicizing progress through the local media Initiating networking between service providers and community systems.
Confirmation/ expansion	Standard activities and policies are in place and community decision makers are involved in the expansion of the intervention. Decisions are also supported through established evaluation and monitoring systems.	Expand and enhance program by: Maintaining and expanding the data management systems Establishing long-term policies regarding the program with local officials Publicizing information about the progress of the program.
Professionalization	The community has a sophisticated knowledge of its needs and an understanding of where efforts should be targeted. Staff are appropriately trained and supervised to run services effectively. Evaluation is strongly embedded within programs and services to test their effectiveness and make modifications when necessary. The community is actively engaged in services and willing to hold agencies accountable for their performance.	Maintain momentum and continue growth by: Diversifying funding resources Continuing with professional training and advanced training Continuing to monitor the program's progress Conducting an external evaluation and using feedback to enhance program development.

Continued overleaf

commissioner must have a firm understanding of the community's needs and resources, know how to work collaboratively to identify priorities, and plan services and establish systems for monitoring performance. These challenges constitute the gap between the positive outcomes achieved by evidence-based interventions in the clinic and a lack of such outcomes when these interventions are implemented in communities.

Fortunately, a number of frameworks are now available to provide commissioners with the knowledge and skills needed to overcome many of the challenges associated with the commissioning process. CTC, OBA and *Common Language* are three examples of effective frameworks for conducting a needs assessment and commissioning services. Research suggests that when these frameworks are used, positive community changes can be achieved. However, before these frameworks can be used, communities must be ready for change.

An evidence-based intervention cannot make a community ready for change, but an individual or a small team of dedicated practitioners can. The guidelines in this chapter provide an overview of the steps involved in effectively commissioning and implementing evidence-based family services. Other resources include:

1   The National Implementation Research Network website: http://www.fpg.unc. edu/~nirn/default.cfm
2   The Rand *Getting to Outcomes 2004* manual: http://www.rand.org/pubs/technical_ reports/TR101/index.html
3   The Center for Excellence in Outcomes website: http://www.c4eo.org.uk/help.aspx
4   The Commissioning Support Program at: http://www.commissioningsupport.org.uk/

Box 7.9: Key points

- A portfolio of evidence-based parenting interventions implemented at scale can achieve positive outcomes for parents and children at the community level.
- Community-level impacts are most likely if multiple evidence-based interventions are implemented at multiple levels of need, within a developmental framework.
- Evidence from the United States and Norway suggests that a portfolio of evidence-based interventions can effectively reduce antisocial behavior and child maltreatment rates.
- Evidence suggests that the implementation of a portfolio of evidence-based interventions also results in community-wide savings.
- Commissioning boards should include representation from all agencies involved in the delivery of children's services.
- The commissioning process should begin with a thorough assessment of community-level needs or 'outcomes'.
- Once community needs are thoroughly assessed, specific priority groups can be identified.
- Needs should also be identified through consultation with parents and children. The best way of consulting parents is through door-to-door surveys.
- Needs should also be mapped against available services identified via an area-wide service audit.
- A good commissioning strategy should be based upon local needs and linked to national indicators via local priorities.

- A good commissioning strategy should also include a mixture of preventive and remedial services.
- A good commissioning strategy should include the specifics of how services will be delivered and who will deliver them, and include an implementation action plan.
- Commissioning arrangements should be determined before commissioning takes place and should be clear and transparent.
- Evidence-based parenting interventions will not be effective unless they are implemented effectively.
- Agencies delivering evidence-based parenting interventions frequently need to undergo structural changes to implement evidence-based interventions effectively.
- In order to maintain program effectiveness, host agencies should also develop systems for increasing staff competence. These systems include recruitment processes, pre-service training, coaching and supervision and staff performance evaluations.
- Host agencies must also implement organizational systems for sustaining evidence-based parenting interventions. These systems include decision support data systems, policies and procedures related to the implementation of parenting interventions and ongoing processes for making sure that funding and staff are available to deliver the intervention.
- It frequently takes four years or more before evidence-based parenting interventions are consistently effective.
- Communities and agencies are unlikely to effectively implement evidence-based interventions until they are ready to do so. Readiness refers to awareness that evidence-based interventions are needed and effective.

Note

1   By evidence-based we refer to program models with evidence of a strong short- and/or long-term outcome through at least one well-designed and -implemented RCT.

8 Moving the agenda forward

Past achievements and future challenges

Progress to date

Evidence-based practice as we know it today has its roots in Archibald Cochrane's monograph *Effectiveness and Efficiency: Random Reflections on Health Services*, published in 1972. In this seminal work, Cochrane proposed that, given that resources are always limited, resources should be put towards interventions which have been shown through properly designed research to be effective. In particular, Cochrane stressed the need to consider evidence from randomized controlled trials (RCTs) whenever possible, as the RCT design is the most rigorous way of measuring the effectiveness of an intervention.

In the 38 years since *Effectiveness and Efficiency* was originally published, the field of evidence-based practice has gained a steady momentum – witnessing major advances in how we gather evidence and measure outcomes. Ongoing research in the fields of developmental psychology and therapeutic practice have improved our knowledge of how interventions work and the ways in which specific intervention outcomes improve children's developmental trajectories. This knowledge has been used to develop standardized instruments which now make it possible to assess the extent to which family interventions are achieving the outcomes they were designed to achieve. Research can now also shed light on how best to train practitioners so that they can effectively engage parents and teach them the skills necessary to optimally support their children's wellbeing. The increased use of RCTs and systematic reviews has additionally helped policy makers and practitioners to identify interventions with a high probability of improving outcomes for individual families and entire communities.

Thanks to these major advances, a rapidly growing number of evidence-based services are available for parents and children. Parenting interventions have a particularly high potential for improving a wide range of child outcomes, including children's school achievement, their behavior and their emotional wellbeing. Several of these programs have an established track record of over 25 years, consistently resulting in significant parent and child benefits which have been shown to be sustainable for ten years or more.

While knowledge of how to commission and effectively implement parenting interventions is still advancing, a number of promising frameworks now exist to help commissioners meet their community's needs through appropriate evidence-based interventions. Evidence-based programs are now also starting to develop sophisticated support systems to facilitate the implementation process. Research suggests that when evidence-based parenting interventions are implemented effectively at scale, a variety of cost savings can be achieved.

Ongoing challenges

Despite this positive progress, evidence-based parenting interventions are the exception and not the rule in most communities. For example, Klett-Davies et al. (2008) observed that the majority of local authority expenditure on parenting interventions in England is directed towards interventions which lack any evidence of effectiveness, despite the fact that most directors of children's services believe that evidence of an intervention's effectiveness is an important reason for commissioning it. Many of these directors of children's services believe that evidence-based parenting interventions are expensive and cite the lack of consistent funding as a primary reason for not commissioning them. However, findings from a recent study involving the cost of parenting programs within the UK suggest that many non-evidence-based programs are just as expensive to deliver as evidence-based ones, if not more so (Puig-Peiró et al. 2010).

Practical barriers

Cost is just one of a number of practical barriers to the implementation of evidence-based parenting services. Additional barriers to the delivery of evidence-based parenting interventions include the sheer hard work involved in the implementation process. As the research described in Chapter 7 suggests, practitioners and service managers wishing to implement evidence-based services face numerous challenges in setting them up and getting them running. These challenges include structural and organizational changes to meet the requirements of the intervention, finding practitioners with the skills and qualifications to deliver them, obtaining buy-in from partner agencies, establishing effective referral routes and developing effective monitoring systems. Findings from the ongoing evaluation of the National Academy for Parenting Practitioners (NAPP) training offer suggest that many practitioners experience difficulty implementing parenting groups because the obstacles in setting them up are too difficult to overcome (Asmussen et al. 2010). Although some evidence-based interventions now provide an extensive package of implementation support through purveyor organizations, this support does not reduce the actual amount of work involved in successfully implementing and sustaining an evidence-based parenting intervention.

An additional barrier to the widespread use of evidence-based parenting interventions is the fact that the kinds of interventions currently available apply to a relatively limited set of child and parent outcomes. Although a number of programs addressing children's behavior are available to choose from, relatively few parenting interventions address other aspects of children's development, including their physical health and educational attainment (Stewart-Brown 2008). In addition, a relatively small number of evidence-based interventions are available for subgroups of parents who are harder to reach and are often considered more vulnerable (Klett-Davies et al. 2008). These groups include parents who have a mental health or substance misuse problem, ethnic minority families and parents with learning disabilities.

Fortunately, it is likely that the variety of evidence-based interventions will increase in the years to come. Research suggests that a growing number of interventions are currently being developed to address differing family structures and developmental issues. Examples of such programs include *Family Foundations* (described in Box 3.7), which supports the coparenting relationship, *Marriage and Parenting in Stepfamilies* (DeGarmo and Forgatch 2007), which supports stepfamilies and *Parenting Under Pressure* (Dawe and Harnett 2007), which supports children of substance-misusing parents. A wide variety of interventions addressing other aspects of children's development are also currently undergoing RCT trials. These interventions include parenting programs which tackle children's obesity, children's achievement and childhood mental health problems. Hopefully, many of these newer interventions will demonstrate improved outcomes for parents and children once they have completed efficacy and effectiveness trials.

Conceptual barriers

While the practical issues listed above are indeed significant barriers to the implementation of evidence-based interventions, they can be overcome through additional resources, funding and policies which support the use of evidence-based services. However, a number of conceptual barriers also exist which are likely to be more difficult to surmount. These barriers include a lack of consensus on what constitutes evidence-based practice and an overall lack of understanding of why an evidence base (particularly RCT evidence) is important. Brownson et al. (2009) observe that this is likely related to the fact that very few policy makers, service managers and practitioners outside the field of medicine receive training in the principles of evidence-based practice. Brownson et al. further note that many of the competencies required to understand and commission evidence-based services are cross-disciplinary. For example, community assessment is a skill learned through community planning, whereas evaluation is a skill learned through the post-graduate study of evaluation and research.

Brownson et al. additionally observe that evidence-based practice involves a set of skills, such as literature searching and critical appraisal, which are specific to evidence-based practice. Because evidence-based practice is relatively new, most practitioners will not have learned these skills during their formal education. The authors also note that some skills, such as collaborative interagency working, are not learned through education and can be learned only on the job.

A second conceptual barrier to the use of evidence-based parenting interventions is that they pose a threat to locally developed programs which presumably better reflect the needs of local parents. The fundamental assumption here is that locally developed interventions are as effective (if not more so) as evidence-based interventions developed elsewhere, but have not had the resources to undergo a proper evaluation.

The extent to which the above assumption is true can be known only if locally developed interventions subject themselves to sufficiently rigorous evaluations. However, there is good reason to believe that many locally developed programs are not likely to be effective. Recall from Chapter 1 that Barlow et al. (2007) observed that many of the local parenting services delivered through the *Sure Start* initiative resulted in few positive benefits for parents and children. More recent evidence from the *Commissioning Toolkit* additionally suggests that programs that have not undergone an evaluation are significantly more likely to have a poorly defined target population, non-evidence-based program content and inadequate training materials (Asmussen 2010). From this perspective, it is likely that the process of evaluation is an important step in an intervention's development. Parenting interventions that have not undergone an evaluation have also not had the opportunity for objective reflection on the benefits and drawbacks of their activities and therefore are unlikely to fully understand the ways in which their interventions are and are not effective.

A third conceptual barrier to the widespread adoption of evidence-based parenting interventions is that many academics and practitioners still question the fundamental value of RCT evidence. In this respect, Midgley (2009) has observed that while evidence-based practice is attracting an increasing number of followers, it also has a number of very vocal detractors. These evidence-based practice 'rejecters' go beyond the ethical and practical concerns summarized in Chapter 2 by arguing that RCT evidence is fundamentally flawed (Oakley 2006). These arguments include the notion that RCT evidence overly excludes other forms of evidence (Cartwright et al. 2009, Holmes et al. 2006) and that RCTs are not relevant because they lack external validity (Hammersley 2005). More cynical skeptics additionally charge that an emphasis on RCT evidence is nothing more than a strategy used by ambitious researchers to acquire political power and financial gain (Lather 2004).

Additional arguments against the use of RCTs include the idea that their use (and the use of similarly rigorous designs) constitutes a **positivistic approach** to knowledge generation that may be appropriate for medical treatments, but not for social interventions (Morrison 2001). The basic premise here is that the assumptions underpinning evidence-based practice are too narrow and therefore interfere with practitioners' knowledge of social phenomena (Gray and McDonald 2006). More specifically, a reliance on research evidence constricts practitioners' ability to think critically about their cases and make morally sensitive judgments when providing social care to families (Hammersley 2005, Lather 2004, Upshur 2006).

Oakley (2006) observes that the extent to which these 'resistance' arguments are accepted has to do with one's faith in the validity of empirical research in the first place, rather than any specific arguments against the use of randomization or a control group for reducing bias in research designs. Based on postmodernist thinking, these arguments propose that within the fields of mental health, social work and education, evidence cannot be obtained through scientific methods, but through 'situated' knowledge that is best gained through practical experience within local settings (Staller 2006). This perspective is particularly dominant in the field of social work, which has been strongly influenced by the 'postpositivistic' perspective that emphasizes collaborative methods of knowing over logical paradigms (Heineman 1981, Tyson 1995). Thus, there is a paradigmatic clash between postpositivistic approaches and 'industrialized' evidence-based methods which include standardized measures, systematic reviews and logic models. Despite this clash, a growing number of social workers and academics observe similarities between the two perspectives (particularly in the application of professional judgment) and a number of recent efforts have been made to reconcile evidence-based principles with postpostivistic social work practice (Blom 2009, Maynard 2007, Plath 2006, Regehr et al. 2007, Rosen 2003).

A fourth conceptual issue inhibiting the implementation of evidence-based parenting interventions is the belief that parenting is a private matter that should not be the subject of government or professional intervention (Bristow 2010, James 2009). These arguments are rooted in the belief that adults should be allowed to make their 'own decisions about how to live [their] personal lives and raise [their] children' (Bristow 2010) and assert that government parenting policies undermine parental confidence by intensifying anxieties about 'virtually every aspect of children's lives' (Furedi *Society Today* 15 September 2009).

These arguments are based, in part, in suspicions regarding governments' motivation for supporting parents. For example, Furedi (2008, 2009) suggests that the 'politicization' of parenting is, in fact, a method used by government to blame parents for societal problems rather than search for solutions within government-based enterprises, such as education and employment. Gillies takes this argument one step further by suggesting that government support for parenting is 'driven by a moral agenda that seeks to regulate and control the behavior of marginalized families' (2005: 71). Some have even implied that the field of developmental psychology is as much a political enterprise as it is a science (Burman 2008).

It should be noted that none of these arguments is based upon evidence, but instead on an analysis of political discourse which assumes that parenting policies are underpinned by a hidden government agenda and a belief that 'parenting science' is 'utter rubbish' (Bristow 2010). In this respect, any form of empirical evidence is rendered as invalid, and personal opinions – in the form of 'gut feelings' – are privileged over the accumulation of knowledge across multiple scientific disciplines.

Evidence aside, these arguments seldom entertain the perspective that the government has a genuine interest in helping parents and that parenting support is offered, in part, in response to parents who actively seek childrearing advice. For example, findings from a 2006 UK poll observed that 72 per cent of parents with children under the age of 16 have watched at least one parenting program and 83 per cent of these individuals found the information they provided to be helpful (Ipsos MORI 2006). In a more recent UK government survey, over two-thirds of all parents said that they accessed parenting support within the past twelve months and 97 per cent of these parents found these services to be useful (Peters et al. 2010). Other studies also suggest that many parents, especially those who are experiencing difficulties with their children, want additional support and prefer it if they know the support is evidence-based (Flynn 2005, Patterson et al. 2002, Ralph et al. 2003). With the exception of Parenting Orders, parents are not forced to access these services, but make adult decisions to attend them on their own.

Evidence-based parenting support is necessary

Despite highly publicized arguments claiming that parenting support is 'utter rubbish', the best evidence suggests that the demand is much higher than the supply (Kavanagh et al. 2010, O'Connell et al. 2009). As noted in Chapter 1, 10 to 20 per cent of children will have a diagnosable mental health disorder before they reach adulthood. However, the best estimates observe that between 40 and 80 per cent will not receive the support they need and research consistently suggests that the costs of not receiving this support are psychologically and financially high (Scott et al. 2001). Most would agree that governments have a responsibility to support the wellbeing of families and protect children. When there is now a high amount of evidence that childhood mental health problems can be prevented and cured it would be unethical not to continue to provide effective interventions to parents and children who need and want them.

Evidence-based parenting services are also necessary because they have built-in methods for ensuring accountability. As mentioned in Chapter 6, financial, retail, health and educational enterprises all have predetermined outcomes (e.g. profits, health improvements and grades) that allow their stakeholders to monitor progress and ensure accountability. Up until recently, social interventions have had difficulty identifying relevant outcomes and measuring them effectively. Measures now exist, however, to assess whether family-based interventions are effective and provide value for money. These measures should be used to develop services and ensure that they are consistently delivered to a high standard (Garralda 2009, Hogan 2003).

A third reason why evidence-based interventions are necessary is because the process of establishing the evidence base ensures the longevity of a quality program. As the example of *Head Start* in Chapter 2 suggests, rigorously collected, outcome-based information about the efficacy of an intervention provides an objective starting point for considering whether a service should be sustained or decommissioned. Had it not been for *Head Start*'s initial positive evidence, it is unlikely that the program would still be in operation today.

Evidence-based parenting work is rewarding

One point not sufficiently covered in this book is the fact that while most practitioners find evidence-based parenting work extremely challenging, they also find it highly rewarding. Findings from the NAPP training offer suggest that over 95 per cent of those trained through the offer were highly satisfied with what they learned and over half said that it positively influenced their daily practice (Asmussen et al. 2010). Qualitative studies involving practitioners' perceptions of evidence-based parenting work also note increases in job satisfaction through the implementation of evidence-based interventions. For example, Barnes et al. (2008) report high levels of enthusiasm among nurses delivering FNP and Ogden et al. (2009) observe increased job satisfaction among practitioners implementing PMTO. Findings from both of these studies suggest that practitioners' increased job satisfaction is related to the higher levels of supervision they see and visible improvements in the families they work with.

Moving forward

The field of evidence-based parenting practice has virtually exploded over the last 25 years. Multiple interventions now exist that effectively support the needs of children and parents. Examples from the US, UK, Australia and Norway all suggest that when local and national governments support evidence-based parenting interventions, cost savings for schools and communities can be achieved.

Despite these achievements, much more needs to be accomplished. Although a growing number of communities are now taking evidence-based interventions to scale, the vast majority of children still do not have access to evidence-based mental health services. In an effort to expand the availability of evidence-based interventions, Weisz and Kazdin (2010) make the following recommendations:

- Evidence-based interventions need to be developed in areas where there are current gaps
- Evidence-based interventions should better reflect the developmental needs of children and teenagers
- Theoretical models require further refinement and development to further inform the development of treatment models
- The scope of many treatment models should be extended to address co-occurring mental health difficulties
- The scope and duration of treatment outcomes should be considered through more in-depth, longitudinal research
- The understanding of how practitioner characteristics and therapeutic alliances contribute to treatment outcomes should be improved
- The understanding of how various models interact with family and child demographic characteristics should be expanded
- More research is required to investigate the necessary and sufficient conditions for ensuring treatment efficacy
- Methods for evaluating the 'mechanisms of change' within treatment models should be developed
- The impact of interventions under ideal conditions should be further investigated
- Methods for transporting and disseminating evidence-based interventions within new populations and contexts should be developed and tested.

The research presented in this book also suggests that more work is required to understand the cost-benefits of parenting programs and the extent to which practitioners can be better supported to understand and deliver evidence-based interventions.

Conclusion

Evidence-based parenting support presents multiple challenges at multiple levels. Practitioner-level challenges include understanding the theories and methods underpinning evidence-based interventions so that they can be delivered with fidelity. Agency-level challenges include the motivation and knowledge to install and implement parenting interventions effectively. Community-level challenges involve knowing how to assess community needs and commission interventions to meet these needs. Government-level challenges include policies, training and funding to develop and sustain the infrastructures necessary for evidence-based research and practice. There is no question that a great deal of coordinated effort and financial investment is required to overcome each of these challenges. But the research presented in this book suggests that the pay-back from these efforts is high. When appropriate investments in evidence-based parenting support are made, entire societies will benefit.

Box 8.1: Key points

- Over the past 40 years there have been significant advances in the field of evidence-based practice. These include the increased use of randomized controlled trials to establish an evidence base, the use of systematic reviews to understand the overall effectiveness of intervention models and an increase in the number of standardized instruments available to measure outcomes.
- There has been a dramatic increase in the availability of evidence-based parenting interventions.
- Much more is known about how to effectively commission and implement evidence-based social interventions.
- A number of practical challenges exist to the adoption of evidence-based parenting interventions. These include sustainable funding, the variety of interventions available and the sheer effort required to implement interventions effectively.
- A number of conceptual barriers also exist in the adoption of evidence-based parenting interventions. These include a lack of knowledge of what constitutes an evidence base, a belief that local interventions are more likely to be effective than those with an established evidence base, fundamental skepticism regarding the use of RCTs and resistance to government interference in parenting matters.
- Research suggests that a growing number of parents seek and want evidence-based advice and services.
- Evidence-based interventions have mechanisms within them to improve accountability and service quality.
- Many practitioners find the implementation of evidence-based parenting interventions personally rewarding.

Acronyms

APSAC	American Professional Society on the Abuse of Children
ASBO	AntiSocial Behaviour Order
C4EO	Center for Excellence and Outcomes
CAF	*Common Assessment Framework*
CBCL	*Child Behavioral Checklist*
CBT	cognitive behavioural therapy
CDSR	Cochrane Database of Systematic Reviews
CDSS	computerized decision-support system
COS	*Circle of Security*
CPP	*Child–Parent Psychotherapy*
CPPRG	Conduct Problems Prevention Research Group
CSAP	Center for Substance Abuse Prevention
CSP	Commissioning Support Program
CSR	Comprehensive Spending Review
CTC	*Communities That Care*
DfES	Department for Education and Skills
ECM	*Every Child Matters*
FAST	*Families and Schools Together*
FFT	*Functional Family Therapy*
FIMP	Fidelity of Implementation rating system
FIP	Family Intervention Projects
GIS	geographic information system
HFA	*Healthy Families America*
HIPPY	*The Home Instruction Program for Preschool Youngsters*
IOM	Institute of Medicine
IPP	*Infant–Parent Psychotherapy*
IY	*Incredible Years*
MCQ	Maternal Confidence Questionnaire
MLSPC	Minnesota Longitudinal Study of Parents and Children
MST	*Multisystemic Therapy*
MTFC	*Multi-dimensional Treatment Foster Care*
NAPP	National Academy for Parenting Practitioners
NBAS	Neonatal Behavioral Assessment Scale
NFP	*Nurse–Family Partnership*
NICE	National Institute for Health and Clinical Excellence
NIRN	National Implementation Research Network

NIT	National Implementation Team
NREPP	National Registry of Effective Prevention Programs
OBA	*Outcome-based Accountability*
OSLC	Oregon Social Learning Centre
PALS	Primary Age Learning Study
PAT	*Parents as Teachers*
PCT	personal construct theory
PEIPS	*Parenting Early Intervention Pathfinders*
PET	Parent Effectiveness Training
PIER	Physician's Information and Education Resource
PMTO	*Parent Management Training–Oregon*
PPET	*Parenting Programme Evaluation Tool*
PPI	psycho-educational parenting intervention
RCCP	*Resolving Conflict Creative Program*
RCT	randomized controlled trial
REBT	Rational Emotive Behavioral Therapy
RET	Rational Emotive Theory
SAMHSA	Substance Abuse and Mental Health Services Administration
SCIE	Social Care Institute for Excellence
SDQ	Strengths and Difficulties Questionnaire
SFSC	*Strengthening Families, Strengthening Communities*
SMART	Specific, Measurable, Achievable, Realistic, Time-limited
SPOKES	*Supporting Parents on Kids' Education in Schools*
SPR	Society for Prevention Research
SSLP	*Sure Start* Local Programme
TAC	Team Around the Child
VIPP	*Video-feedback Intervention to Promote Positive Parenting*
WSIPP	Washington State Institute for Public Policy
YOT	Youth Offending Team

Glossary

A

accommodate   a technique used in family therapy in which the therapist joins with the family and adapts to their style of interacting with one another.

action research   the use of research to develop an intervention, service or organization.

activating events (A)   in Rational Emotive Theory (part of the ABC model) activating events are what trigger **beliefs** and **emotional consequences**.

active listening   listening carefully to what someone is saying and mirroring back key phrases and ideas.

actualizing tendency   the inherent human capacity to maximize personal potential.

alignment   the way in which family members come together or split when carrying out specific activities. There are functional alignments, as well as dysfunctional alignments, such as triangulation or detouring.

alliance-based motivation   one of the principles of change of *Functional Family Therapy*. The therapist creates a trustworthy, hopeful and supportive environment for the family members, which should increase their motivation to change maladaptive emotional reactions and beliefs.

ambivalent/resistant attachment   one of the three patterns of attachment identified by Ainsworth and her colleagues. These children show distress when their mother leaves during the reunion episode, but are surprisingly angry when she returns.

amygdala   a part of the limbic system within the brain involved with emotion regulation and memory.

analysis of variance   a set of statistical tests which helps to compare the means of two or more groups or to analyze the effect of a categorical variable on the mean scores. These tests examine whether a certain variable (or being in a certain group) has a significant effect on the scores, and if yes, what percentage of the variability in the scores can be explained by that certain variable (or group belongingness).

analytic study   research designs involving a comparison group.

authoritarian parenting   one of the three parenting styles identified by Diane Baumrind where parents manage their children's behavior within strict boundaries and rarely involve them in decision making processes.

authoritative parenting   one of the three parenting styles identified by Diane Baumrind where parents maintain high standards for their children's behavior but encourage independent thinking and democratic decision making.

avoidant attachment   one of the three patterns of attachment identified by Ainsworth and her colleagues. These children do not appear as stressed as the other children when their mother leaves and avoid their mother when she returns.

axon   a part of a brain cell that carries electro-chemical impulses away from the cell body and towards other cells.

B

basic research   preliminary research conducted to understand the potential of an intervention – i.e. to determine whether a randomized controlled trial is worth conducting.

Beck Depression Inventory   a standardized assessment tool use to diagnose depression in adults and children.

behavior potential   the potential to engage in a particular behavior in a given environment.

beliefs (B)   in Rational Emotive Theory (part of the ABC model) beliefs are firmly held ideas that interpret **activating events**, or occurrences in life, and determine **emotional consequences**.

benefit–cost analysis   see cost–benefit analysis.

benefit realization   a continuous process of monitoring the progress of financial and non-financial benefits of a program or project. This is done by checking results on a real-time basis and making adjustments accordingly.

blamer   one of four dysfunctional communication stances identified by V. Satir in stress situations, whereby people feel isolated and try to compensate for this by trying to take charge.

blinding   a method used to reduce bias in randomized controlled trials that refers to a participant's or researcher's lack of knowledge regarding treatment assignment.

bonds   close relationships between family members, including emotional and physical attachment.

buffering   processes used to insulate the family system from outside influences.

C

case series trial   a study that tracks the outcomes of patients participating in an intervention.

chaos   a crucial aspect of V. Satir's change model of family therapy, representing the state of discomfort after a powerful **foreign element** has been introduced, which can create an opportunity for re-arrangement of the system.

choice corollary   one of the eleven corollaries of Personal Construct Theory, referring to the choice to expand or change one's personal constructs or keep to a former construct.

cluster randomization   sampling that involves the selection of a random subset of groups or communities.

coalitions   a structural component of a family which describes the way two or more members of a family collude with each other against other members in order to influence a specific decision-making process and its outcomes.

cognitive restructuring   a process of Rational Emotive Behavioural Therapy (REBT) whereby the client and therapist consider the extent to which beliefs are rational, beneficial and necessary, and if not, choose and learn new thinking patterns that are more flexible and positive.

cohort study a research design that prospectively follows comparison groups of participants (cohorts) over a period of time, which can be months, years or decades.

commonality corollary one of the eleven corollaries of Personal Construct Theory – the sharing of common personal constructs, based upon a similar upbringing and culture.

co-morbid refers to psychological disorders that occur together. Examples include ADHD and conduct disorder, substance misuse and depression, etc.

competency drivers organizational processes that aim to improve staff performance. These include staff recruitment and selection processes, training, coaching, supervision and performance evaluation.

conceptual shift a therapeutic effort of moving the focus of family therapy from an individual perspective (emphasizing the individuals themselves) to an inter-individual perspective (emphasizing the relationships between individuals).

concurrent controlled trial a type of non-randomized controlled trial, which can involve concurrent or historic samples, where the participant or practitioner determines allocation to the control or treatment group.

congruence internal and external consistency, or lack of distortions of feeling and experience, that is likely to result in psychological wellbeing. In humanistic psychology, it is a match between the real and self ideal.

congruent (communication) clear, free-flowing communication patterns. In this type of communication, thoughts and emotions are shared without projecting them onto others, which helps to avoid manipulations, and there is no contradiction between verbal and non-verbal expressions.

construct (or personal construct) is a theory or idea of reality developed by individuals to understand and interpret external events and phenomena.

construct validity refers to the extent to which a measure is an accurate reflection of the concept being measured.

construction corollary one of the eleven corollaries of Personal Construct Theory – 'a person anticipates events by construing their replications'. This means that previous experience serves as a basis for interpreting events.

constructive alternativism in Personal Construct Theory, the differential experience of reality based on people's different constructs. Alternative constructs can provide different explanations of the same behavior or events.

constructs in Personal Construct Theory, one's ideas about reality that are based on observation or experience. One discovers and modifies constructs in a manner similar to the scientific method of experimentation used by researchers. Experiences are in turn interpreted through existing constructs.

content validity refers to the extent to which a measure adequately captures all aspects of the concept being measured.

control group (also referred to as comparison group) a set of study participants not receiving the intervention under investigation. They may instead be given either a **placebo**, an alternative treatment or no treatment.

core components mechanisms of change or active ingredients of evidence-based programs that include components such as the program's content (e.g. the use of incentive plans based on social learning theory), activities (e.g. homework or role play) and processes (e.g. the quality of the relationship between the parent and practitioner).

core constructs in Personal Construct Theory, ideas that are basic to one's **core role structure** – i.e. an individual's beliefs about him- or herself as a person.

core role structure in Personal Construction Theory, one's sense of self and integrity.

corpus callosum   a region of white matter responsible for communication between the brain's left and right hemispheres.

correlational study   a study that determines to what extent two variables, traits, or attributes are related to one another through covariance or statistical regression.

cortisol   is a steroid hormone released in response to stress.

cost–benefit analysis   a method of economic evaluation that measures the potential benefits of a proposed program in monetary terms and compares them with its costs.

criterion validity   refers to the extent to which a measure is a good predictor of the trait it is measuring either now or in the future.

critical appraisal   the process of systematically assessing the quality of a piece of research.

critical period   a limited period during an organism's development in which appropriate stimulation from the external environment is required in order for specific developmental processes to take place. If this stimulation is not provided, optimal development will not occur and permanent damage may result.

cross-sectional (design)   research method that involves observation or measurement of differentiated study groups at the same point or points in time. Often used to study developmental trends and delayed outcomes by observing subjects differentiated by age. Conclusions drawn must take into consideration the assumption that groups are otherwise similarly matched.

cybernetics   the study of communication and control mechanisms in complex systems (such as biological or mechanical systems). These systems are goal oriented; in order to maintain the homeostasis, they use negative and positive feedback loops. It has influenced family system theory in relation to complexity and interdependence of parts of the family system, as well as communication of information between the parts of the system.

cycle of evaluation   a cyclical process by which evaluation is used to develop an intervention, service or organization – characterized by the use of baseline data to understand trends, plan activities, implement them and review their success or failure. Findings from the review are used to initiate a new evaluation cycle.

D

defense mechanisms   a variety of coping strategies used to manage conscious and unconscious conflict. These techniques may be healthy or unhealthy, depending upon how they are applied.

demographics   characteristics used to profile a population. Demographic characteristics typically include gender, race, age, disability status, education, income, family structure and employment status.

dendrite   a branched part of a brain cell that receives electro-chemical impulses into the cell body. Some dendrites can also release chemo-electrical impulses from the nerve body.

descriptive statistics   the set of statistics that is used to summarize the patterns or trends in the dataset, or to describe sample characteristics.

descriptive study   an observational study that does not involve a control group. Descriptive studies can use either statistical or qualitative methods to describe observations and relationships, but they cannot verify whether a treatment is effective.

detouring   takes place when two or more family members hold an excluded member responsible for problems occurring between the other family members.

dichotomy corollary   one of the eleven corollaries of Personal Construct Theory

– referring to people's tendency to organize constructs around dichotomous poles, such as 'good' versus 'bad', 'big' versus 'small', 'smart' versus 'stupid'.

differential attrition bias   a bias that occurs when post-treatment change is assessed with data collected only from those who complete the treatment.

differential susceptibility   refers to differences between children with respect to their vulnerability to environmental risks, as well as their ability to receive benefits from enriching circumstances, including high-quality parenting support.

diffuse boundaries   a term used in structural family therapy to refer to personal boundaries between family members that require family members to be overly responsible or involved with one another. Diffuse boundaries can involve family members taking responsibility for each other's feelings or behaviors.

disengaged family structure   rigid family structures where members live separate, distinct, private lives with high autonomy.

disorganized/disoriented attachment   one of the three patterns of attachment identified by Ainsworth and her colleagues. The behavior of these children frequently lacks any coherent organization. Babies also often act as if they are frightened when their mothers return during the reunion phase of the **strange situation.**

dosage   the amount and intensity of the treatment provided.

double-blind   a method used to reduce bias in studies where both the participants and researchers are blind to who was assigned to the treatment and control groups.

E

ecological model   theory that emphasizes the impact of multiple environmental systems on human development. These systems include the individual, family, school, community and society.

effect size   an index of the magnitude of difference in outcome between **treatment groups** and **control groups**.

effectiveness trial   determines the effectiveness of a treatment within a real-world, community-based setting.

efficacious (programs)   interventions demonstrating a significant effect through at least two randomized controlled trials conducted under ideal conditions. The effect has been observed with a sufficiently large sample that is representative of the program's target population, via standardized measures and statistical analyses.

efficacy trial   a randomized controlled trial used to determine the efficacy of a treatment under ideal conditions.

ego   the portion of the psyche that regulates sexual and aggressive impulses with the demands of the super-ego – coordinating the psyche into a coherent whole.

eligibility criteria   subject characteristics necessary for participation in research or intervention.

eligibility requirements   characteristics required for participation in an intervention. Examples of eligibility requirements include the children's age range, the parents' gender, the complexity of their problems, etc.

emotional consequences (C)   in Rational Emotive Theory (part of the ABC model) emotional consequences are feelings that result from the interpretation of **activating events**, or occurrences in life, by one's **beliefs**.

empathy   a therapeutic quality which enables the therapist to understand the client's concerns and feelings from the client's perspective.

empirical (empirically)   research conducted to test a hypothesis.

enactment   a technique used in family therapy which encourages family members to revisit or re-enact a commonly occurring issue within the family.

enmeshed family structure   refers to a lack of healthy boundaries between family members, where family members are over-involved in each other's lives.

evidence-based   an intervention or program underpinned with evidence of its efficacy. Evidence-based most commonly applies to interventions underpinned by randomized controlled trial evidence.

evidence-based practice   consultation of research evidence to inform treatment decisions.

exclusion criteria   criteria used to identify who is not eligible for a treatment.

exosystem   a term derived from the ecological model referring to the system immediately surrounding the family, including parents' employers and community resources.

expectancy   an individual's perception that a specific behavior will lead to a specific outcome.

experience corollary   one of the eleven corollaries of Personal Construct Theory assuming that constructs are modified based on life experiences.

experience-dependent   a type of synaptic connection that occurs on account of environmental influences. Brain development through this process is not predetermined genetically and relies upon an individual's unique interaction with the environment.

experience-expectant   a type of synaptic connection that is due to genetically determined processes that are triggered by environmental factors, such as exposure to light and sound.

experimental study   a carefully controlled study involving random assignment to a control group and a treatment group to study the effects of a treatment.

external validity   refers to the extent to which inferences based on a specific study can be generalized to other populations and conditions.

externalizing problem/difficulties   mental health problems that manifest themselves through outward behavior, most often involving negative or aggressive acts.

extinction   behaviors which cease because they are no longer reinforced.

extrinsic rewards: rewards that come from the external environment.

F

face validity   refers to the extent to which a measure accurately reflects what it intends to measure in a common-sense way.

family life chronology   a technique used to gather information about the family at the initial stage of a therapy.

family mapping   a therapeutic technique used to understand substructures within family systems – including alliances and coalitions.

family narrative   family stories that help to understand families' histories, communication patterns, the way the family system is organized and operates.

fidelity   the correspondence between an intervention's model and the way in which it is implemented.

fixed-ratio schedules   in operant conditioning, the provision of rewards at fixed intervals.

focus group   a group interview model, administered to a subset of the target population.

foreign element   part of V. Satir's change model. It is something that did not exist in the old system (i.e., **old status quo**), which has been stable for a certain amount of time; but once introduced, it has a power to disrupt the old system.

fragmentation corollary one of the eleven corollaries of Personal Construct Theory – individuals often hold personal constructs and beliefs which may contradict one another.

free association a technique of **psychodynamic** therapy in which patients are invited to relate the thoughts that spontaneously come into their mind during a therapy session and to try their best not to censor any ideas.

full implementation refers to a fully operational intervention, delivered by competent staff to families from the appropriate target population.

fundamental postulate in Personal Construct Theory, the idea that an individual's activities are informed by the constructs he uses to anticipate and explain what happens in his daily life.

G

genogram pictorial display of relationships between family members, representing the historical, emotional, communicative aspects of these relationships as well as their quality.

grey matter concentrations of brain tissue consisting primarily of cell bodies, dendrites and non-myelinated axons.

H

hippocampus an important region of the brain's limbic system, thought to be involved in emotion regulation, long-term memory and spatial regulation.

historic control a non-randomized design where the outcomes of individuals participating in a treatment are then compared to outcomes from a comparable sample in the past who did not receive the treatment.

hysteria a psychological condition brought on by extreme **neurosis** that involves the perception of symptoms of physiological disease or debilitation which have no underlying physical cause. Examples include hysterical blindness, paralysis and deafness.

I

iatrogenic effect unintentional and harmful effects of a treatment.

id unconscious part of the psyche that operates off the **pleasure principle** to fulfill sexual and aggressive drives.

imagery a category of cognitive behavioral therapy techniques that can be used for the purposes of distraction, motivation or relaxation.

I-messages direct statements that clearly affirm what an individual wants or thinks. A method of addressing behavior without assigning blame.

implementation effectiveness the conditions under which an intervention is acceptable to the target population and remains effective.

inclusion criteria a set of conditions that must be met by an individual or a family in order to participate in an intervention.

incongruence a lack of internal and external consistency that is likely to result in psychological maladjustment. In humanistic psychology, it is a mismatch between the real and the self ideal.

indicated prevention strategies, services or interventions that target individuals who have been screened as being at risk for a specific behavioral or emotional problem.

individual corollary one of the eleven corollaries of Personal Construct Theory suggesting that experiences shared between individuals will still be interpreted differently, based upon individuals' previous histories of similar events.

inferential statistics a set of statistics that allows the making of inferences about a population from a sample through testing hypotheses.

initial implementation the first stage of an intervention's implementation within a host agency, where practitioners and managers learn how to implement the intervention as they implement it the first time.

innovation occurs after an intervention has been in operation for a period of time and is in the process of expanding to meet the requirements of new settings or target populations.

input financial, human or physical resources applied to a service or intervention.

installation involves making structural changes within host agencies to adopt and effectively implement an evidence-based intervention.

integration and practice the stage a family goes through after **transformation** in V. Satir's change theory of family therapy, when family members start to become comfortable with new perceptions and feelings brought forward during the transformation, and even start to get excited about the change.

intention-to-treat (design) research method in which analysis is based upon the initial treatment intent as opposed to the treatment as administered. This means assessing pre- and post-treatment outcomes in treatment subjects, regardless of whether they completed the treatment.

inter-item reliability refers to the extent to which items included in a standardized questionnaire to measure the same concept are, in fact, related to each other.

internal validity refers to an evaluation design's ability to infer cause and effect.

internalizing problems/difficulties mental health problems that manifest themselves through inward, negative thoughts and feelings. Internalizing problems include depression and anxiety.

inter-observer reliability refers to the extent to which different researchers (interviewers, observers, etc.) achieve the same results with the same measure.

intrinsic reward an internal positive reinforcement for behavior, such as greater self-esteem, personal pride or personal integrity.

irrelevant person one of four dysfunctional communication stances identified by V. Satir, whereby a person can become easily confused in stressful situations and might not be sure of what to do. Instead of trying to take a positive action, these people generally try to distract others.

J

join the effort of a therapist to establish a rapport with the family to enter the family system.

juvenile parents a term used in family therapy to refer to parents who act immaturely in relation to their children, often placing the children in the parenting role.

L

lateral ventricles two of four ventricles of the brain containing cerebral spinal fluid. This fluid is thought to cushion and protect the brain.

law of effect attributions of causality made through trial and error learning.

learned helplessness   the belief that personal actions or abilities will not result in desired changes. Learned helpless behavior involves giving up before trying.

locus of control   people's general beliefs regarding the extent to which events are within one's personal control or due to external forces, including luck, fate and favoritism.

logic model   an explanation of an intervention in terms of its inputs (resources), activities, outputs (immediate effect of the intervention) and intended outcomes.

longitudinal study   a research design that involves repeated observations or measures of the same group of people over an extended period of time. Often used to track developmental trends or delayed outcomes.

M

macrosystem   a term derived from the ecological model referring to one's culture, religion, race, socio-economic status and society.

magnetic resonance imaging (MRI)   radiological medical imaging techniques used to display the internal structure and function of the body.

matching   one of the principles of *Functional Family Therapy* where the therapist matches his or her style to the style of the family.

mean   the sum of a series of values divided by the number of values.

meditation   a cognitive behavioral technique that involves deep concentration, which accentuates detachment from physical states and from feelings and thoughts.

merging   seeking contact within family systems.

mesosystem   a term derived from the ecological model referring to the systems immediately surrounding the family, including schools, church, friends, neighborhoods, etc.

meta-effect size   the statistical combination of effect sizes produced by statistically combining the effect sizes from multiple studies. Believed to be a more powerful estimate of the true effect size for an intervention than one calculated in a single study.

meta-review   a systematic review of the research literature which includes the effect sizes of similar interventions and combines them to produce a meta-effect (see **meta-effect size** above).

microsystem   a term derived from the ecological model referring to the immediate layer of environmental influence in which interactions with parents, caregivers and friends take place. The child actively influences his or her family and neighborhood while these environments simultaneously influence him or her.

midpointing   a term used in *Functional Family Therapy* to describe the desire to maintain a balance between the distance and the closeness among family members.

mimesis   a technique used by a family therapist to integrate him- or herself into the family system by adopting the style in which family members interact with one another.

mindfulness technique   a form of cognitive therapy that emphasizes an awareness of what is happening in the present moment in order to reduce the negative thinking associated with depression and substance misuse.

modulation corollary   one of the eleven corollaries of Personal Construct Theory which asserts that some personal **constructs** are more open to change than others.

moral anxiety   an unpleasant psychological state brought on by overwhelming feelings of shame or guilt caused by an over-involved **super-ego**.

myelin   an insulating material that covers neuronal **axons**. The myelin sheath increases the speed with which a neural impulse is transmitted along an axon.

myelination   the formation of a myelin sheath around the axon.

N

negative automatic thoughts   excessively negative emotional responses related to firmly established maladaptive thinking patterns.

negative cognitive triad   three negative thought schemas: 1) I am defective or inadequate, 2) all of my experiences result in defeats or failure and 3) the future is hopeless.

negative punishment   in operant conditioning, the removal of rewarding consequences to discourage behavior.

negative reinforcement   in operant conditioning, the removal of aversive consequences to encourage a behavior.

neglecting parenting   a style of parenting whereby parents either dismiss or detach themselves from their children or are disengaged and uninvolved, although they may still provide their basic needs.

neurogenesis   the formation of new brain cells.

neuron   a brain cell made up of a cell body, information in-putting **dendrites** and an information out-putting **axon**. Neurons transmit information through electro-chemical signaling.

neurosis   maladaptive thinking and behavior related to the inappropriate use of defense mechanisms in response to perceived threats.

neurotic anxiety   an unpleasant psychological state brought on by fear of being overwhelmed by id-related impulses. One feels on the verge of losing their temper, rationality or even their mind.

neurotransmitters   cellular chemicals found in **neurons**. These chemicals may be released into a synapse and connect with other cells in order to transmit a signal.

new status quo   the last stage in V. Satir's change model of family therapy, where previously foreign knowledge becomes part of a family's new reality, accepted and internalized by all members of the family.

norm-referenced standardized measure   a type of **standardized measure** that compares individual performance to a population-based average.

null hypothesis   the hypothesis that the observed outcome could naturally occur by chance.

O

object relations   a theory of child development that assumes that children's behavior is driven by a desire to interact and be with 'primary' objects – i.e. the child's parents.

observational study   a study in which systematic observations of activities are made as they are happening naturally without any experimental manipulation.

obtainable change goals   an aspect of *Functional Family Therapy* which identifies significant yet achievable behavioral change within the family.

old status quo   a concept of V. Satir's change model of family therapy, representing a stable system where the events are predictable, familiar, and comfortable. Things might stay the same for a long time in this status quo, where members know what to do and how to do it.

olfactory bulb   a part of the brain responsible for the processing of odors.

operant conditioning   the learned modification of voluntary behavior based on expected consequences. Either reinforcement or punishment can **shape** a behavior.

operationalize   to transform an abstract, theoretical construct into an observable and concrete level where it can be directly measured as an indicator of the theoretical construct.

organization corollary one of the eleven corollaries of Personal Construct Theory assuming that constructs are organized into super- and subordinate concepts, with some ideas falling under the umbrella of others.

organization drivers organizational-level components which contribute to the effective delivery of evidence-based interventions. These include data management systems to support decision making, facilitative administrative supports that include policies and procedures to support the implementation process, and systems interventions, which involve processes for ensuring that resources remain available to support the ongoing implementation of the intervention.

outcome the primary short- and long-term goals of an intervention.

output the product of a project or intervention. The term output can refer to activities or people participating in the activities.

P

p value the probability value of whether a statistical outcome is greater than what would occur by chance.

parent–child subsystem the subsystem of a family involving a parent and child.

parental subsystem the subsystem which is created between parents after the birth of the first child, with a focus on parental roles and tasks.

partnership an approach to therapeutic work that involves the client and practitioner working collaboratively within the context of individual or group therapy.

peer review a process by which research articles are reviewed by a panel of experts in a field of study who consider the validity of research methods, results and conclusions to determine whether the study is worthy of publication.

performancebased contracts are service contracts in which payment is explicitly linked to the agency implementing the service meeting pre-specified performance indicators.

peripheral parent family structure a family structure whereby one parent maintains a role exterior to other family members.

permeable in Personal Construct Theory, the extent to which a person's construct system is open to re-interpretation or re-construction.

permissive parenting one of three styles of parenting identified by Diane Baumrind as having few behavioral expectations of the child.

placater one of four dysfunctional communication stances identified by V. Satir, whereby individuals are always concerned about how they will be perceived, and are likely to avoid conflicts by agreeing or apologizing quickly.

placebo a treatment that is physiologically or psychologically inert and without directly beneficial effects, yet is known to improve symptoms, in comparison to receiving no intervention.

pleasure principle the idea that humans are internally and unconsciously motivated to seek pleasure and avoid pain by pursuing instinctual drives which demand immediate gratification without consideration of what the longer-term consequences may be.

positive punishment in operant conditioning, the use of aversive consequences to discourage behavior.

positive reinforcement in operant conditioning, the use of rewarding consequences to encourage behavior.

positivistic approach an approach to knowledge that heavily relies on **empirical** research evidence and the description of observable and measurable phenomena.

post-hoc   refers to the analysis of research findings after an experiment has concluded – for patterns in the data that were anticipated ahead of time.

power   the level of authority of each family member through their decision-making ability.

preconscious   the portion of the psyche that is unconscious, but is not repressed and can be brought into conscious thinking.

prefrontal cortex   the upper front region of the brain involved in planning, decision making and moderating impulsive behavior.

presenting problem   the behavioral or mental health problems of an individual family member which represents dysfunction within the family system.

primary maternal preoccupation   the period of early motherhood marked by a particular focus upon the baby during which she intuitively identifies with her infant in order to meet his or her physical and emotional needs.

primary process thinking   the use of internal images, fantasies or dreams to reduce **id**-related tensions. This mode of thought can partially but not fully satisfy unconscious drives.

primary survival triad   a hallmark of Satir's human validation process model, which represents the mother, father, child triad.

process use   the benefits of the actual evaluation process, rather than the results of the evaluation itself. Process use benefits can include learning a new skill, improved shared organizational knowledge and the opportunity to reflect on organizational activities.

program evaluation   the ongoing evaluation of an intervention as it is implemented at scale.

psychodynamic theory   ideas pertaining to the underlying forces that drive human emotions and behavior, founded on principles set forth by Sigmund Freud. Psychological processes are thought to be determined by a constant interplay between conscious and unconscious motivations.

psychological situation   strong and subjective differences between people in their interpretations of environments based upon their previous experiences and personal values.

purveyor   a centralized organization responsible for supporting the implementation of evidence-based interventions.

Q

qualitative method   a research method that produces non-numerical information, including observations, interviews and **focus groups**.

quantitative method   research methods that produce numerical data that can be used in statistical analyses.

quasi-experimental study   an experimental design that does not use randomization to assign participants to a treatment and control group.

R

randomized controlled trial (RCT)   study design in which participants are randomly assigned to either one or more treatment groups and a control group to determine the efficacy of a treatment. The use of randomization ensures that known or unknown confounding factors are evenly distributed across intervention groups.

range corollary   one of the eleven corollaries of Personal Construct Theory that observes that **constructs** are limited in their range of application, depending upon the specificity of the corollary.

reach   proportion of the population receiving a service or intervention.

realistic anxiety   an unpleasant psychological state brought on by realistic fears that stem from normal life situations.

reality principle   the concept that the human **ego** tests reality and delays gratification of instinctual drives until the appropriate environmental conditions are found.

reciprocal determinism   the idea that, as environments influence behavior, behaviors, in turn, influence environments.

re-construe   in Personal Construct Theory, the process of modifying **constructions** when experiences do not match expectations.

reflecting   the act of mirroring back key phrases and ideas to a client during therapy without interpreting them or offering advice.

reflective diary   the use of written diaries to gather research information. Reflective diaries can be written by the participants about their own experiences or by the researcher as a reflection of the data collection process.

reframing   a therapeutic technique used by therapists to offer an alternative interpretation of an event or behavior. This is done to help family members' adopt alternative viewpoints and reduce negativity between family members.

reinforcement value   the desirability of the consequences for specific behaviors.

relaxation   a cognitive behavioral technique that involves relaxing on self-cue in the face of a stimulus or situation one finds aversive.

reperception of situation   a cognitive behavioral technique that involves taking a new perspective on stimuli that formerly controlled one's behavior.

respect   genuine regard, caring for a client as an individual with a valid perspective and believing that the client is capable of positive change.

rigid boundaries   refers to strong boundaries between the family and the external world, as well as strong boundaries between family subsystems.

role play   a therapeutic technique in which a client attempts to act as another family member, in order to understand differences in perspectives.

S

sample   a subset of a population participating in a research study.

secondary process thinking   the ego's use of realistic, logical thought processes to manage pleasure-seeking impulses made by the **id**.

secure attachment   one of the three attachment categories identified by Ainsworth, whereby children use their mother as a secure base from which to explore the room, show distress when their mother leaves, but are easily comforted when she returns.

secure base   a central concept to attachment theory that indicates the infant's ability to use attachment figures as a base from which to explore the outside world.

selective prevention   strategies, services or interventions aimed at specific groups of children or parents who may be at risk of having future difficulties.

self-efficacy   the belief that one can personally master a particular task or activity.

self-monitoring   an important component of cognitive behavioral interventions, which consists of self-observing and reflecting upon one's behaviors and the recording of the observed findings.

self-statements   statements people make to themselves to guide their feelings, thoughts and behavior.

semi-structured interview   a conversational interview technique involving the use of predetermined questions, as well as unplanned questions, so that interviewers can fully understand interviewees' response to the question, as well as explore key issues.

separating   a construct used in *Functional Family Therapy* to describe the distancing behaviors between family members so that they can gain independence from each other.

service level agreement   a formal agreement that defines the level of a service between an agency delivering the service and its clients.

shape   in operant conditioning, to teach new behaviors through the use of reinforcement.

sibling subsystem   the family subsystem involving brothers and sisters, but not parents.

significance tests   statistical calculations to determine whether the observed difference between the treatment and control group is greater than what might happen by chance.

simple regression   a statistical test that estimates the relationship between two variables by examining if the scores for one of these variables depend on the scores of the other variable.

sleeper effect   the delayed or unexpected effects of an intervention.

sociality corollary   one of the eleven corollaries of Personal Construct Theory – the process by which people relate to and influence each other's construction process.

Socratic method   a form of inquiry and debate based on asking and answering questions from opposite points of view in order to promote more rational thinking.

spousal subsystem   a family subsystem involving the relationship between the adult couple.

standard deviation   a measure of the variation of data around its **mean**. A standard deviation can be calculated as follows:

$$s = \sqrt{\frac{1}{N-1} \sum_{i=1}^{N} (x_i - \bar{x})^2}$$

standardized measures   questionnaires and assessment tools that have been psychometrically tested as valid and reliable.

statistical power   the probability of not committing a type II error (accepting the null hypothesis when it is false).

statistical significance   a result where the observed difference between the treatment and control group is greater than what might happen by chance.

strange situation   a natural observational paradigm created by Mary Ainsworth to activate children's attachment behaviors. The strange situation involves a phase where the mother and child play together in the presence of a stranger. This is followed by a brief phase when the mother leaves the child alone in the room. This is followed by a reunion episode when the mother returns to her child.

subjective (subjectively)   a personal interpretation of an event, behavior or information.

subjective omnipotence   the infant's belief that his or her own wish creates the object of desire.

successive approximation   in operant conditioning, a process by which animals may be taught new behaviors that do not come naturally to them, by successively rewarding related behaviors.

summaries   are systems managed by health care organizations that integrate the best available evidence (from studies, systematic reviews, etc.) to inform practice decisions about a specific health problem.

super-ego   a part of the psyche informed by internalized judgments of right and wrong, good and bad that are informed by the morals and standards of parents and society.

super-reasonable person   one of four dysfunctional communication stances that V. Satir identified. People with this communication type generally have problems controlling their emotions and showing them. When faced with stressful situations, they act like computers, using a rigid logic, avoiding emotions and trying to be super-cool.

sustainability   systems (quite often financial) to help services maintain efficacy in the advent of large organizational and staff changes.

synapse   the space between brain cells, or **neurons**, through which **neurotransmitters** diffuse from one cell to another in order to communicate a brain signal.

synaptic overproduction   brain development process that entails the creation of a vast number of neuronal connections throughout the brain, most of which are later extinguished; occurs prenatally and during the first three years of life; connections are made stronger, weaker or lost according to environmental exposure (learning).

synaptic pruning   a process during which redundant and unnecessary synaptic connections that are not used wither and die.

synaptogenesis   the formation of new synapses.

synopses   academic journals that provide information on important advances in evidence-based practice on a regular basis.

systematic desensitization   a type of behavioral therapy often used in the treatment of anxieties and phobias, involving the successive use of relaxation techniques to calm clients as they are systematically exposed to increasingly fearful situations.

systematic (literature) review   use of consistent and transparent methods to systematically search for, appraise and summarize all of the published information surrounding a specific topic.

T

target population   the group of individuals possessing the characteristics and circumstances for which an intervention is designed.

terminal button   part of a neuron located at the distal tip of the **axon** where neurotransmitter chemicals are released into a **synapse** to communicate with other neurons.

test/retest reliability   the extent to which a test administered to the same subjects at two time points will result in the same outcome.

theory of change   a theory that links an intervention's theoretical basis to its inputs, outputs and short- and long-term outcomes.

therapeutic alliance   the working relationship formed between a mental health professional and a client within the context of ongoing therapy.

thought stopping   a cognitive behavioral technique that involves literally stopping the ideas when negative thoughts, worries or compulsions enter consciousness.

threats to internal validity   factors that confound an evaluation design's ability to infer cause and effect.

time diary   a written diary used for research, with the purpose of collecting detailed data on how participants use their time.

time out   a form of discipline whereby a child is removed from the environment in which he or she is misbehaving. This is used to calm children down and/or stop negative behavior from being reinforced.

tracking   a technique used in family therapy whereby the therapist actively keeps track of themes, ideas and words that repeat themselves during the course of therapy.

transference   the unconscious redirection of feelings from one person to another unrelated person. For example, a client may transfer feelings he or she had towards their father to their therapist.

transformation   a stage in family therapy where family members realize how their specific behaviors and patterns of interaction contributed to ongoing problems. This understanding enables them to make choices about their behavior that will allow them to go forward in the process of positive change.

treatment group   the set of study participants receiving the intervention under investigation.

triangulation   two family members align themselves against a third family member.

t-test   a statistical test that compares the means of two samples.

type I error   rejecting the null hypothesis when it is true (i.e. concluding a treatment is effective when it is not).

type II error   accepting the null hypothesis when it is false (i.e. concluding that the treatment is not effective when it is).

U

unconditional positive regard   affirming acceptance of an individual under any and all circumstances.

unconscious   characteristic of mental processes that occur beyond one's awareness. May include feelings, skills, perceptions and thoughts.

undifferentiated symbiosis   the infant's illusion that he/she and mother are one being.

uninvolved parents   a term used in family therapy to refer to parents who appear uninterested in their children and show very little emotion towards them.

universal prevention   strategies, services or interventions made available to all members of the population within a specific target group.

V

variable schedules   in operant conditioning, the use of rewards for behavior in a non-fixed and often unpredictable format.

vicious cycle   one event leads to another event which in turn aggravates the first event; and eventually creates a complex set of mutually reinforcing events.

video diary   subjects provide information about their thoughts, feelings and experiences through the use of video-tapes rather than a written diary.

W

white matter   concentration of brain matter consisting primarily of myelinated axons.

wish fulfillment   the process by which one forms internal representations of objects to reduce **id**-related drives in an attempt to gain short-term satisfaction. Primarily occurs on an unconscious level as a form of **primary process thinking**.

References

Aber, J. L., Jones, S. M., Brown, J. L., Chaudry, N. and Samples, F. (1998) 'Resolving conflict creatively: Evaluating the developmental effects of a school-based violence prevention program in neighborhood and classroom context', *Development and Psychopathology*, 10(2), 187–213.

Abidin, R. R. (1995) *Parenting Stress Index: Professional Manual*, 3rd edn, New York, NY: Psychological Assessment Resources, Inc.

Ainsworth, M. D. S., Bell, S. M. and Stayton, D. J. (1971) 'Individual differences in strange situation behaviour of one-year-olds', in Schaffer, H. R. and Ciba Foundation (eds.) *The Origins of Human Social Relations*, London; New York, NY: Academic Press, 17–57.

Ainsworth, M. D. S., Blehar, M. C., Waters, E. and Wall, S. (1978) *Patterns of Attachment: A Psychological Study of the Strange Situation*, Hillsdale, NJ: Lawrence Erlbaum Associates.

Alexander, J. F. (2009) 'Levels of qualifications of practitioners in FFT'. E-mail (26 May).

Alexander, J. F. and Parsons, B. V. (1973) 'Short-term behavioral intervention with delinquent families: Impact on family process and recidivism', *Journal of Abnormal Psychology*, 81(3), 219–225.

Alexander, J. F. and Parsons, B. V. (1982) *Functional Family Therapy*, Monterey, CA: Brooks/Cole Publishing Company.

Alexander, J. F., Barton, C., Schiavo, R. S. and Parsons, B. V. (1976) 'Systems behavioral intervention with families of delinquents: Therapist characteristics, family behavior, and outcome', *Journal of Consulting and Clinical Psychology*, 44(4), 656–664.

Allen, G. (2011) 'Early intervention: The next steps', London: HM Government.

Allen, J. P., Hauser, S. T., Bell, K. L. and O'Connor, T. G. (1994) 'Longitudinal assessment of autonomy and relatedness in adolescent–family interactions as predictors of adolescent ego development and self-esteem', *Child Development*, 65(1), 179–194.

Allison, S., Stacey, K., Dadds, V., Roeger, L., Wood, A. and Martin, G. (2003) 'What the family brings: Gathering evidence for strengths-based work', *Journal of Family Therapy*, 25(3), 263–284.

Angold, A., Costello, E. J., Messer, S. C., Pickles, A., Winder, F. and Silver, D. (1995) 'Development of a short questionnaire for use in epidemiological studies of depression in children and adolescents', *International Journal of Methods in Psychiatric Research*, 5(4), 237–249.

Annapolis Coalition on the Behavioral Health Workforce (2007) *An Action Plan for Behavioral Health Workforce Development: A Framework for Discussion*, Rockville, MD: Department of Health and Human Services.

Aos, S. (2006) *Evidence-Based Public Policy Options to Reduce Future Prison Construction, Criminal Justice Costs, and Crime Rates*, Olympia, WA: Washington State Institute for Public Policy.

Aos, S. (2009) 'Using evidence-based public policy to reduce incarceration, crime, and criminal justice costs'. Online. Available HTTP: http://video.google.com/videoplay?docid=-2702910829423493079 (accessed 2 August 2009).

Aos, S. (2010) 'Improve outcome and save money: Evidence-based programs, picking them, passing them, doing them, and holding them accountable', paper presented at *Blueprints for Violence Prevention* in San Antonio, TX, 9 April 2010.

Aos, S., Barnoski, R. and Lieb, R. (1998) *Watching the Bottom Line: Cost-effective Interventions for Reducing Crime in Washington*, Olympia, WA: Washington State Institute for Public Policy.

Aos, S., Lieb, R., Mayfield, J., Miller, M. and Pennucci, A. (2004) *Benefits and Costs of Prevention and Early Intervention Programs for Youth*, Olympia, WA: Washington State Institute for Public Policy.

Aos, S., Phipps, P., Barnoski, R. and Lieb, R. (2001) *The Comparative Costs and Benefits of Programs to Reduce Crime*, Olympia, WA: Washington State Institute for Public Policy.

APA (American Psychological Association) (2002) 'Criteria for evaluating treatment guidelines', *American Psychologist*, 57(12), 1052–1059.

Appleton, P. L. and Minchom, P. E. (1991) 'Models of parent partnership and child-development centers', *Child Care Health and Development*, 17(1), 27–38.

Appleyard, K., Egeland, B., van Dulman, M. H. M. and Sroufe, A. L. (2005) 'When more is not better: The role of cumulative risk and child behavior outcome', *Journal of Child Psychology and Psychiatry*, 46, 235–245.

Arnold, D. S., O'Leary, S. G., Wolff, L. S. and Acker, M. M. (1993) 'The parenting scale: A measure of dysfunctional parenting in discipline situations', *Psychological Assessment*, 2, 137–144.

Arthur, W., Bennett, W., Stanush, P. L. and McNelly, T. L. (1998) 'Factors that influence skill decay and retention: A quantitative review and analysis', *Human Performance*, 11(1), 57–101.

Asmussen, K. (2010) 'Understanding the Quality of Parenting Programmes: Findings from the Commissioning Toolkit', London: The National Academy for Parenting Research, unpublished.

Asmussen, K., Puga, F. and Eryigit, S. (2010) '"The National Academy for Parenting Practitioners" Training Offer Phases 1 & 2: Factors that Contribute to the Implementation of Evidence Based Parenting Groups', London: National Academy for Parenting Research, unpublished.

Astuto, J. and Allen, L. (2009) 'Home visitation and young children: An approach worth investing in?', *Social Policy Report*, 23(4), 1–21.

Aubel, J. (1999) *Participatory Program Evaluation Manual*, Claverton, MD: The Child Survival Technical Support Project (CSTS).

Audit Commission (2008) *Are We There Yet? Improving Governance and Resource Management in Children's Trusts*, London: Audit Commission.

Aveyard, H. and Sharp, P. (2009) *A Guide to Evidence-Based Practice in Health and Social Care*, New York, NY: Open University Press.

Axford, N., Berry, V., Little, M. and Morpeth, L. (2006) 'Developing a common language in children's services through research-based inter-disciplinary training', *Social Work Education*, 25(2), 161–176.

Backer, T. E. (2001) *Finding the Balance: Program Fidelity and Adaptation in Substance-Abuse Prevention: A State of the Art Review*, Rockville, MD: Center for Substance Abuse Prevention.

Baird, A. A., Gruber, S. A., Fein, D. A., Maas, L. C., Steingard, R. J., Renshaw, P. F., Cohen, B. M. and Yurgelun-Todd, D. A. (1999) 'Functional magnetic resonance imaging of facial affect recognition in children and adolescents', *Journal of the American Academy of Child and Adolescent Psychiatry*, 38(2), 195–199.

Bakermans-Kranenburg, M. J., van IJzendoorn, M. H. and Juffer, F. (2003) 'Less is more: Meta-analyses of sensitivity and attachment interventions in early childhood', *Psychological Bulletin*, 129(2), 195–215.

Ball, M. (2002) *Getting Sure Start Started*, London: The National Evaluation of Sure Start.

Bandler, R., Grinder, J. and Satir, V. (1976) *Changing with Families: A Book about Further Education for Being Human*, Palo Alto, CA: Science and Behavior Books.

Bandura, A. (1977) *Social Learning Theory*, Englewood Cliffs, NJ: Prentice Hall.

Bandura, A. (1986) *Social Foundations of Thought and Action: A Social Cognitive Theory*, Prentice-Hall Series in Social Learning Theory, Englewood Cliffs, NJ: Prentice-Hall.

Bandura, A. (1994) 'Self-efficacy', in V. S. Ramachaudran (ed.) *Encyclopedia of Human Behavior*, vol. 4, New York: Academic Press, 71–81.

Bandura, A. and Walters, R. H. (1963) *Social Learning and Personality Development*, New York, NY: Holt, Rinehart, & Winston.

Bandura, A., Ross, D. and Ross, S. A. (1961) 'Transmission of aggression through imitation of aggressive models', *Journal of Abnormal and Social Psychology*, 63(3), 575–582.

Bandura, A., Ross, D. and Ross, S. A (1963) 'Imitation of film-mediated aggressive models', *Journal of Abnormal Psychology*, 66(1), 3–11.

Banmen, J. (2002) 'The Satir model: Yesterday and today', *Contemporary Family Therapy*, 24(1), 7–22.

Barlow, J., Coren, E. and Stewart-Brown, S. (2001) *Systematic Review of the Effectiveness of Parenting Programmes in Improving Maternal Psychosocial Health*, Oxford: Health Services Research Unit.

Barlow, J., Coren, E. and Stewart-Brown, S. (2002) 'Meta-analysis of the effectiveness of parenting programmes in improving maternal psychosocial health', *British Journal of General Practice*, 52(476), 223–233.

Barlow, J., Kirkpatrick, S., Wood, D., Ball, M. and Stewart-Brown, S. (2007) *Family and Parenting Support in Sure Start Local Programmes*, London: NESS.

Barnard, K. E. (1998) 'Developing, implementing, and documenting interventions with parents and young children', *Zero to Three*, 18(4), 23–29.

Barnes, J., Ball, M., Meadows, P., McLeish, J. and Belsky, J. (2008) *Nurse–Family Partnership Programme: First Year Pilot Sites Implementation in England*, London: DCSF.

Barnett, W. (1995) *Lives in the Balance: Age 27 Benefit-cost Analysis of the High/Scope Perry Preschool Program*, Ypsilanti, MI: High/Scope Press.

Barnoski, R. (2002) *Washington State's Implementation of Functional Family Therapy for Juvenile Offenders: Preliminary Findings*, Olympia, WA: Washington State Institute for Public Policy.

Barnoski, R. (2004) *Outcome Evaluation of Washington State's Research-based Programs for Juvenile Offenders*, Olympia, WA: Washington State Institute for Public Policy.

Barrett, H. (2007) *Evaluating Evaluations: Evaluating Recent Evaluations of Sure Start, Home-Start and Primary Age Learning Study*, London: National Family and Parenting Institute.

Baumrind, D. (1971) 'Current patterns of parental authority', *Developmental Psychology*, 4(1), 1–103.

Baumrind, D. (1978) 'Parental disciplinary patterns and social competence in children, *Youth & Society*, 9(3), 239–276.

Baumrind, D. (1991) 'The influence of parenting style on adolescent competence and substance use', *The Journal of Early Adolescence*, 11(1), 56–95.

Beck, A. T., Steer R. A. and Brown, G. K. (1996) *Manual for the Beck Depression Inventory-II*, San Antonio, TX: Psychological Corporation.

Beck, A. T., Brown, G., Epstein, N. and Steer, R. A. (1988) 'An inventory for measuring clinical anxiety: Psychometric properties', *Journal of Consulting and Clinical Psychology*, 56(6), 893–897.

Beckett, C., Kallitsoglou, A., Doolan, M., Ford, T. and Scott, S. (2010) 'Helping Children Achieve: Summary of the Study 2007–2010', London: National Academy for Parenting Research, unpublished.

Beckett, C., Maughan, B., Rutter, M., Castle, J., Colvert, E., Groothues, C., Kreppner, J., Stevens, S., O'Connor, T. G. and Sonuga-Barke, E. J. S. (2006) 'Do the effects of early severe deprivation on cognition persist into early adolescence? Findings from the English and Romanian adoptees study', *Child Development*, 77(3), 696–711.

Beebe, B. (2000) 'Coconstructing mother–infant distress: The microsynchrony of maternal impingement and infant avoidance in the face-to-face encounter', *Psychoanalytic Inquiry*, 20(3), 421–440.

Belfer, M. L. (2008) 'Child and adolescent mental disorders: The magnitude of the problem across the globe', *Journal of Child Psychology and Psychiatry*, 49(3), 226–236.

Belsky, J., Crnic, K. and Gable, S. (1995) 'The determinants of coparenting in families with toddler boys – spousal differences and daily hassles', *Child Development*, 66(3), 629–642.

Belsky, J. and de Haan, M. (2010) 'Annual research review: Parenting and children's brain development: The end of the beginning', *Journal of Child Psychology and Psychiatry*. Online. Available HTTP: http://onlinelibrary.wiley.com/doi/10.1111/j.1469-7610.2010.02281.x/abstract (accessed 27 January 2011).

Belsky, J., Melhuish, E. and Barnes, J. (2007) *The National Evaluation of Sure Start: Does Area-Based Early Intervention Work?*, Bristol: Policy Press.

Belsky, J., Melhuish, E., Barnes, J., Leyland, A. H., Romaniuk, H. and National Evaluation Sure Start Team (2006) 'Effects of *Sure Start* local programmes on children and families: Early findings from a quasi-experimental, cross sectional study', *British Medical Journal*, 332(7556), 1476–1478.

Belsky, J., Putman, S. and Crnic, K. (1996) 'Coparenting, parenting and early emotional development', *New Directions for Child and Adolescent Development*, 74, 45–55.

Benassi, V. A., Sweeney, P. D. and Dufour, C. L. (1988) 'Is there a relation between locus of control orientation and depression?', *Journal of Abnormal Psychology*, 97(3), 357–367.

Bentovim, A. (2006) 'Therapeutic interventions with children who have experienced sexual and physical abuse in the UK', in C. McAuley, P. J. Pecora and W. Rose (eds.) *Enhancing the Well-Being of Children and Families through Effective Interventions*, London: Jessica Kingsley, 143–157.

Berkel, C., Mauricio, A. M., Schoenfelder, E. and Sandler, I. N. (2010) 'Putting the pieces together: An integrated model of program implementation', *Prevention Science*. Online. Available HTTP: http://www.springerlink.com/content/p006g4608861w2t8/ (accessed 1 November 2010).

Berlin, L. J. (2005) 'Interventions to enhance early attachments: The state of the field today', in L. J. Berlin, Y. Ziv, L. Amaya-Jackson and M. Greenberg (eds.) *Enhancing Early Attachments: Theory, Research, Intervention and Policy*, New York, NY: Guilford Press, 3–33.

Berlin, L. J., Ziv, Y., Amaya-Jackson, L. and Greenberg, M. T. (2005) *Enhancing Early Attachments: Theory, Research, Intervention and Policy*, New York, NY: Guilford Press.

Bhabra, S. and Ghate, D. (2004) *Parent Information Point: Evaluation of the Pilot Phase*, London: National Family and Parenting Institute.

Biehal, N. (2005) *Working with Adolescents: Supporting Families, Preventing Breakdown*, London: British Association for Adoption and Fostering.

Biehal, N. (2006) 'Support for young people and their families in the community in the UK', in C. McAuley, P. J. Pecora and W. Rose (eds.) *Enhancing the Well-Being of Children and Families through Effective Interventions*, London: Jessica Kingsley, 91–102.

Bignold, S., Cribb, A. and Ball, S. J. (1995) 'Befriending the family: An exploration of a nurse–client relationship', *Health & Social Care in the Community*, 3(3), 173–180.

Birmingham City Council (2007) *A Brighter Future for Children and Young People*. Online. Available HTTP: http://ebriefing.bgfl.org/bcc_ebrief/content/resources/resource.cfm?id=4314&key=&zz=201009 19145327568&zs=n (accessed 19 September 2010).

Blair, T. (2006) 'A failed test of leadership', *Guardian*, 5 October.

Blakely, C. H., Mayer, J. P., Gottschalk, R. G., Schmitt, N., Davidson, W. S., Roitman, D. B. and Emshoff, J. G. (1987) 'The fidelity–adaptation debate: Implications for the implementation of public-sector social programs', *American Journal of Community Psychology*, 15(3), 253–268.

Blakemore, S. J. and Choudhury, S. (2006) 'Brain development during puberty: State of the science', *Developmental Science*, 9(1), 11–14.

Blase, K. A., Fixsen, D. L., Duda, M. A., Metz, A. J., Naoom, S. F. and van Dyke, M. K. (2010) 'Implementing and sustaining evidence-based programmes: Have we got a sporting chance?', paper presented at *Blueprints for Violence Prevention* in San Antonio, TX, 10 April 2010.

Blom, B. (2009) 'Knowing or un-knowing? That is the question in the era of evidence-based social work practice', *Journal of Social Work*, 9(2), 158–177.

Bor, W., Sanders, M. R. and Markie-Dadds, C. (2002) 'The effects of the Triple P-Positive Parenting Program on preschool children with co-occurring disruptive behavior and attentional/hyperactive difficulties', *Journal of Abnormal Child Psychology*, 30(6), 571–587.

Bordin, E. S. (1979) 'The generalizability of the psychoanalytic concept of the working alliance', *Psychotherapy: Theory, Research and Practice*, 16(3), 252–260.

Bordin, E. S. (1980) 'Of human bonds that bind or free', paper presented at the Annual Meeting of the Society for Psychotherapy, Pacific Grove, CA, June 1980.

Bordin, E. S. (1994) 'Theory and research in the therapeutic working alliance: New directions', in A. O. Horvarth and L. S. Greenberg (eds.) *The Working Alliance: Theory, Research and Practice*, New York: Wiley, 13–37.

Borkovec, T. D. and Castonguay, L. G. (1998) 'What is the scientific meaning of empirically supported therapy?', *Journal of Consulting and Clinical Psychology*, 66(1), 136–142.

Bosquet, M. and Egeland, B. (2001) 'Associations among maternal depressive symptomatology, state of mind and parent and child behaviors: Implications for attachment-based interventions', *Attachment & Human Development*, 3(2), 173–99.

Bower, P., Rowland, N. and Hardy, R. (2003) 'The clinical effectiveness of counselling in primary care: A systematic review and meta-analysis', *Psychological Medicine*, 33(2), 203–215.

Bowlby, J. (1969) *Attachment and Loss*, New York, NY: Basic Books.

Bowlby, J. (1988) *A Secure Base: Parent–Child Attachment and Healthy Human Development*, New York: Basic Books.

Braun, D., Davis, H. and Mansfield, P. (2006) *How Helping Works: Towards a Shared Model of Process*. London: Parentline Plus.

Braver, S. L., Griffin, W. A. and Cookston, J. T. (2005) 'Prevention programs for divorced non-resident fathers', *Family Court Review*, 43(1), 81–96.

Brazelton, T. B. (1979) 'Behavioral competence of the newborn infant', in J. K. Gardner (ed.) *Readings in Developmental Psychology*, Boston, MA: Little, Brown and Company, 79–90.

Brazelton, T. B. and Nugent, J. K. (1995) *Neonatal Behavioral Assessment Scale (NBAS)*, 3rd edn, London: Mac Keith Press.

Brestan, E. V. and Eyberg, S. M. (1998) 'Effective psychosocial treatments of conduct-disordered children and adolescents: 29 years, 82 studies, and 5,272 kids', *Journal of Clinical Child Psychology*, 27(2), 180–189.

Bright, J. I., Baker, K. D. and Neimeyer, R. A. (1999) 'Professional and paraprofessional group treatments for depression: A comparison of cognitive-behavioral and mutual support interventions', *Journal of Consulting and Clinical Psychology*, 67(4), 491–501.

Bristow, J. (2010) 'Bringing up baby is not an exact science'. Online. Available HTTP: http://www.spiked-online.com/index.php/site/article/9660 (accessed 30 October 2010).

Broderick, C. B. (1993) *Understanding Family Process: Basics of Family Systems Theory*, Newbury Park, CA: SAGE Publications.

Brody, G. H., Beach, S. R. H., Philibert, R. A., Chen, Y. F., Lei, M. K., Murry, V. M. and Brown, A. C. (2009) 'Parenting moderates a genetic vulnerability factor in longitudinal increases in youths' substance use', *Journal of Consulting and Clinical Psychology*, 77(1), 1–11.

Brody, G. H., Dorsey, S., Forehand, R. and Armistead, L. (2002) 'Unique and protective contributions of parenting and classroom processes to the adjustment of African American children living in single-parent families', *Child Development*, 73(1), 274–286.

Brody, G., Ge, X., Katz, J. and Arias, I. (2000) 'A longitudinal analysis of internalization of parental alcohol-use norms and adolescent alcohol use', *Applied Developmental Science*, 4(2), 71–79.

Brody, G. H., Kogan, S. M., Chen, Y. F. and Murry, V. M. (2008) 'Long-term effects of the Strong African American Families Program on youths' conduct problems', *Journal of Adolescent Health*, 43(5), 474–481.

Brody, G. H., Neubaum, E. and Forehand, R. (1988) 'Serial marriage: A heuristic analysis of an emerging family form', *Psychological Bulletin*, 103(2), 211–222.

Bronfenbrenner, U. (1974) *A Report on Longitudinal Evaluations of Preschool Programs: Is Early Intervention Effective?*, vol. 2, Washington, DC: Department of Health, Education and Welfare.

Bronfenbrenner, U. (1979) *The Ecology of Human Development: Experiments by Nature and Design*, Cambridge, MA: Harvard University Press.

Bronfenbrenner, U., Condry, J. C. and Russell Sage Foundation (1970) *Two Worlds of Childhood: U.S. and U.S.S.R.*, New York, NY: Russell Sage Foundation.

Brookes, S. J., Summers, J. A., Thornburg, K. R., Ispa, J. M. and Lane, V. J. (2006) 'Building successful home visitor–mother relationships and reaching program goals in two Early Head Start programs: A qualitative look at contributing factors', *Early Childhood Research Quarterly*, 21(1), 25–45.

Brownson, R. C., Fielding, J. E. and Maylahn, C. A. (2009) 'Evidence-based public health: A fundamental concept for public health practice', *Annual Review of Public Health*, 30, 175–201.

Budd, K. S. (2005) 'Assessing parenting capacity in a child welfare context', *Children and Youth Services Review*, 27(4), 429–444.

Bulik, C. M., Berkman, N. D., Brownley, K. A., Sedway, J. A. and Lohr, K. N. (2007) 'Anorexia nervosa treatment: A systematic review of randomized controlled trials', *International Journal of Eating Disorders*, 40(4), 310–320.

Bumbarger, B. K. 'Evidence-based programs: moving from "lists" to public health impact', paper presented at *Blueprints for Violence Prevention* in San Antonio, TX, 9 April 2010.

Buri, J. R., Louiselle, P. A., Misukanis, T. M. and Mueller, R. A. (1988) 'Effects of parental authoritarianism and authoritativeness on self-esteem', *Personality and Social Psychology Bulletin*, 14(2), 271–282.

Burman, E. (2008) *Deconstructing Developmental Psychology*, 2nd edn, London: Routledge.

Campbell, D. T. (1957) 'Factors relevant to the validity of experiments in social settings', *Psychological Bulletin*, 54(4), 297–312.

Campbell, S. and Markesinis, B. (2002) *Review of Anti-Social Behaviour Orders*, London: Home Office Research Development and Statistics Directorate.

Carlson, M. J., Pilkauskas, N. V., McLanahan, S. S. and Brooks-Gunn, J. (2009) 'Couples as partners and parents over children's early years'. Online. Available HTTP: http://crcw.princeton.edu/workingpapers/WP09–12-FF.pdf (accessed 22 October 2009).

Cartwright, N., Goldfinch, A. and Howick, J. (2009) 'Evidence-based policy: Where is our theory of evidence?', *Journal of Children's Services*, 4(4), 6–14.

Castro, F. G., Barrera, M. and Martinez, C. R. (2004) 'The cultural adaptation of prevention interventions: Resolving tensions between fidelity and fit', *Prevention Science*, 5(1), 41–45.

Chaffin, M. (2004) 'Is it time to rethink healthy start/healthy families', *Child Abuse and Neglect*, 28(6), 589–595.

Chaffin, M., Hanson, R., Saunders, B. E., Nichols, T., Barnett, D., Zeanah, C., Berliner, L., Egeland, B., Newman, E., Lyon, T., LeTourneau, E. and Miller-Perrin, C. (2006) 'Report of the APSAC task force on attachment therapy, reactive attachment disorder, and attachment problems', *Child Maltreatment*, 11(1), 76–89.

Chamberlain, P., Leve, L. D. and DeGarmo, D. S. (2007) 'Multidimensional treatment foster care for girls in the juvenile justice system: 2-year follow-up of a randomized clinical trial', *Journal of Consulting and Clinical Psychology*, 75(1), 187–193.

Chambless, D. L. and Hollon, S. D. (1998) 'Defining empirically supported therapies', *Journal of Consulting and Clinical Psychology*, 66(1), 7–18.

Chinman, M., Inm, P. and Wandersman, A. (2004) *Getting to Outcomes 2004: Promoting Accountability through Methods and Tools for Planning, Implementation and Evaluation*, Santa Monica, CA: RAND Corporation.

Christensen, A. and Jacobson, N. S. (1994) 'Who (or what) can do psychotherapy: The status and challenge of nonprofessional therapies', *Psychological Science*, 5(1), 8–14.

Cicchetti, D. and Lynch, M. (1993) 'Toward an ecological/transactional model of community violence and child maltreatment: Consequences for children's development', *Psychiatry*, 56(1), 96–118.

Cicchetti, D. and Rizley, R. (1981) 'Developmental perspectives on the etiology, intergenerational transmission, and sequelae of child maltreatment', *New Directions for Child and Adolescent Development*, 11, 31–55.

Cicchetti, D., Rogosch, F. A. and Toth, S. L. (2006) 'Fostering secure attachment in infants in maltreating families through preventive interventions', *Development and Psychopathology*, 18(3), 623–649.

Cicirelli, V. (1969) *The Impact of Head Start: An Evaluation of the Effects of Head Start on Children's Cognitive and Affective Development*, Athens, OH: Westinghouse Learning Corporation, Ohio University.

Cleveland, M. J., Gibbons, F. X., Gerrard, M., Pomery, E. A. and Brody, G. H. (2005) 'The impact of parenting on risk cognitions and risk behavior: A study of mediation and moderation in a panel of African American adolescents', *Child Development*, 76(4), 900–916.

Cohen, M. A. (2005) *The Costs of Crime and Justice*, New York: Routledge.

Cohen, N. J., Muir, E., Lojkasek, M., Muir, R., Parker, C. J., Barwick, M. and Brown, M. (1999) 'Watch, wait, and wonder: Testing the effectiveness of a new approach to mother–infant psychotherapy', *Infant Mental Health Journal*, 20(4), 429–451.

Coleman, J. and Roker, D. (2007) 'Working with parents of young people: Setting the scene', in D. Roker and J. Coleman (eds.) *Working with Parents of Young People: Research, Policy and Practice*, London: J. Kingsley Publishers, 15–26.

Collins, W. A. and Laursen, B. (2004) 'Parent–adolescent relationships and influences', in R. M. Lerner, and L. Steinberg (eds.) *Handbook of Adolescent Psychology*, Chichester: Wiley, 331–361.

Collishaw, S., Maughan, B., Goodman, R. and Pickles, A. (2004) 'Time trends in adolescent mental health', *Journal of Child Psychology and Psychiatry*, 45(8), 1350–1362.

Collishaw, S., Maughan, B., Natarajan, L. and Pickles, A. (2010) 'Trends in adolescent emotional problems in England: A comparison of two national cohorts twenty years apart', *Journal of Child Psychology and Psychiatry*, 51(8), 885–894.

Collishaw, S., Pickles, A., Messer, J., Rutter, M., Shearer, C. and Maughan, B. (2007) 'Resilience to adult psychopathology following childhood maltreatment: Evidence from a community sample', *Child Abuse & Neglect*, 31(3), 211–229.

Connell, J. P., Spencer, M. B. and Aber, J. L. (1994) 'Educational risk and resilience in African-American youth – context, self, action, and outcomes in school', *Child Development*, 65(2), 493–506.

Cook, T. D. and Campbell, D. T. (1979) *Quasi-Experimentation: Design and Analysis Issues for Field Settings*, Chicago, IL: Rand McNally College Publishing Company.

Cookston, J. T., Braver, S. L., Grivvin, W. A., De Luse, S. R. and Miles, J. C. (2006) 'Effects of the Dads for Life intervention on interparental conflict and coparenting in the two years after divorce', *Family Process*, 46(1), 123–137.

Costello, E. J., Mustillo, S., Erkanli, A., Keeler, G. and Angold, A. (2003) 'Prevalence and development of psychiatric disorders in childhood and adolescence', *Archives of General Psychiatry*, 60(8), 837–844.

Coulton, C. J., Crampton, D. S., Irwin, M., Spilsbury, J. C. and Korbin, J. E. (2007) 'How neighborhoods influence child maltreatment: A review of the literature and alternative pathways', *Child Abuse & Neglect*, 31(11–12), 1117–1142.

Coulton, C. J., Korbin, J. E. and Su, M. (1999) 'Neighborhoods and child maltreatment: A multi-level study', *Child Abuse & Neglect*, 23(11), 1019–1040.

Coulton, C. J., Korbin, J. E., Su, M. and Chow, J. (1995) 'Community-level factors and child maltreatment rates', *Child Development*, 66(5), 1262–1276.

Courtney, R., Ballard, E., Fauver, S., Gariota, M. and Holland, L. (1996) 'The partnership model: Working with individuals, families, and communities toward a new vision of health', *Public Health Nursing*, 13(3), 177–186.

Cox, A. D. (1993) 'Befriending young mothers', *British Journal of Psychiatry*, 163(1), 6–18.

Cox, A. D., Pound, A., Mills, M., Puckering, C. and Owen, A. L. (1991) 'Evaluation of a home visiting and befriending scheme for young mothers: Newpin', *Journal of the Royal Society of Medicine*, 84(4), 217–220.

Cox, H. and Hughes, R. (2007) *Effective Practice in Commissioning in Children's Services*, London: PA Consulting Group.

CPPRG (Conduct Problems Prevention Research Group) (1992) 'A developmental and clinical model for the prevention of conduct disorder: The Fast-Track Program', *Development and Psychopathology*, 4(4), 509–527.

CPPRG (Conduct Problems Prevention Research Group) (1999) 'Initial impact of the Fast Track prevention trial for conduct problems: II. Classroom effects', *Journal of Consulting and Clinical Psychology*, 67(5), 648–57.

CPPRG (Conduct Problems Prevention Research Group) (2007) 'Fast Track randomized controlled trial to prevent externalizing psychiatric disorders: Findings from grades 3 to 9', *Journal of the American Academy of Child and Adolescent Psychiatry*, 46(10), 1250–62.

Creer, T. L., Holroyd, K. A., Glasgow, R. E. and Smith, T. W. (2004) 'Health psychology', in M. J. Lambert (ed.) *Bergin and Garfield's Handbook of Psychotherapy and Behaviour Change*, New York: John Wiley & Sons, 697–742.

Crozier, M., Rokutani, L., Russett, J., Godwin, E. and Banks, G. (2010) 'A multisite program evaluation of Families and Schools Together (FAST): Continued evidence of a successful multifamily community-based prevention program', *School Community Journal*, 20(1), 187–208.

CSP (2009) 'Good commissioning: Principles and practice. The Commissioning Support Program'. Online. Available HTTP: http://www.commissioningsupport.org.uk (accessed 1 November 2010).

Cui, M., Conger, R. D., Bryant, C. M. and Elder, G. H. (2002) 'Parental behavior and the quality of adolescent friendships: A social-contextual perspective', *Journal of Marriage and the Family*, 64(3), 676–689.

Cuijpers, P., van Straten, A., Andersson, G. and van Oppen, P. (2008) 'Psychotherapy for depression in adults: A meta-analysis of comparative outcome studies', *Journal of Consulting and Clinical Psychology*, 76(6), 909–922.

Cummings, E., Davies, P. T. and Simpson, K. (1994) 'Marital conflict, gender, and children's appraisals and coping efficacy as mediators of child adjustment', *Journal of Family Psychology*, 8(2), 141–141.

Currie, J. and Thomas, D. (1995) 'Does Head Start make a difference?', *American Economic Review*, 85(3), 341–364.

Dahl, R. E. and Hariri, A. R. (2005) 'Lessons from G. Stanley Hall: Connecting new research in biological sciences to the study of adolescent development', *Journal of Research on Adolescence*, 15(4), 367–382.

Dane, A. V. and Schneider, B. H. (1998) 'Program integrity in primary and early secondary prevention: Are implementation effects out of control', *Clinical Psychology Review*, 18(1), 23–45.

Darling, R. B. (2000) *The Partnership Model in Human Services: Sociological Foundations and Practices*, New York: Kluwer Academic/Plenum Publishers.

Davidson, K., Scott, J., Schmidt, U., Tata, P., Thornton, S. and Tyrer, P. (2004) 'Therapist competence and clinical outcome in the prevention of parasuicide by manual assisted cognitive behaviour therapy trial: The POPMACT study', *Psychological Medicine*, 34(5), 855–863.

Davies, P. T. and Cummings, E. M. (1998) 'Exploring children's emotional security as a mediator of the link between marital relations and child adjustment', *Child Development*, 69(1), 124–139.

Davies, P. T., Harold, G. T., Goeke-Morey, M. C., Cummings, E. M., Shelton, K. and Rasi, J. A. (2002) 'Child emotional security and interparental conflict', *Monographs of Society for Research in Child Development*, 67(3), i–v, vii–viii, 1–115.

Davis, D. (2004) *Child Development: A Practitioner's Guide*, New York, NY: Guilford Press.

Davis, E. P. and Sandman, C. A. (2010) 'The timing of prenatal exposure to maternal cortisone and psychosocial stress is associated with human infant cognitive development', *Child Development*, 81(1), 131–148.

Davis, E. P., Townsend, E. L., Gunnar, M. R., Georgieff, M. K., Guiang, S. F., Cifuentes, R. F. et al. (2004) 'Effects of prenatal corticosteroid exposure on regulation of stress physiology in healthy premature infants', *Psychoneuroendocrinology*, 29(29), 1028–1036

Davis, H., Day, C. and Bidmead, C. (2002) *Working in Partnership with Parents: The Parent Adviser Model*, London: Psychological Corporation.

Dawe, S. and Harnett, P. (2007) 'Reducing potential for child abuse among methadone-maintained parents: Results from a randomized controlled trial', *Journal of Substance Abuse Treatment*, 32(4), 381–390.

Dawes, M., Davies, P., Gray, A., Mant, J., Seers, K., and Snowball, R. (2005) *Evidence-based Practice: A Primer for Health Care Professionals*, 2nd edn, London: Elsevier.

Day, C., Kowalenko, S., Ellis, M., Dawe, S., Harnett, P. and Scott, S. (in press) 'The Helping Families Program: A new parenting intervention for children with severe and persistent conduct problems', *Child and Adolescent Mental Health*.

DCSF (2010) *Sure Start Children's Centres*. Online. Available HTTP: http://www.dcsf.gov.uk/everychild-matters/earlyyears/surestart/whatsurestartdoes/ (accessed 19 September 2010).

De Bellis, M. D. and Keshavan, M. S. (2003) 'Sex differences in brain maturation in maltreatment-related pediatric post-traumatic stress disorder', *Neuroscience and Biobehavioral Reviews*, 27(1–2), 103–117.

De Bellis, M. D., Keshavan, M. S., Clark, D. B. et al. (1999b) 'Developmental traumatology, part II: Brain development', *Biological Psychiatry*, 45(10), 1271–1284.

De Bellis, M. D., Baum, A., Birmaher, B., Keshavan, M., Eccard, C. H., Boring, A. M. et al. (1999a) 'A. E. Bennett Research Award, Developmental traumatology part I: Biological stress systems', *Biological Psychiatry*, 45(10), 1259–1270.

De Bellis, M. D., Keshavan, M. S., Shifflett, H., Iyenager, S., Beers, S., Hall, J. and Moritz, G. (2002) 'Brain structures in pediatric maltreatment-related posttraumatic stress disorder: A sociodemographically matched study', *Biological Psychiatry*, 52(10), 1066–1078.

Decker, S. L. (2008) 'Intervention psychometrics: Using norm-referenced methods for treatment planning and monitoring', *Assessment for Effective Intervention*, 34(1), 52–61.

DeGarmo, D. S. and Forgatch, M. S. (2007) 'Efficacy of parent training for stepfathers: From playful spectator and polite stranger to effective stepfathering', *Parenting – Science and Practice*, 7(4), 331–355.

Dembo, M. H., Sweitzer, M. and Lauritzen, P. (1985) 'An evaluation of group parent education: Behavioral, PET, and Adlerian programs', *Review of Educational Research*, 55(2), 155–200.

Deoni, S. C. L., Mercure, E., Basi, A., Gasston, D., Thomson, A., Johnson, M., Williams S. C. R. and Murphy D. G. M. (2011) 'Mapping infant brain myelination', *The Journal of Neuroscience*, 31(2), 784–791.

DfES (2004) *Every Child Matters: Change for Children*, Nottingham: DfES Publications.

DfES (2006) *Parenting Support Guidance for Local Authorities in England*, Nottingham: DfES Publications.

DfES (2007) *Every Parent Matters*, Nottingham: DfES Publications.

Dishion, T. J. and Andrews, D. W. (1995) 'Preventing escalation in problem behaviors with high-risk young adolescents – immediate and 1-year outcomes', *Journal of Consulting and Clinical Psychology*, 63(4), 538–548.

Dishion, T. J., McCord, J. and Poulin, F. (1999) 'When interventions harm: Peer groups and problem behavior', *American Psychologist*, 54(9), 755–764.

Dmitrieva, J., Chen, C. S., Greenberger, E. and Gil-Rivas, V. (2004) 'Family relationships and adolescent psychosocial outcomes: Converging findings from Eastern and Western cultures', *Journal of Research on Adolescence*, 14(4), 425–447.

Dodge, K. A. (2009) 'Community intervention and public policy in the prevention of antisocial behavior', *Journal of Child Psychology and Psychiatry*, 50(1–2), 194–200.

DoH/DfES (2004a) *National Service Framework for Children, Young People and Maternity Services*, London: Department of Health.

DoH/DfES (2004b) *National Service Framework for Children, Young People and Maternity Services. Core Standards*, London: Department of Health.

Donaldson, S. I., Graham, J. W. and Hansen, W. B. (1994) 'Testing the generalizability of intervening mechanism theories: Understanding the effects of adolescent drug use prevention interventions', *Journal of Behavioral Medicine*, 17(2), 195–216.

Donaldson, S. I., Graham, J. W., Piccinin, A. M. and Hansen, W. B. (1995) 'Resistance-skills training and onset of alcohol-use: Evidence for beneficial and potentially harmful effects in public schools and in private Catholic schools', *Health Psychology*, 14(4), 291–300.

Dornbusch, S. M., Ritter, P. L., Leiderman, P. H., Roberts, D. F. and Fraleigh, M. J. (1987) 'The relation of parenting style to adolescent school performance', *Child Development*, 58(5), 1244–1257.

Drake, E., Aos, S. and Miller, M. (2009) 'Evidence-based public policy options to reduce crime and criminal justice costs: Implications in Washington State', *Victims and Offenders*, 4(12) 170–196.

Dretzke, J., Davenport, C., Frew, E., Barlow, J., Stewart-Brown, S., Bayliss, S., Taylor, R. S., Sandercock, J. and Hyde, C. (2009) 'The clinical effectiveness of different parenting programmes for children with conduct problems: A systematic review of randomised controlled trials', *Child and Adolescent Psychiatry and Mental Health*, 3(1), 7.

Duggan, A., Fuddy, L., Burrell, L., Higman, S., McFarlane, E., Windham, A. and Sia, C. (2004a) 'Randomized trial of a statewide home visiting program to prevent child abuse: Impact in reducing parental risk factors', *Child Abuse & Neglect*, 28(6), 625–645.

Duggan, A., McFarlane, E., Fuddy, L., Burrell, L., Higman, S., Windham, A. and Sia, C. (2004b) 'Randomized trial of a statewide home visiting program: Impact in preventing child abuse and neglect', *Child Abuse & Neglect*, 28(6), 597–622.

Durlak, J. A. and DuPre, E. P. (2008) 'Implementation matters: A review of research on the influence of implementation on program outcomes and the factors affecting implementation', *American Journal of Community Psychology*, 41(3–4), 327–350.

Duyme, M., Arseneault, L., and Bumaret, A. C. (2004) ' Environmental influences on intellectual abilities in childhood: Findings from a longitudinal adoption study', in P. L. Chase-Lansdale, K. Kiernan, and R. J. Friedman (eds.) *Human Development across Lives and Generations: The Potential for Change*, New York, NY: Cambridge University Press, 278–292.

Eames, C., Daley, D., Hutchings, J., Whitaker, C. J., Jones, K., Hughes, J. C. and Bywater, T. (2009) 'Treatment fidelity as a predictor of behaviour change in parents attending group-based parent training', *Child Care Health and Development*, 35(5), 603–612.

Eckenrode, J., Campa, M., Luckey, D. W., Henderson, C. R., Cole, R., Kitzman, H., Anson, E., Sidora-Arcoleo, K., Powers, J. and Olds, D. (2010) 'Long-term effects of prenatal and infancy nurse home visitation on the life course of youths: 19-year follow-up of a randomized trial', *Archives of Pediatrics & Adolescent Medicine*, 164(1), 9–15.

Edwards, A., Barnes, M., Plewis, I. and Morris, K. (2006) *Working to Prevent the Social Exclusion of Children and Young People: Final Lessons from the National Evaluation of the Children's Fund*, Research Report No. 734, Nottingham: DfES Publications.

Edwards, R. T., Ceilleachair, A., Bywater, T., Hughes, D. A. and Hutchings, J. (2007) 'Parenting programme for parents of children at risk of developing conduct disorder: Cost effectiveness analysis', *British Medical Journal*, 334(7595), 682–685.

Edwards, R. W., Jumper-Thurman, P., Plested, B. A., Oetting, E. R. and Swanson, L. (2000) 'Community readiness: Research to practice', *Journal of Community Psychology*, 28(3), 291–307.

Egeland, B. (2009) 'Attachment-based intervention and prevention programs for young children'. Online. Available HTTP: http://www.child-encyclopedia.com/pages/PDF/EgelandANGxp_rev.pdf (accessed 3 October 2010).

Ehrenberg, M. F., Gearing-Small, M., Hunter, M. A. and Small, B. J. (2001) 'Childcare task division and shared parenting attitudes in dual-earner families with young children', *Family Relations*, 50(2), 143–153.

Eisenberg, N. (1990) 'Prosocial development in early and mid-adolescence', in R. Montemayor, G. R Adams and T. P. Gullotta (eds.) *From Childhood to Adolescence: A Transitional Period*, Newbury Park, CA: Sage.

Eisenberg, N., Morris, A. S., McDaniel, B. and Spinrad, T. L. (2004) 'Moral cognitions and prosocial responding in adolescence', in R. M. Lerner, and L. Steinberg (eds.) *Handbook of Adolescent Psychology*, Chichester: Wiley, 155–188.

Eisler, I., Simic, M., Russell, G. F. M. and Dare, C. (2007) 'A randomised controlled treatment trial of two forms of family therapy in adolescent anorexia nervosa: A five-year follow-up', *Journal of Child Psychology and Psychiatry*, 48(6), 552–560.

Elbert, T., Pantev, C., Wienbruch, C., Rockstroh, B. and Taub, E. (1995) 'Increased cortical representation of the fingers of the left hand in string players', *Science*, 270(5234), 305–307.

Elliott, D. S. and Mihalic, S. (2004) 'Issues in disseminating and replicating effective prevention programs', *Prevention Science*, 5(1), 47–53.

Elliott, R., Greenberg, L. S. and Lietaer, G. (2004) 'Research on experiential psychotherapies', in M. J. Lambert (ed.) *Bergin and Garfield's Handbook of Psychotherapy and Behaviour Change*, New York: John Wiley and Sons, 493–540.

Ellis, A. (1989) 'The history of cognition in psychotherapy', in A. Freeman, K. M. Simon, L. E. Beutler and H. Arkowitz (eds.) *Comprehensive Handbook of Cognitive Therapy*, New York: Plenum Publishing, 5–19.

Ellis, A. (2003) 'Early theories and practices of rational emotive behavior therapy and how they have been augmented and revised during the last three decades', *Journal of Rational-Emotive and Cognitive-Behaviour Therapy*, 21(3–4), 219–243.

Emshoff, J., Blakely, C., Gray, D., Jakes, S., Brounstein, P., Coulter, J. and Gardner, S. (2003) 'An ESID case study at the federal level', *American Journal of Community Psychology*, 32(3–4), 345–357.

Ensink, K. and Mayes, L. C. (2010) 'The development of mentalisation in children from a theory of mind perspective', *Psychoanalytic Inquiry*, 30(4), 301–337.

Epstein, N. B., Baldwin, L. and Bishop, D. S. (1983) 'The McMaster Family Assessment Device', *Journal of Marital and Family Therapy*, 9(2), 171–180.

Ernst, C. C., Grant, T. M., Streissguth, A. P. and Sampson, P. D. (1999) 'Intervention with high-risk alcohol and drug-abusing mothers: II. Three-year findings from the Seattle model of paraprofessional advocacy', *Journal of Community Psychology*, 27(1), 19–38.

Evans, D. (2003) 'Hierarchy of evidence: A framework for ranking evidence evaluating healthcare interventions', *Journal of Clinical Nursing*, 12(1), 77–84.

Fairbairn, W. R. D. (1952) *Psychoanalytic Studies of the Personality*, London: Tavistock Publications.

Fairbairn, W. R. D. (1986) 'A revised psychopathology of the psychoses and psychoneuroses', *International Journal of Psycho-Analysis*, 22, 250–279, 1941; reprinted in P. Buckley (ed.) *Essential Papers on Object Relations*, New York, NY: New York University Press, 71–101.

Feinberg, M. (2002) 'Coparenting and the transition to parenthood: A framework for prevention', *Clinical Child & Family Psychology Review*, 5(3), 73–195.

Feinberg, M. E. (2003) 'The internal structure and ecological context of coparenting: A framework for research and intervention', *Parenting-Science and Practice*, 3(2), 95–131.

Feinberg, M. E., Jones, D. E., Kan, M. L. and Goslin, M. (2010) 'Effects of a transition to parenthood program on parents, parenting and children', *Journal of Family Psychology*, 24(5), 532–542.

Feinberg, M. E., Jones, D., Greenberg, M. T., Osgood, D. W. and Bontempo, D. (2010) 'Effects of the Communities That Care model in Pennsylvania on change in adolescent risk and problem behaviors', *Prevention Science*, 11(2), 163–171.

Feinberg, M. E. and Kan, M. L. (2008) 'Family foundations at child age one year: Effects on observed coparenting, parenting, and child self-regulation', *Prevention Science*, 10(3), 276–285.

Feinstein, A. R. (1985) *Clinical Epidemiology: The Architecture of Clinical Research*, Philadelphia, PA: WB Saunders Company.

Feldman, J. and Kazdin, A. (1995) 'Parent management training for oppositional and conduct problem children', *The Clinical Psychologist*, 48(4), 3–5.

Fetterman, D. M. and Wandersman, A. (2005) *Empowerment Evaluation Principles in Practice*, New York: Guilford Press.

Field, F. (2010) *The Foundation Years: Preventing Poor Children Becoming Poor Adults*, London: Cabinet Office.

Fixsen, D. L., Blase, K. A., Naoom, S. F. and Wallace, F. (2009) 'Core implementation components', *Research on Social Work Practice*, 19(5), 531–540.

Fixsen, D. L., Naoom, S. F., Blase, K. A., Friedman, R. M. and Wallace, F. (2005) *Implementation Research: A Synthesis of the Literature*, Tampa, FL: University of South Florida, Louis de la Parte Florida Mental Health Institute, The National Implementation Research Network.

Fixsen, D. L., Blase, K. A., Duda, M. A., Naoom, S. F. and Van Dyke, M. (2010) 'Implementation of evidence-based treatments for children and adolescents: Research findings and their implications for the future', in J. R. Weisz and A. E. Kazdin (eds.) *Evidence-Based Psychotherapies for Children and Adolescents*, 2nd edn, London: The Guilford Press, 435–451.

Flavell, S. W., Cowan, C. W., Kim, T. K., Greer, P. L., Lin, X., Paradis, S. et al. (2006) 'Activity-dependent regulation of MEF2 transcription factors suppresses excitatory synapse number', *Science*, 311(5763), 1008–1012.

Flay, B. R. (1986) 'Efficacy and effectiveness trials (and other phases of research) in the development of health promotion programs', *Preventive Medicine*, 15(5), 451–474.

Flay, B. R., Biglan, A., Boruch, R. F., Castro, F. G., Gottfredson, D., Kellam, S., Moscicki, E. K., Schinke, S., Valentine, J. C. and Ji, P. (2005) 'Standards of evidence: Criteria for efficacy, effectiveness and dissemination', *Prevention Science*, 6(3), 151–175.

Floyd, F. J. and Zmich, D. E. (1991) 'Marriage and the parenting partnership: Perceptions and interactions of parents with mentally-retarded and typically-developing children', *Child Development*, 62(6), 1434–1448.

Flynn, L. M. (2005) 'Family perspectives on evidence-based practice', *Child and Adolescent Psychiatric Clinics of North America*, 14(2), 217–224.

Fonagy, P. (1997) 'Attachment and theory of mind: Overlapping constructs?', *Association for Child Psychology and Psychiatry Occasional Papers*, 14, 31–40.

Fonagy, P., Steele, M., Moran, G., Steele, H. and Higgitt, A. (1993) 'Measuring the ghost in the nursery: An empirical study of the relation between parents' mental representations of childhood experiences and their infants' security of attachment', *Journal of the American Psychoanalytic Association*, 41(4), 957–989.

Fonagy, P., Steele, M., Steele, H., Moran, G. S. and Higgitt, A. C. (1991) 'The capacity for understanding mental states – the reflective self in parent and child and its significance for security of attachment', *Infant Mental Health Journal*, 12(3), 201–218.

Fonagy, P., Target, M., Cottrell, D., Phillips, J. and Kurtz, A. (2002) *What Works for Whom?: A Critical Review of Treatments for Children and Adolescents*, New York: Guilford Press.

Ford, C. A., Pence, B. W., Miller, W. C., Resnick, M. D., Bearinger, L. H., Pettingell, S. and Cohen, M. (2005) 'Predicting adolescents' longitudinal risk for sexually transmitted infection – Results from the national longitudinal study of adolescent health', *Archives of Pediatrics & Adolescent Medicine*, 159(7), 657–664.

Forehand, R. and Kotchick, B. A. (2002) 'Behavioral parent training: Current challenges and potential solutions', *Journal of Child and Family Studies*, 11(4), 377–384.

Forgatch, M. S. and Patterson, G. R. (2010) 'Parent management training – Oregon model: An intervention for antisocial behavior in children and adolescents', in J. R. Weisz and A. E. Kazdin (eds.) *Evidence-based Psychotherapies for Children and Adolescents*, 2nd edn, New York: Guilford Press, 159–178.

Forgatch, M. S., Patterson, G. R. and DeGarmo, D. S. (2005) 'Evaluating fidelity: Predictive validity for a measure of competent adherence to the Oregon model of parent management training', *Behavior Therapy*, 36(1), 3–13.

Forgatch, M. S., Patterson, G. R., Degarmo, D. S. and Beldavs, Z. G. (2009) 'Testing the Oregon delinquency model with 9-year follow-up of the Oregon Divorce Study', *Development and Psychopathology*, 21(2), 637–660.

Foster, E. M., Dodge, K. A. and Jones, D. (2003) 'Issues in the economic evaluation of prevention programs', *Applied Developmental Science*, 7(2), 76–86.

Fox, S. E., Levitt, P. and Nelson III, C. A. (2010) 'How the timing and quality of early experiences influence the development of brain architecture', *Child Development*, 81(1), 28–40.

Fraiberg, S., Adelson, E. and Shapiro, V. (1980) 'Ghosts in the nursery: A psychoanalytic approach to the problem of impaired infant–mother relationships', *Journal of the American Academy of Child Psychiatry*, 14(3), 387–421, 1975; reprinted in S. Fraiberg (ed.) *Clinical Studies in Infant Mental Health: The First Year of Life*, New York, NY: Basic Books.

Freud, S. (1911) 'Formulations regarding the two principles of mental functioning', *Collected Papers, Vol. IV*, New York: Basic Books, 1959.

Freud, S. (1924) *A General Introduction to Psychoanalysis*, New York: Boni and Liveright.

Freud, S. (1933) *New Introductory Lectures on Psychoanalysis*, W. J. H. Sproutt (trans.), New York: Norton.

Freud, S. (1940) 'An outline of psychoanalysis', *International Journal of Psychoanalysis*, 21(1), 27–84.

Freud, S. (1948) *Beyond the Pleasure Principle*, London: The Hogarth Press.

Freud, S. (1953) *The Interpretation of Dreams*, J. Strachey (trans.), London: Hogarth Press.

Freud, S. (1959) *Collected Papers*, Vols. I – V, New York: Basic Books.

Frick, P. (1991) 'The Alabama Parenting Questionnaire', University of Alabama, unpublished.

Friedman, M. (2005) *Trying Hard is Not Good Enough. How to Produce Measurable Improvements for Customers and Communities*, Victoria, British Columbia: Trafford Publishing.

Frosch, C. A., Mangelsdorf, S. C. and McHale, J. L. (2000) 'Marital behavior and the security of preschooler–parent attachment relationships', *Journal of Family Psychology*, 14(1), 144–161.

Fuhrman, T. and Holmbeck, G. N. (1995) 'Contextual-moderator analysis of emotional autonomy and adjustment in adolescence', *Child Development*, 66(3), 793–811.

Fuligni, A. J. and Eccles, J. S. (1993) 'Perceived parent-child relationships and early adolescents' orientation toward peers', *Developmental Psychology*, 29(4), 622–632.

Furedi, F. (2008) *Paranoid Parenting: Why ignoring the experts may be best for your child*, London: Continuum UK.

Furedi, F. (2009) *Intensive Parenting*, Frank Furedi. Online. Available HTTP: http://www.frankfuredi.com/index.php/site/article/328 (accessed 30 October 2010).

Garbarino, J. and Crouter, A. (1978) 'Defining community context for parent–child relations – correlates of child maltreatment', *Child Development*, 49(3), 604–616.

Garbarino, J. and Sherman, D. (1980) 'High-risk neighborhoods and high-risk families: The human ecology of child maltreatment', *Child Development*, 51(1), 188–198.

Garces, E., Thomas, D. and Currie, J. (2002) 'Longer-term effects of Head Start', *American Economic Review*, 92(4), 999–1012.

Garralda, E. M. (2009) 'Accountability of specialist child and adolescent mental health services', *British Journal of Psychiatry*, 194(5), 389–391.

George, C. (1996) 'A representational perspective of child abuse and prevention: Internal working models of attachment and caregiving', *Child Abuse & Neglect*, 20(5), 411–424.

Gerris, J. R. M., van As, N. M. C., Wells, P. M. A. and Jansson, J. M. A. M. (1998) 'From parent education to family empowerment', in L. L'Abato (ed.) *Family Psychotherapy: The Relational Roots of Dysfunctional Behaviour*, New York: The Guildford Press, 401–426.

Ghate, D., Asmussen, K., Tian, Y. and Hauari, H. (2008) *On Track Phase Two National Evaluation: Reducing risks and increasing resilience. How did On Track work?* Research Report No. 35, London: DCSF.

Ghate, D. and Hazel, N. (2004) *Parenting in Poor Environments: Key Messages for Policy Makers from a New National Study*, London: Department of Health.

Ghate, D. and Ramella, M. (2002) *Positive Parenting: The National Evaluation of the Youth Justice Board's Parenting Programme*, London: Youth Justice Board.

Gibaud-Wallston, J. and Wandersman, L. (1978) 'Development and utility of the Parenting Sense of Competence Scale', paper presented at the meeting of the American Psychological Association in Toronto.

Gibbs, L. E. (2003) *Evidence-based Practice for the Helping Professions: A Practical Guide with Integrated Multimedia*, Pacific Grove, CA: Brooks/Cole-Thomson Learning.

Giedd, J. N. (2004) 'Structural magnetic resonance imaging of the adolescent brain', *Annals of New York Academy of Sciences*, Adolescent Brain Development: Vulnerabilities and Opportunities, 1021, 77–85.

Gillies, V. (2005) 'Meeting parents' needs? Discourses of "support" and "inclusion" in family policy', *Critical Social Policy*, 25(1), 70–90.

Glass, N. (1999) '*Sure Start*: The development of an early intervention programme for young children in the United Kingdom', *Children and Society*, 13(4), 257–264.

Goldenberg, I. and Goldenberg, H. (1996) *Family Therapy: An Overview*, 4th edn, Pacific Grove, CA: Brooks/Cole.

Gomby, D. S. (1999) 'Understanding evaluations of home visitation programs', *Future of Children*, 9(1), 27–43.

Gomby, D. S. (2007) 'The promise and limitations of home visiting: Implementing effective programs', *Child Abuse & Neglect*, 31(8), 793–799.

Gomby, D., Culross, P. and Behrman, R. (1999) 'Home visiting: Recent program evaluations: Analysis and recommendations', *The Future of Children*, 9(1), 4–26.

Goodman, R. (1997) 'The strengths and difficulties questionnaire: A research note', *Journal of Child Psychology and Psychiatry and Allied Disciplines*, 38(5), 581–586.

Gordon, D. A. (2000) 'Parent training via CD-ROM: Using technology to disseminate effective prevention practices', *Journal of Primary Prevention*, 21(2), 227–251.

Gordon, D. A. and Arbuthnot, J. (1988) 'The use of paraprofessionals to deliver home-based family therapy to juvenile delinquents', *Criminal Justice and Behavior*, 15(3), 364–378.

Granic, I. and Patterson, G. R. (2006) 'Toward a comprehensive model of antisocial development: A dynamic systems approach', *Psychological Review*, 113(1), 101–131.

Grant, T. M., Ernst, C. C. and Streissguth, A. P. (1996) 'An intervention with high-risk mothers who abuse alcohol and drugs: The Seattle Advocacy Model', *American Journal of Public Health*, 86(12), 1816–1817.

Grant, T., Ernst, C. C., Pagalilauan, G. and Streissguth, A. (2003) 'Postprogram follow-up effects of paraprofessional intervention with high-risk women who abused alcohol and drugs during pregnancy', *Journal of Community Psychology*, 31(3), 211–222.

Gray, M. and McDonald, C. (2006) 'Pursuing good practice? The limits of evidence-based practice', *Journal of Social Work*, 6(1), 7–20.

Green, H., McGinnity, A., Meltzer, H., Ford, T. and Goodman, R. (2005) *Mental Health of Children and Young People in Great Britain, 2004*, New York: NY: Palgrave Macmillan.

Green, J. (2006) 'Annotation: The therapeutic alliance – a significant but neglected variable in child mental health treatment studies', *Journal of Child Psychology and Psychiatry*, 47(5), 425–435.

Greenberg, M. T. (1999) 'Attachment and psychopathology in childhood', in J. Cassidy and P. R. Shaver (eds.) *Handbook of Attachment: Theory, Research, and Clinical Applications*, New York, NY: Guilford Press, 469–496.

Greenberg, M. T., Kusche, C. A., Cook, E. T. and Quamma, J. P. (1995) 'Promoting emotional competence in school-aged children: The effects of the PATHS curriculum', *Development and Psychopathology*, 7(1), 117–136.

Greenough, W. T. and Black, J. E. (1992) 'Induction of brain structure by experience: Substrates for cognitive development', in M. R. Gunnar and C. A. Nelson (eds.) *Developmental Behavioral Neuroscience*, Hillsdale, NJ: Lawrence Erlbaum Associates, 155–200.

Grimes, D. A. and Schulz, K. F. (2002a) 'An overview of clinical research: The lay of the land', *Lancet*, 359(9300), 57–61.

Grimes, D. A. and Schulz, K. F. (2002b) 'Bias and causal associations in observational research', *Lancet*, 359(9302), 248–252.

Grolnick, W. S. and Farkas, M. (2002) 'Parenting and the development of children's self-regulation', in M. H. Bornstein (ed.) *The Handbook of Parenting: Practical Issues in Parenting*, vol. 5, New Jersey, NJ: Lawrence Erlbaum, 89–110.

Grotevant, H. D. and Cooper, C. R. (1998) 'Individuality and connectedness in adolescent development: Review and prospects for research on identity, relationships and context', in E. Skoe and A. von der Lippe (eds.) *Personality Development in Adolescence: A Cross National and Life Span Perspective*, London: Routledge, 3–37.

Gunnar, M. and Quevedo, K. (2007) 'The neurobiology of stress and development', *Annual Review of Psychology*, 58, 145–173.

Gutteling, B. M., de Weerth, C. and Buitelaar, J. K. (2005) 'Prenatal stress and children's cortisol reaction to the first day of school', *Psychoneuroendocrinology*, 30(6), 541–549.

Haggerty, K. P. and Spoth, R. (2010) 'Recruiting parents into blueprint model parenting programs: What we've learned and lessons from the field', paper presented at *Blueprints for Violence Prevention*, San Antonio, TX, 10April 2010.

Haggerty, K. P., MacKenzie, E. P., Skinner, M. L., Harachi, T. W. and Catalano, R. F. (2006) 'Participation in "Parents Who Care": Predicting program initiation and exposure in two different program formats', *Journal of Primary Prevention*, 27(1), 47–65.

Hamilton, C. E. (2000) 'Continuity and discontinuity of attachment from infancy through adolescence', *Child Development*, 71(3), 690–694.

Hammersley, M. (2005) 'Is the evidence-based practice movement doing more good than harm? Reflections on Iain Chalmers' case for research-based policy making and practice', *Evidence and Policy*, 1(1), 85–100.

Hardiker, P., Exton, K. and Barker, M. (1991) 'The social policy contexts of prevention in child care', *British Journal of Social Work*, 21(4), 341–359.

Harpaz-Rotem, I., Leslie, D. and Rosenheck, R. A. (2004) 'Treatment retention among children entering a new episode of mental health care', *Psychiatric Services*, 55(9), 1022–1028.

Haskins, R., Paxson, C. and Brooks-Gunn, J. (2009a) 'Home visiting programs: An example of social science influencing policy', *Social Policy Report. Society for Research in Child Development*, 23(9), 7.

Haskins, R., Paxson, C. and Brooks-Gunn, J. (2009b) 'Social science rising: A tale of evidence shaping public policy', *The Future of Children*, 19(2), 1–7.

Hauser, S. T., Powers, S. I., Noam, G. G., Jacobson, A. M., Weiss, B. and Follansbee, D. J. (1984) 'Familial contexts of adolescent ego development', *Child Development*, 55(1), 195–213.

Hawkins, J. D. and Catalano, R. F. (1992) *Communities that Care: Action for Drug Abuse Prevention*, San Francisco, CA: Jossey-Bass Inc.

Hawkins, J. D., Brown, E. C., Oesterle, S., Arthur, M. W., Abbott, R. D. and Catalano, R. F. (2008) 'Early effects of Communities That Care on targeted risks and initiation of delinquent behavior and substance use', *Journal of Adolescent Health*, 43(1), 15–22.

Haynes, R. B. (2006) 'Of studies, syntheses, synopses, summaries, and systems: The "5S" evolution of information services for evidence-based healthcare decisions', *Evidence-Based Medicine*, 11(6), 162–164.

Haynes, R., Devereaux, P. J. and Guyatt, G. H. (2002) 'Clinical expertise in the era of evidence-based medicine and patient choice', *Evidence-Based Medicine*, 7(2), 36–38.

Head, B. W. (2008) 'Three lenses of evidence-based policy', *Australian Journal of Public Administration*, 67(1), 1–11.

Hebbeler, K. M. and Gerlach-Downie, S. G. (2002) 'Inside the black box of home visiting: A qualitative analysis of why intended outcomes were not achieved', *Early Childhood Research Quarterly*, 17(1), 28–51.

Heineman, M. B. (1981) 'The obsolete scientific imperative in social-work research', *Social Service Review*, 55(3), 372–397.

Hellend, H. (2009) 'Developing and implementing an integrated suite of evidence-based programmes in Norway', paper presented at *Investing in Children* in London, 24 February 2009.

Henggeler, S. W. and Schaeffer, C. (2010) 'Treating serious antisocial behavior using multisystemic therapy', J. R. Weisz and A. E. Kazdin (eds.) *Evidence-Based Psychotherapies for Children and Adolescents*, 2nd edn, New York: Guilford Press, 259–276.

Henggeler, S. W., Melton, G. B., Brondino, M. J., Scherer, D. G. and Hanley, J. H. (1997) 'Multisystemic therapy with violent and chronic juvenile offenders and their families: The role of treatment fidelity in successful dissemination', *Journal of Consulting and Clinical Psychology*, 65(5), 821–833.

Henggeler, S. W., Mihalic, S. F., Rone, L., Thomas, C. and Timmons-Mitchell, J. (1998) *Multisystemic Therapy: Blueprints for Violence Prevention, Book Six*, Boulder, CO: Center for the Study and Prevention of Violence, Institute of Behavioral Science, University of Colorado at Boulder.

Henrich, C. (2004) 'Head Start as a national laboratory', in E. Zigler and S. J. Styfco (eds.) *The Head Start Debates: Are We Failing the Children Most at Risk? 53 of America's Leading Experts Weigh In*, Baltimore, MD: Paul H. Brookes Publishing, 517–532.

Henricson, C. (1999) *Teenagers' attitudes to parenting: A survey of young people's experiences of being parented and their views on how to bring up children*, London: National Family and Parenting Institute.

Higgins, J. and Green, S. (2008) *Cochrane Handbook for Systematic Reviews of Interventions: Cochrane Book Series*, Chichester, England; Hoboken, NJ: Wiley-Blackwell.

HM Government (2004) *Children Act 2004*, London: The Stationery Office.

HM Treasury (1998) *Comprehensive Spending Review: Cross-departmental Review of Provision for Young Children*, London: The Stationery Office.

HM Treasury (2002) *Spending Review*, London: The Stationery Office.

HM Treasury (2005) *Support for Parents: The Best Start for Children*, London: The Stationery Office.

Hoagwood, K. E. and Cavaleri, M. A. (2010) 'Ethical issues in child and adolescent psychosocial treatment research', in J. R. Weisz and A. E. Kazdin (eds.) *Evidence-based Psychotherapies for Children and Adolescents*, 2nd edn, New York, NY: Guilford Press, 10–28.

Hoffman, K. T., Marvin, R. S., Cooper, G. and Powell, B. (2006) 'Changing toddlers' and preschoolers' attachment classifications: The circle of security intervention', *Journal of Consulting and Clinical Psychology*, 74(6), 1017–1026.

Hogan, M. F. (2003) 'The President's New Freedom Commission: Recommendations to transform mental health care in America', *Psychiatric Services*, 54(11), 1467–1474.

Hollon, S. D. and Beck, A. T. (2004) 'Cognitive and cognitive behavioural therapies', in M. J. Lambert (ed.) *Bergin and Garfield's Handbook of Psychotherapy and Behaviour Change*, New York: John Wiley and Sons, 447–492.

Holmbeck, G. N., Devine, K. A. and Bruno, E. F. (2010) 'Developmental issues and considerations in research and practice', in J. R. Weisz and A. E. Kazdin (eds.) *Evidence-based Psychotherapies for Children and Adolescents*, 2nd edn, New York: Guilford Press, 28–45.

Holmes, D., Murray, S. J., Perron, A. and Rail, G. (2006) 'Deconstructing the evidence-based discourse in health sciences: Truth, power and fascism', *International Journal of Evidence Based Healthcare*, 4(3), 180–186.

Home Office (1998) *Supporting Families*, London: The Stationery Office.

Horvath, A. O. (1994) 'Research on the alliance', in A. O. Horvath and L. S. Greenberg (eds.) *The Working Alliance: Theory, Research and Practice*, New York: Wiley, 259–286.

Horvath, A. O. and Bedi, R. P. (2002) 'The alliance', in J. C. Norcross (ed.) *Psychotherapy Relationships that Work: Therapist Contributions and Responsiveness to Patients*, New York: Oxford University Press, 37–69.

Horvath, A. O. and Greenberg, L. S. (1989) 'Development and validation of the Working Alliance Inventory', *Journal of Counseling Psychology*, 36(2), 223–233.

Huey, S. J., Henggeler, S. W., Brondino, M. J. and Pickrel, S. G. (2000) 'Mechanisms of change in multisystemic therapy: Reducing delinquent behavior through therapist adherence and improved family and peer functioning', *Journal of Consulting and Clinical Psychology*, 68(3), 451–467.

Hull, D. (2010) 'How many journal articles have been published (ever)?'. Online. Available HTTP: http://duncan.hull.name/2010/07/15/fifty-million/ (accessed 30 September 2010).

Hunter, B. (2001) 'Emotion work in midwifery: A review of current knowledge', *Journal of Advanced Nursing*, 34(4), 436–444.

Hutchings, J., Bywater, T., Daley, D., Gardner, F., Whitaker, C., Jones, K., Eames, C. and Edwards, R. T. (2007) 'Parenting intervention in *Sure Start* services for children at risk of developing conduct disorder: Pragmatic randomised controlled trial', *British Medical Journal*, 334(7604), 1158–1158.

Hutchings, J., Lane, E., Owen, R. E. and Gwyn, R. (2004) 'The introduction of the Webster-Stratton Incredible Years Classroom Dinosaur School Programme in Gwynedd, North Wales: A pilot study', *Educational and Child Psychology*, 21(4), 4–15.

Huttonlocher, P. R. (1990) 'Morphometric study of human cerebral cortex development', *Neuropsychologica*, 28(6), 517–527.

Huttonlocher, P. R. (1997) 'Regional differences in the synaptogenesis in human cerebral cortex', *The Journal of Comparative Neurology*, 387(2), 167–178.

IOM (Institute of Medicine) (2001) *Crossing the Quality Chasm: A New Health System for the 21st Century*, Washington, DC: National Academy Press.

IOM (Institute of Medicine) (2003) *Health Professions Education: A Bridge to Quality*, Washington, DC: National Academies Press.

IOM (Institute of Medicine) (2006) *Improving the Quality of Health Care for Mental and Substance-Use Conditions: Quality Chasm Series*, Washington, DC: National Academies Press.

Ipsos MORI (2006) 'Happy Families?'. Online. Available HTTP: http://ipsos-rsl.com/researchpublications/researcharchive/poll.aspx?oItemId=348 (accessed 31 October 2010).

Itzhaky, H. and Bustin, E. (2003) 'Strengths and pathological perspectives in community social work', *Journal of Community Practice*, 10(3), 61–73.

Jackson, C. and Dickinson, D. M. (2009) 'Developing parenting programs to prevent child health risk behaviors: A practice model', *Health Education Research*, 24(6), 1029–1042.

Jaffee, S. R., Caspi, A., Moffitt, T. E., Polo-Tomas, M. and Taylor, A. (2007) 'Individual, family, and neighborhood factors distinguish resilient from non-resilient maltreated children: A cumulative stressors model', *Child Abuse & Neglect*, 31(3), 231–253.

Jaffee, S. R., Harrington, H. L., Cohen, P. and Moffitt, T. E. (2005) 'Cumulative prevalence of psychiatric disorder in youths', *Journal of the American Academy of Child and Adolescent Psychiatry*, 44(5), 406–407.

James, C. (2009) *Ten Years of Family Policy: 1999–2009*, London: The Family and Parenting Institute.

Jenkins, V., Farewell, D., Batt, L., Maughan, T., Branston, L., Langbridge, C., Parlor, L., Farewell, V. and Fallowfield, L. (2010) 'The attitudes of 1066 patients with cancer towards participation in randomized controlled trials', *British Journal of Cancer*, 103(12), 1801–1807.

Joyce, B. R. and Showers, B. (2002) *Student Achievement through Staff Development*, 3rd edn, Alexandria, VA: Association for Supervision and Curriculum Development.

Juffer, F., Bakermans-Kranenburg, M. J. and van Ijzendoorn, M. H. (2005) 'The importance of parenting in the development of disorganized attachment: Evidence from a preventive intervention study in adoptive families', *Journal of Child Psychology and Psychiatry*, 46(3), 263–274.

Juffer, F., Bakermans-Kranenburg, M. J. and van Ijzendoorn, M. H. (2008) *Promoting Positive Parenting: An Attachment-based Intervention*, New York, NY: Lawrence Erlbaum Associates.

Kalinauskiene, L., Cekuoliene, D., van Ijzendoorn, M. H., Bakermans-Kranenburg, M. J., Juffer, F. and Kusakovskaja, I. (2009) 'Supporting insensitive mothers: The Vilnius randomized control trial of video-feedback intervention to promote maternal sensitivity and infant attachment security', *Child Care Health and Development*, 35(5), 613–623.

Kaminski, J. W., Valle, L. A., Filene, J. H. and Boyle, C. L. (2008) 'A meta-analytic review of components associated with parent training program effectiveness', *Journal of Abnormal Child Psychology*, 36(4), 567–589.

Kandel, E. R. and Schwartz, J. H. (1985) *Principles of Neural Science*, 2nd edn, New York, NY: Elsevier.

Karoly, L., Kilburn, M. and Cannon, J. (2005) *Early Childhood Interventions: Proven Results, Future Promise*, Santa Monica, CA: Rand Corporation.

Kavanagh, J. E., Brooks, E., Dougherty, S., Gerdes, M., Guevara, J. and Rubin, D. (2010) 'Meeting the mental health needs of children', *Evidence into Action*, 2, 1–10.

Kazak, A. E., Hoagwood, K., Weisz, J. R., Hood, K., Kratochwill, T. R., Vargas, L. A. and Banez, G. A. (2010) 'A meta-systems approach to evidence-based practice for children and adolescents', *American Psychologist*, 65(2), 85–97.

Kazdin, A. E. (1990) 'Premature termination from treatment among children referred for antisocial behavior', *Journal of Child Psychology and Psychiatry and Allied Disciplines*, 31(3), 415–425.

Kazdin, A. E. (1990) 'Psychotherapy for children and adolescents', *Annual Review of Psychology*, 41, 21–54.

Kazdin, A. E. (2005) *Parent Management Training: Treatment for Oppositional, Aggressive, and Antisocial Behavior in Children and Adolescents*, New York, NY: Oxford University Press.

Kazdin, A. E., Holland, L. and Crowley, M. (1997a) 'Family experience of barriers to treatment and premature termination from child therapy', *Journal of Consulting and Clinical Psychology*, 65(3), 453–463.

Kazdin, A. E., Holland, L., Crowley, M. and Breton, S. (1997b) 'Barriers to treatment participation scale: Evaluation and validation in the context of child outpatient treatment', *Journal of Child Psychology and Psychiatry and Allied Disciplines*, 38(8), 1051–1062.

Kazdin, A. E., Marciano, P. L. and Whitley, M. K. (2005) 'The therapeutic alliance in cognitive-behavioral treatment of children referred for oppositional, aggressive, and antisocial behavior', *Journal of Consulting and Clinical Psychology*, 73(4), 726–730.

Kazdin, A. E. and Mazurick, J. L. (1994) 'Dropping out of child-psychotherapy – distinguishing early and late dropouts over the course of treatment', *Journal of Consulting and Clinical Psychology*, 62(5), 1069–1074.

Kazdin, A. E., Mazurick, J. L. and Bass, D. (1993) 'Risk for attrition in treatment of antisocial children and families', *Journal of Clinical Child Psychology*, 22(1), 2–16.

Kazdin, A. E. and Whitley, M. K. (2006) 'Pretreatment social relations, therapeutic alliance, and improvements in parenting practices in parent management training', *Journal of Consulting and Clinical Psychology*, 74(2), 346–355.

Kazdin, A. E., Whitley, M. and Marciano, P. L. (2006) 'Child–therapist and parent–therapist alliance and therapeutic change in the treatment of children referred for oppositional, aggressive, and antisocial behavior', *Journal of Child Psychology and Psychiatry*, 47(5), 436–445.

Kelley, A., Schochet, T. and Landry, C. (2004) 'Risk taking and novelty seeking in adolescence: Introduction to part I', *Annals of the New York Academy of Sciences* (Adolescent Brain Development: Vulnerabilities and Opportunities), 1021, 27–32.

Kelly, G. A. (1963) *A Theory of Personality: The Psychology of Personal Constructs*, London: W.W. Norton and Company.

Kelsch, W., Sim, S. and Lois, C. (2010) 'Watching synaptogenesis in the adult brain', *Annual Review of Neuroscience*, 33, 131–149.

Kertes, D. A., Donzella, B., Talge, N. M., Garvin, M. C., van Ryzin, M. J. and Gunnar, M. R. (2009) 'Inhibited temperament and parent emotional availability differentially predict young children's cortisol responses to novel social and non-social events', *Developmental Psychobiology*, 51(7), 421–532.

Kessler, R. C., Berglund, P., Demler, O., Jin, R., Merikangas, K. R. and Walters, E. E. (2005) 'Lifetime prevalence and age-of-onset distributions of DSM-IV disorders in the national comorbidity survey replication', *Archives of General Psychiatry*, 62(7), 593–602.

Kessler, R. C., Chiu, W. T., Demler, O. and Walters, E. E. (2005) 'Prevalence, severity, and comorbidity of 12-month DSM-IV disorders in the National Comorbidity Survey Replication', *Archives of General Psychiatry*, 62(6), 617–627.

Kitzman, H., Olds, D. L., Henderson, C. R., Hanks, C., Cole, R., Tatelbaum, R., McConnochie, K. M., Sidora, K., Luckey, D. W., Shaver, D., Engelhardt, K., James, D. and Barnard, K. (1997) 'Of prenatal and infancy home visitation by nurses on pregnancy outcomes, childhood injuries, and repeated childbearing trial – A randomized controlled trial', *JAMA – Journal of the American Medical Association*, 278(8), 644–652.

Klett-Davies, M., Skaliotis, E. and Wollny, I. (2008) *Mapping and Analysis of Parenting Services in England: Assessing Needs and Patterns of Spending*, London: The Family and Parenting Institute.

Klietz, S. J., Bourduin, C. M. and Schaeffer, C. M. (2010) 'Cost-benefit analysis of multisystemic therapy with serious and violent juvenile offenders', *Journal of Family Psychology*, 24(5), 657–666.

Knudson, E. I. (2004) 'Sensitive periods in the development of the brain and behavior', *Journal of Cognitive Neuroscience*, 16(8), 1412–1425.

Knutson, N. M., Forgatch, M. S. and Rains, L. A. (2003) *Fidelity of Implementation Rating System (FIMP): The Training Manual for PMTO*, Eugene, OR: Oregon Social Learning Center.

Kobak, R., Cassidy, J., Lyons-Ruth, K. and Ziv, Y. (2006) 'Attachment and developmental psychopathology', in D. Cicchetti and D. J. Cohen (eds.) *Developmental Psychopathology*, 2nd edn, New Jersey: John Wiley & Sons, 333–369.

Koffman, L. (2008) 'Holding parents to account: Tough on children, tough on the causes of children?', *Journal of Law and Society*, 35(1), 113–130.

Korbin, J. E., Coulton, C. J. and Chard, S. (1998) 'Impoverishment and child maltreatment in African American and European American communities', *Development and Psychopathology*, 10(2), 215–233.

Korfmacher, J., O'Brien, R., Hiatt, S. and Olds, D. (1999) 'Differences in program implementation between nurses and paraprofessionals providing home visits during pregnancy and infancy: A randomized trial', *American Journal of Public Health*, 89(12), 1847–1851.

Kochanska, G. (2002) 'Mutually responsive orientation between mothers and their young children: A context for the early development of conscience', *Current Directions in Psychological Science*, 11(6), 191–195.

Kratochwill, T. R., McDonald, L., Levin, J. R., Bear-Tibbetts, H. Y. and Demaray, M. K. (2004) 'Families and Schools Together: an experimental analysis of a parent-mediated multi-family group program for American Indian children', *Journal of School Psychology*, 42(5), 359–383.

Kratochwill, T. R., McDonald, L., Levin, J. R., Scalia, P. A. and Coover, G. (2009) 'Families and schools together: An experimental study of multi-family support groups for children at risk', *Journal of School Psychology*, 47(4), 245–265.

Kreppner, J. M., Rutter, M., Beckett, C., Castle, J., Colvert, E., Groothues, C., Hawkins, A., O'Connor, T. G., Stevens, S. and Sonuga-Barke, E. J. S. (2007) 'Normality and impairment following profound early institutional deprivation: A longitudinal follow-up into early adolescence', *Developmental Psychology*, 43(4), 931–946.

Lambert, M. J., Bergin, A. E. and Garfield, S. L. (2004) 'Introduction and historical overview', in M. J. Lambert (ed.) *Bergin and Garfield's Handbook of Psychotherapy and Behavior Change*, 5th edn, New York: John Wiley and Sons, 3–15.

Lamborn, S. D. and Steinberg, L. (1993) 'Emotional autonomy redux: Revisiting Ryan and Lynch', *Child Development*, 64(2), 483–499.

Laming, W. H. (2003) *The Victoria Climbié Inquiry: Report of an Inquiry*, London: Stationery Office.

Landgraf, J. M., Abetz, L. and Ware, J. E. (1996) *The CHQ User's Manual*, Boston: The Health Institute, New England Medical Centre.

Lather, P. (2004) 'This IS your father's paradigm: Government intrusion and the case of qualitative research in education', in J. Satterthwaite, E. Atkinson and W. Moore (eds.) *The Disciplining of Education: New Languages of Power and Resistance*, Stoke on Trent: Trentham Books, 21–36.

Laurent, H. K., Kim, H. K. and Capaldi, D. M. (2008) 'Prospective effects of interparental conflict on child attachment security and the moderating role of parents' romantic attachment', *Journal of Family Psychology*, 22(3), 377–388.

Lee, V. E. and Loeb, S. (1995) 'Where do Head Start attendees end up? One reason why preschool effects fade out', *Educational Evaluation and Policy Analysis*, 17(1), 62–82.

Lee, V. E., Schnur, E. and Brooks-Gunn, J. (1988) 'Does Head Start work? A 1-year follow-up comparison of disadvantaged children attending Head Start, no preschool, and other preschool programs', *Developmental Psychology*, 24(2), 210–222.

Lee, V. E., Brooks-Gunn, J., Schnur, E. and Liaw, F. R. (1990) 'Are Head Start effects sustained? A longitudinal follow-up comparison of disadvantaged children attending Head Start, no preschool, and other preschool programs', *Child Development*, 61(2), 495–507.

Lewis, J. (2011) 'From *Sure Start* to Children's Centres: An analysis of policy change in English early years programmes', *Journal of Social Policy*, 40(1), 71–88.

Li, Z. (2007) 'Non-randomized trial', in R. D'Agostino, L. M. Sullivan and J. Massaro (eds) *Wiley Encyclopedia of Clinical Trials*, Hoboken: John Wiley & Sons, Inc.

Lieberman, A. F. (1991) 'Attachment theory and infant–parent psychotherapy: Some conceptual, clinical and research considerations', in D. Cicchetti and S. L. Toth (eds.) *Rochester Symposium on Developmental Psychopathology: Models and Integrations*, Rochester, NY: University of Rochester Press, 261–287.

Lieberman, A. F. (1992) 'Infant parent psychotherapy with toddlers', *Development and Psychopathology*, 4(4), 559–574.

Lieberman, A. F. and Pawl, J. H. (1988) 'Clinical applications of attachment theory', in J. Belsky and T. Nezworski (eds.) *Clinical Implications of Attachment*, Hillsdale, NJ: Erlbaum, 325–351.

Lieberman, A. F., Briscoe Smith, A., Gosh Ippen, C. and Van Horn, P. (2006) 'Violence in infancy and early childhood: Relationship-based treatment and evaluation', in A. F. Lieberman and R. DeMartino (eds.) *Intervention for Children Exposed to Violence*, New Brunswick, NJ: Johnson & Johnson Pediatric Institute, 65–83.

Lieberman, A. F., Ippen, C. G. and Van Horn, P. (2006b) 'Child–parent psychotherapy: 6-month follow-up of a randomized controlled trial', *Journal of the American Academy of Child and Adolescent Psychiatry*, 45(8), 913–918.

Lieberman, A. F., Van Horn, P. and Ippen, C. G. (2005) 'Toward evidence-based treatment: Child–parent psychotherapy with preschoolers exposed to marital violence', *Journal of the American Academy of Child and Adolescent Psychiatry*, 44(12), 1241–1248.

Lindsay, G., Davies, H., Band, S., Cullen, M., Cullen, S., Strand, S., Hasluck, C., Evans, R. and Stewart-Brown, S. (2008) *Parenting Early Intervention Pathfinder Evaluation*, Research Report No. 36, Nottingham: DCSF.

Linehan, M. (1993) *Skills Training Manual for Treating Borderline Personality Disorder*, New York, NY: Guilford Press.

Lloyd, E. (1999). What works in Parenting Education. Barnardo's. Online. Available HTTP: http://www.barnardos.org.uk/what_works_in_parenting_education__1999_-_summary.pdf (Accessed 05 April 2011).

Loeber, R. (1990) 'Development and risk-factors of juvenile antisocial-behavior and delinquency', *Clinical Psychology Review*, 10(1), 1–41.

Loman, M. N. and Gunnar, M. R. (2010) 'Early experience and the development of stress reactivity and regulation in children', *Neuroscience and Biobehavioral Reviews*, 34(6), 867–876.

Love, J. M., Kisker, E. E., Ross, C., Raikes, H., Constantine, J., Boller, K., Brooks-Gunn, J., Chazan-Cohen, R., Tarullo, L. B., Brady-Smith, C., Fuligni, A. S., Schochet, P. Z., Paulsell, D. and Vogel, C. (2005) 'The effectiveness of early Head Start for 3-year-old children and their parents: Lessons for policy and programs', *Developmental Psychology*, 41(6), 885–901.

Lovibond, S. H. and Lovibond, P. F. (1995) *Manual for the Depression Anxiety Stress Scales*, Sydney: Psychology Foundation.

Ludwig, J. and Miller, D. L. (2007) 'Does Head Start improve children's life chances? Evidence from a regression discontinuity design', *Quarterly Journal of Economics*, 122(1), 159–208.

Lyons-Ruth, K. and Jacobvitz, D. (1999) 'Attachment disorganization: Unresolved loss, relational violence, and lapses in behavioral and attentional strategies', in J. Cassidy and P. R. Shaver (eds.) *Handbook of Attachment: Theory, Research, and Clinical Applications*, New York, NY: Guilford Press, 520–554.

Maccoby, E. E. (1980) *Social Development: Psychological Growth and the Parent-Child Relationship*, New York: Harcourt Brace Jovanovich.

Maccoby, E. E. (1992) 'The role of parents in the socialization of children: An historical overview', *Developmental Psychology*, 28(6), 1006–1017.

Maccoby, E. E. and Martin, J. A. (1983) 'Socialization in the context of the family: Parent–child interaction', in P. H. Mussen and E. M. Hetherington (eds.) *Handbook of Child Psychology*, 4th edn, New York, NY: Wiley, 1–101.

Main, M., Kaplan, N. and Cassidy, J. (1985) 'Security in infancy, childhood, and adulthood: A move to the level of representation', *Monographs of the Society for Research in Child Development*, 50(1–2), 66–104.

Main, M. and Solomon, J. (1986) 'Discovery of a new, insecure-disorganized/disoriented attachment pattern', in M. Yogman and B. Brazelton (eds.) *Affective Development in Infancy*, Norwood, NJ: Ablex.

March, J. S. (1997) *Multidimensional Anxiety Scale for Children: Technical Manual*, Toronto: Multi-Health Systems.

Markie-Dadds, C. and Sanders, M. R. (2006) 'A controlled evaluation of an enhanced self-directed behavioural family intervention for parents of children with conduct problems in rural and remote areas', *Behaviour Change*, 23(1), 55–72.

Martinez, C. R. and Forgatch, M. S. (2002) 'Adjusting to change: Linking family structure transitions with parenting and boys' adjustment', *Journal of Family Psychology*, 16(2), 107–117.

Marvin, R. S. (2000) 'The Circle of Security Project: An attachment theory-based intervention', The FHL Foundation. Online. Available HTTP: http://128.121.62.12/Marvin_Evid_Tx.htm (accessed 3 October 2010).

Maynard, B. R. (2007) 'To EBP or not to EBP? Social work's dilemma with evidence-based practice', *PRAXIS*, 7, 5–15.

McBride, B. A. and Rane, T. R. (1998) 'Parenting alliance as a predictor of father involvement: An exploratory study', *Family Relations*, 47(3), 229–236.

McCartney, K. and Rosenthal, R. (2000) 'Effect size, practical importance, and social policy for children', *Child Development*, 71(1), 173–180.

McCord, J. (1978) 'A thirty-year follow-up of treatment effects', *American Psychologist*, 33(3), 284–289.

McCurdy, K. and Daro, D. (2001) 'Parent involvement in family support programs: An integrated theory', *Family Relations*, 50(2), 113–121.

McDonald, L. and Sayger, T. (1998) 'Impact of a family and school based prevention program on protective factors for high risk youth', *Drugs & Society*, 12(1), 61–85.

McDonald, L., Billingham, S., Conrad, T., Morgan, A., O, N. and Payton, E. (1997) 'Families and Schools Together (FAST). Integrating community development with clinical strategies', *Families in Society – the Journal of Contemporary Human Services*, 78(2), 140–155.

McDonald, L., Moberg, D., Brown, R., Rodriguez-Espiricueta, I., Flores, N., Burke, M. and Coover, G. (2006) 'After-school multifamily groups: A randomized controlled trial involving low-income, urban, Latino children', *Children and Schools*, 28(1), 25–34.

McGorry, P. D., Purcell, R., Hickie, I. B. and Jorm, A. F. (2007) 'Investing in youth mental health is a best buy', *Medical Journal of Australia*, 187(7), S5–S7.

McGuigan, W. M., Katzev, A. R. and Pratt, C. C. (2003) 'Multi-level determinants of retention in a home-visiting child abuse prevention program', *Child Abuse & Neglect*, 27(4), 363–380.

McHale, J. P., Kuersten-Hogan, R. and Rao, N. (2004) 'Growing points for coparenting theory and research', *Journal of Adult Development*, 11(3), 221–234.

McHale, J. P., Lauretti, A., Talbot, J. and Pouquette, C. (2002) 'Retrospect and prospect in the psychological study of coparenting and family group process', in J. P. McHale and W. S. Grolnick (eds.) *Retrospect and Prospect in the Psychological Study of Families*, Mahwah, NJ: Lawrence Erlbaum Associates, 127–166.

McHale, J. P. and Rasmussen, J. L. (1998) 'Coparental and family group-level dynamics during infancy: Early family precursors of child and family functioning during preschool', *Development and Psychopathology*, 10(1), 39–59.

McKey, R., Condelli, L., Ganson, H., Barrett, B., McConkey, C. and Plantz, M. (1985) *The Impact of Head Start on Children, Families and Communities: Final Report on the Head Start Evaluation, Synthesis, and Utilization Project (DHHS Pub. No. ODHS 85-31193)*, Washington, DC: US Government Printing Office.

McMahon, R. J. and Forehand, R. L. (2003) *Helping the Noncompliant Child: Family-based Treatment for Oppositional Behavior*, 2nd edn, New York: Guilford Press.

McNaughton, S., Glynn, T. and Robinson, V. (1987) *Pause, Prompt and Praise: Effective Tutoring for Remedial Reading*, Birmingham: Positive Products.

Meadows, P. (2001) *Guidance for Sure Start Local Evaluators and Programme Managers on the Estimation of Cost Effectiveness on a Local Level*, London: The National Evaluation of *Sure Start*.

Meadows, P. (2007) 'The costs and benefits of *Sure Start* Local Programmes', in J. Belsky, E. Melhuish and J. Barnes (eds.) *The National Evaluation of Sure Start: Does Area-based Early Intervention Work?*, Bristol: Policy Press, 113–130.

Mehta, M. A., Golembo, N. I., Nosarti, C., Colvert, E., Mota, A., Willliams, S. C. R., Rutter, M. and Sonuga-Barke, E. J. S. (2009) 'Amygdala, hippocampal and corpus callosum size following severe early institutional deprivation: The English and Romanian adoptees study pilot', *The Journal of Child Psychology and Psychiatry*, 50(8), 943–951.

Melhuish, E., Belsky, J., Leyland, A. H., Barnes, J. and National Evaluation of *Sure Start* Research Team (2008) 'Effects of fully-established *Sure Start* Local Programmes on 3-year-old children and their families living in England: A quasi-experimental observational study', *Lancet*, 372(9450), 1641–1647.

Melhuish, E. and Hall, D. (2007) 'The policy background to *Sure Start*', in J. Belsky, E. Melhuish and J. Barnes (eds.) *The National Evaluation of Sure Start: Does Area-based Early Intervention Work?*, Bristol: Policy Press, 3–21.

Melnyk, B. M. and Fineout-Overholt, E. (2010) *Evidence-based Practice in Nursing and Healthcare: A Guide to Best Practice*, Philadelphia, PA: Lippincott Williams & Wilkins.

Mersky, J. P., Berger, L. M., Reynolds, A. J. and Gromoske, A. N. (2009) 'Risk factors for child and adolescent maltreatment: A longitudinal investigation of a cohort of inner-city youth', *Child Maltreatment*, 14(1), 73–88.

Meschke, L. L., Bartholomae, S. and Zentall, S. R. (2002) 'Adolescent sexuality and parent–adolescent processes: Promoting healthy teen choices', *Journal of Adolescent Health*, 31(6), 264–279.

Metz, A. J. R., Blase, K. and Bowie, L. (2007) 'Implementing evidence-based practices: Six "drivers" of success'. Online. Available: http://www.incredibleyears.com/library/items/Child-Trends_6-Success-Drivers_10-07.pdf (accessed 10 October 2010).

Midgley, N. (2009) 'Editorial: Improvers, adapters and rejecters: The link between "evidence-based practice" and "evidence-based practitioners"', *Clinical Child Psychology and Psychiatry*, 14(3), 323–327.

Mihalic, A. (n.d.) 'Implementation fidelity'. Online. Available: http://www.colorado.edu/cspv/blue-prints/Fidelity.pdf (accessed 10 October 2010).

Mihalic, S. (2004) 'The importance of implementation fidelity', Boulder Co: Center for the Study of Prevention Violence.

Mihalic, S. and Irwin, K. (2003) 'Blueprints for violence prevention: From research to real-world settings – factors influencing the successful replication of model programs', *Youth Violence and Juvenile Justice*, 1(4), 307.

Miller, S. and Sambell, K. (2003) 'What do parents feel they need? Implications of parents' perspectives for the facilitation of parenting programmes', *Children and Society*, 27(1), 32–44.

Miller, W. R., Tonigan, J. S. and Longabaugh, R. (1995) *The Drinker Inventory of Consequences (DrInC): An Instrument for Assessing Adverse Consequences of Alcohol Abuse*, NIAAA Project MATCH Monograph Series vol. 4, Bethesda, MD: U.S. Department of Health and Human Services, National Institutes of Health, National Institute on Alcohol Abuse and Alcoholism.

Minuchin, P. (1985) 'Families and individual development: Provocations from the field of family therapy', *Child Development*, 56(2), 289–302.

Minuchin, S. (1974) *Families and Family Therapy*, Cambridge, MA: Harvard University Press.

Minuchin, S. and Fishman, H. C. (1981) *Family Therapy Techniques*, Cambridge, MA: Harvard University Press.

Mischel, W. (1986) *Introduction to Personality: A New Look*, 4th edn, New York: Holt, Rinehart and Winston.

Molnar, B. E., Buka, S. L., Brennan, R. T., Holton, J. K. and Earls, F. (2003) 'A multilevel study of neighborhoods and parent-to-child physical aggression: Results from the project on human development in Chicago neighborhoods', *Child Maltreatment*, 8(2), 84–97.

Moran, P., Ghate, D. and van der Merwe, A. (2004) *What Works in Parenting Support?*, London: Department for Education and Skills.

Morrison, K. (2001) 'Randomized controlled trials for evidence-based education: Some problems judging "what works"', *Evaluation and Research in Education*, 15(2), 69–83.

Moss, E., Cyr, C., Bureau, J. F., Tarabulsy, G. A. and Dubois-Comtois, K. (2005) 'Stability of attachment during the preschool period', *Developmental Psychology*, 41(5), 773–783.

Mrazek, P. and Haggerty, R. (1994) *Reducing Risks for Mental Disorders: Frontiers for Preventive Intervention Research*, Washington, DC: National Academies Press.

Mulrow, C. D. (1994) 'Systematic reviews: Rationale for systematic reviews', *British Medical Journal*, 309(6954), 597–599.

Mulrow, C. D., Cook, D. J. and Davidoff, F. (1997) 'Systematic reviews: Critical links in the great chain of evidence', *Annals of Internal Medicine*, 126(5), 389–391.

Murray, L. and Cooper, P. J. (1997) 'Effects of postnatal depression on infant development', *Archives of Disease in Childhood*, 77(2), 99–101.

Murray, L., Cooper, P. J., Wilson, A. and Romaniuk, H. (2003) 'Controlled trial of the short- and long-term effect of psychological treatment of post-partum depression: 2. Impact on the mother–child relationship and child outcome', *British Journal of Psychiatry*, 182(5), 420–427.

Naidu, T. and Behari, S. (2010) 'The parent–child–therapist alliance: A case study using a strategic approach', *Journal of Child and Adolescent Mental Health*, 22(10), 41–50.

Nation, M., Crusto, C., Wandersman, A., Kumpfer, K. L., Seybolt, D., Morrissey-Kane, E. and Davino, K. (2003) 'What works in prevention: Principles of effective prevention programs', *American Psychologist*, 58(6–7), 449–456.

National Scientific Council on the Developing Child (2004) *Young Children Develop in an Environment of Relationships: Working Paper No. 1*, Center for the Developing Child, Harvard University. Online. Available HTTP: www.developingchild.harvard.edu (accessed 22 January 2011).

National Scientific Council on the Developing Child (2005) *Excessive Stress Disrupts the Architecture of the Developing Brain: Working Paper No. 3*, Center for the Developing Child, Harvard University. Online. Available HTTP: www.developingchild.harvard.edu (accessed 22 January 2011).

National Scientific Council on the Developing Child (2007) *The Timing and Quality of Early Experiences Combine to Shape Brain Architecture: Working Paper No. 5*, Center on the Developing Child, Harvard University. Online. Available HTTP: www.developingchild.harvard.edu (accessed 22 January 2011).

National Scientific Council on the Developing Child (2009) *Maternal Depression Can Undermine the Development of Young Children: Working Paper No. 8*, Center on the Developing Child, Harvard University. Online. Available HTTP: www.developingchild.harvard.edu (accessed 22 January 2011).

NIRN (2008) 'What is implementation?'. Online. Available HTTP: http://www.fpg.unc.edu/~nirn/implementation/01_implementationdefined.cfm (accessed 26 October 2010).

Nock, M. K. and Ferriter, C. (2005) 'Parent management of attendance and adherence in child and adolescent therapy: A conceptual and empirical review', *Clinical Child and Family Psychology Review*, 8(2), 149–166.

Nores, M., Belfield, C. R., Barnett, W. S. and Schweinhart, L. (2005) 'Updating the economic impacts of the High/Scope Perry Preschool Program', *Educational Evaluation and Policy Analysis*, 27(3), 245–261.

Nuttall, C., Goldblatt, P. and Lewis, C. (1998) *Reducing Offending: An Assessment of Research Evidence on Ways of Dealing with Offending Behaviour*, London: Home Office Research and Statistics Directorate.

Oakley, A. (2006) 'Resistances to "new" technologies of evaluation: Education research in the UK as a case study', *Evidence and Policy*, 2(1), 63–87.

O'Connell, M., Boat, T. and Warner, K. (2009) *Preventing Mental, Emotional, and Behavioral Disorders among Young People: Progress and Possibilities*, Washington, DC: National Academies Press.

O'Connell, M. J., Morris, J. A. and Hoge, M. A. (2004) 'Innovation in behavioural health workforce education', *Administration and Policy in Mental Health*, 32(2), 131–165.

O'Connor, C., Small, S. A. and Cooney, S. M. (2007) *Program Fidelity and Adaptation: Meeting Local Needs without Compromising Program Effectiveness. What Works, Wisconsin – Research to Practice, Series 4*, Madison, WI: The University of Wisconsin–Madison and University of Wisconsin Extension.

O'Connor, T. G., Marvin, R. S., Rutter, M., Olrick, J. T. and Britner, P. A. and the English and Romanian Adoptees Study (2003) 'Child parent attachment following early institutional deprivation', *Development and Psychopathology*, 15(1), 19–38.

Office of Head Start (2010) 'Head Start 2010 Fact Sheet'. Online. Available HTTP: http://www.acf. hhs.gov/programs/ohs/about/fy2010.html (accessed 22 September 2010).

Ogden, T., Forgatch, M. S., Askeland, E., Patterson, G. R. and Bullock, B. M. (2005) 'Implementation of parent management training at the national level: The case of Norway', *Journal of Social Work Practice*, 19(3), 317–329.

Ogden, T. and Hagen, K. A. (2008) 'Treatment effectiveness of Parent Management Training in Norway: A randomized controlled trial of children with conduct problems', *Journal of Consulting and Clinical Psychology*, 76(4), 607–621.

Ogden, T., Hagen, K. A., Askeland, E. and Christensen, B. (2009) 'Implementing and evaluating evidence-based treatments of conduct problems in children and youth in Norway', *Research on Social Work Practice*, 19(5), 582–591.

Olds, D. L. (2002) 'Prenatal and infancy home visiting by nurses: From randomized trials to community replication', *Prevention Science*, 3(3), 153–172.

Olds, D. L., Eckenrode, J., Henderson, C. R., Kitzman, H., Powers, J., Cole, R., Sidora, K., Morris, P., Pettitt, L. M. and Luckey, D. (1997) 'Long-term effects of home visitation on maternal life course and child abuse and neglect – Fifteen-year follow-up of a randomized trial', *JAMA – Journal of the American Medical Association*, 278(8), 637–643.

Olds, D. L., Henderson, C. R., Cole, R., Eckenrode, J., Kitzman, H., Luckey, D., Pettitt, L., Sidora, K., Morris, P. and Powers, J. (1998) 'Long-term effects of nurse home visitation on children's criminal and antisocial behavior – 15-year follow-up of a randomized controlled trial', *JAMA – Journal of the American Medical Association*, 280(14), 1238–1244.

Olds, D. L., Hill, P., Robinson, J., Song, N. and Little, C. (2000) 'Update on home visiting for pregnant women and parents of young children', *Current Problems in Pediatrics*, 30(4), 107–41.

Olds, D. L., Kitzman, H., Cole, R. and Robinson, J. A. (1997) 'Theoretical foundations of a program of home visitation for pregnant women and parents of young children', *Journal of Community Psychology*, 25(1), 9–25.

Olds, D. L., Robinson, J., Pettitt, L., Luckey, D. W., Holmberg, J., Ng, R. K., Isacks, K., Sheff, K. and Henderson, C. R. (2004) 'Effects of home visits by paraprofessionals and by nurses: Age 4 follow-up results of a randomized trial', *Pediatrics*, 114(6), 1560–1568.

O'Neill, D., McGilloway, S., Donnelly, M., Bywater, T. and Kelly, P. (2010) *A Cost-benefit Analysis of Early Childhood Intervention: Evidence from an Experimental Evaluation of the Incredible Years Parenting Program*, Maynooth, Ireland: National University of Ireland.

Orlinsky, D. E. and Ronnestad, M. H. (2000) 'Ironies in the history of psychotherapy research: Rogers, Bordin, and the shape of things that came', *Journal of Clinical Psychology*, 56(7), 841–851.

Orrell-Valente, J. K., Pinderhughes, E. E., Valente, E. and Laird, R. D. (1999) 'If it's offered, will they come? Influences on parents' participation in a community-based conduct problems prevention program', *American Journal of Community Psychology*, 27(6), 753–783.

Owen, M. T. and Cox, M. J. (1997) 'Marital conflict and the development of infant–parent attachment relationships', *Journal of Family Psychology*, 11(2), 152–164.

Parker, S. and Zahr, L. K. (1985) *The Maternal Confidence Questionnaire*, Boston, MA: Boston City Hospital.

Parks, G. (2000) 'The High/Scope Perry Preschool Project'. Online. Available HTTP: http://www. ncjrs.gov/html/ojjdp/2000_10_1/contents.html (accessed 3 November 2010).

Parton, N. (2006) '"Every Child Matters": The shift to prevention whilst strengthening protection in children's services in England', *Children and Youth Services Review*, 28(8), 976–992.

Patel, V., Flisher, A. J., Hetrick, S. and McGorry, P. (2007) 'Adolescent Health 3 – Mental health of young people: A global public-health challenge', *Lancet*, 369(9569), 1302–1313.

Patterson, G. R. (1976) 'The aggressive child: Victim and architect of a coercive system', in L. A. Hamerlynck, L. C. Handy and E. J. Mash (eds.) *Behavior Modification and Families*, New York, NY: Brunner-Mazell.

Patterson, G. R. and Chamberlain, P. R. (1988) 'Treatment process: A problem at three levels', in L. C. Wynne (ed.) *The State of the Art in Family Therapy Research: Controversies and Recommendations*, New York: Family Process Press, 189–223.

Patterson, G. R. and Chamberlain, P. R. (1994) 'A functional analysis of resistance during parent training therapy', *Clinical Psychology: Science and Practice*, 1(1), 53–70.

Patterson, G. R., Debaryshe, B. D. and Ramsey, E. (1989) 'A developmental perspective on antisocial-behavior', *American Psychologist*, 44(2), 329–335.

Patterson, G. R. and Forgatch, M. S. (1985) 'Therapist behavior as a determinant for client noncompliance: A paradox for the behavior modifier', *Journal of Consulting and Clinical Psychology*, 53(6), 846–851.

Patterson, G. R., Littman, R. A. and Bricker, W. (1967) 'Assertive behavior in children: A step toward a theory of aggression', *Monographs of the Society for Research in Child Development*, 32(5–6).

Patterson, J., Mockford, C., Barlow, J., Pyper, C. and Stewart-Brown, S. (2002) 'Need and demand for parenting programmes in a general practice', *Archives of Disease in Childhood*, 87(6), 468–471.

Patton, M. Q. (1997) *Utilization-focused Evaluation: The New Century Text*, 3rd edn, Thousand Oaks, CA: Sage Publications.

Payne, A. A. and Eckert, R. (2010) 'The relative importance of provider, program, school, and community predictors of the implementation quality of school-based prevention programs', *Prevention Science*, 11(2), 126–41.

Perry, B. D. (2002) 'Childhood experience and the expression of genetic potential: What childhood neglect tells us about nature and nurture', *Brain and Mind*, 3(1), 79–100.

Perry, B. D., Pollard, R. A., Blakley, T. L., Baker, W. L. and Vigilante, D. (1995) 'Childhood trauma, the neurobiology of adaptation, and "use-dependent" development of the brain: How "states" become "traits"', *Infant Mental Health Journal*, 16(4), 271–291.

Peterander, F. (2004) 'Preparing practitioners to work with families in early childhood intervention', *Educational and Child Psychology*, 21(1), 89–101.

Peters, M., Seeds, K., Edwards, G. and Garnett, E. (2010) *Parental Opinion Survey 2009*, London: Department for Children, Schools and Families.

Petersen, D. J. and Alexander, G. R. (2001) *Needs Assessment in Public Health: A Practical Guide for Students and Professionals*, New York: Kluwer Academic.

Pittman, L. D. and Chase-Lansdale, P. L. (2001) 'African American adolescent girls in impoverished communities: Parenting style and adolescent outcomes', *Journal of Research on Adolescence*, 11(2), 199–224.

Plath, D. (2006) 'Evidence-based practice: Current issues and future directions', *Australian Journal of Social Work*, 59(1), 56–72.

Pollack, S. D., Nelson, C. A., Schlaak, M. L., Roeber, B. J., Wewerke, S. S., Wilk, K. L., Frenn, K. A., Loman, M. N. and Gunnar, M. R. (2010) 'Neurodevelopmental effects of early deprivation in postinstitutionalized children', *Child Development*, 81(1), 224–236.

Powers, S. I., Hauser, S. T., Schwartz, J. M., Noam, G. G. and Jacobson, A. M. (1983) 'Adolescent ego development and family interaction: A structural-developmental perspective', in H. D. Grotevant and C. R. Cooper (eds.) *Adolescent Development in the Family: New Directions for Child Development*, San Francisco, CA: Jossey-Bass, 5–15.

Prinz, R. J. and Jones, T. (2003) 'Family-based interventions', in C. A. Essau (ed.) *Conduct and Oppositional Defiant Disorders: Epidemiology, Risk Factors, and Treatment*, Mahwah, NJ: Lawrence Erlbaum, 279–298.

Prinz, R. J., Sanders, M. R., Shapiro, C. J., Whitaker, D. J. and Lutzker, J. R. (2009) 'Population-based prevention of child maltreatment: The US Triple P system population trial', *Prevention Science*, 10(1), 1–12.

Prinz, R. J. and Miller, G. E. (1996) 'Parental engagement in interventions for children at risk for conduct disorder', in R .D. V. Peters and R. J. McMahon (eds.) *Preventing Childhood Conduct Disorders, Substance Abuse and Delinquency,* Thousand Oaks, CA: Sage.

Puig-Peiró, R., Beecham, J. and Stevens, M. (2010) 'The Costs and Characteristics of the Parenting Programs in the NAPP Commissioners' Toolkit', London: National Academy for Parenting Research, unpublished.

Puma, M., Bell, S., Cook, R. and Heid, C. (2010) 'Head Start impact final report'. Online. Available HTTP: http://www.acf.hhs.gov/programs/opre/hs/impact_study/reports/impact_study/executive_summary_final.pdf (accessed 22 September 2010).

Puma, M., Bell, S., Cook, R., Heid, C., Lopez, M., Zill, N., Shapiro, G., Broene, P., Mekos, D., Rohacek, M., Quinn, L., Adams, G., Friedman, J. and Bernstein, H. (2005) *Head Start Impact Study: First Year Findings*, Washington, DC: U.S. Department of Health and Human Services.

PwC (2010) 'NAPP Parenting Workforce Analysis'. Online. Available HTTP: https://www.cwdcouncil.org.uk/assets/0001/0549/SP155–0910_Parenting_Workforce_Analysis.pdf (accessed 26 October 2010).

PwC (2006) *The Market for Parental and Family Support Services*, Research Report No. RW72, London: DCSF.

Rakic, P. (1988) 'Specification of cerebral cortex area', *Science*, 241(4862), 170–176.

Rakic, P. (1995) 'A small step for the cell, a giant leap for mankind: A hypothesis of neocortical expansion during evolution', *Trends in Neuroscience*, 18(9), 383–388.

Rakic, P. and Sidman, R. L. (1968) 'Supravital DNA synthesis in the developing human and mouse brain', *Journal of Neuropathology and Experimental Neurology*, 27(2), 246–276.

Ralph, A., Toumbourou, J. W., Grigg, M., Mulcahy, R., Carr-Gregg, M. and Sanders, M. R. (2003) 'Early intervention to help parents manage behavioral and emotional problems in early adolescents: What parents want', *Advances in Mental Health*, 3, 156–168.

Redmond, C., Spoth, R. and Trudeau, L. (2002) 'Family- and community-level predictors of parent support seeking', *Journal of Community Psychology*, 30(2), 153–171.

Regehr, C., Stern, S. and Shlonsky, A. (2007) 'Operationalizing evidence-based practice: The development of an institute for evidence-based social work', *Research on Social Work Practice*, 17(3), 408–416.

Reid, M. J., Webster-Stratton, C. and Hammond, M. (2003) 'Follow-up of children who received the Incredible Years intervention for oppositional-defiant disorder: Maintenance and prediction of 2-year outcome', *Behavior Therapy*, 34(4), 471–491.

Resnick, M. D., Bearman, P. S., Blum, R. W., Bauman, K. E., Harris, K. M., Jones, J., Tabor, J., Beuhring, T., Sieving, R. E., Shew, M., Ireland, M., Bearinger, L. H. and Udry, J. R. (1997) 'Protecting adolescents from harm: Findings from the National Longitudinal Study on Adolescent Health', *JAMA – Journal of the American Medical Association*, 278(10), 823–832.

Respect Task Force (2006) *Respect Action Plan*, London: Home Office.

Roberts, C., Mazzucchelli, T., Studman, L. and Sanders, M. R. (2006) 'Behavioral family intervention for children with developmental disabilities and behavioral problems', *Journal of Clinical Child and Adolescent Psychology*, 35(2), 180–193.

Rodgers, K. B. (1999) 'Parenting processes related to sexual risk-taking behaviors of adolescent males and females', *Journal of Marriage and the Family*, 61(1), 99–109.

Rogers, C. R. (1946) 'Significant aspects of client-centred therapy', *American Psychologist*, 1(10), 415–422.

Rogers, C. R. (1951) *Client-centered Therapy: Its Current Practice, Implications, and Theory*, Boston, MA: Houghton Mifflin.

Rogers, C. R. (1957) 'The necessary and sufficient conditions of therapeutic personality change', *Journal of Consulting Psychology*, 21(2), 95–103.

Rollnick, S. and Miller, W. R. (1995) 'What is motivational interviewing?', *Behavioural and Cognitive Psychotherapy*, 23(4), 325–334.

Rosen, A. (2003) 'Evidence-based social work practice: Challenges and promise', *Social Work Research*, 27(4), 197–208.

Rosen, L., Manor, O., Engelhard, D. and Zucker, D. (2006) 'In defense of the randomized controlled trial for health promotion research', *American Journal of Public Health*, 96(7), 1181–1186.

Rosenfeld, G. W. (2008) *Beyond Evidence-based Psychotherapy: Fostering the Eight Sources of Change in Child and Adolescent Treatment*, New York: Routledge.

Rotter, J. B. (1954) *Social Learning and Clinical Psychology*. Englewood Cliffs, NJ: Prentice-Hall.

Rotter, J. B. (1966) 'Generalized expectancies for internal versus external control of reinforcement', *Psychological Monographs*, 80(1), Whole No. 609).

Rubak, S., Sandboek, A., Lauritzen, T. and Christensen, B. (2005) 'Motivational interviewing: A systematic review and meta-analysis', *British Journal of General Practice*, 55(513), 305–312.

Rutter, M. (1979) 'Protective factors in children's responses to stress and disadvantage', *Annals of Academic Medicine Singapore*, 8(3), 324–338.

Rutter, M. (1985) 'Resilience in the face of adversity: Protective factors and resistance to psychiatric-disorder', *British Journal of Psychiatry*, 147, 598–611.

Rutter, M. (1996) 'Transitions and turning points in developmental psychopathology: As applied to the age span between childhood and mid-adulthood', *International Journal of Behavioral Development*, 19(3), 603–626.

Rutter, M. (2000) 'Psychosocial adversity: Risk, resilience and recovery', in J. M. Richman and M. W. Fraser (eds.) *The Context of Youth Violence: Resilience, Risk and Protection*, Westport, CT: Greenwood Press, 13–42.

Rutter, M. (2006) 'Is *Sure Start* an effective preventive intervention?', *Child and Adolescent Mental Health*, 11(3), 135–141.

Rutter, M. (2007) '*Sure Start* local programmes: An outsider's perspective', in J. Belsky, J. Barnes, and E. Melhuish (eds.) *The National Evaluation of Sure Start: Does Area-based Early Intervention Work?*, Bristol: Policy Press, 197–211.

Rutter, M., O'Connor, T. G. and English Romanian Adoptees Study (2004) 'Are there biological programming effects for psychological development? Findings from a study of Romanian adoptees', *Developmental Psychology*, 40(1), 81–94.

Rutter, M. and Smith, D. J. (1995) *Psychosocial Disorders in Young People: Time Trends and Their Causes*, Chichester: John Wiley and Sons.

Rutter, M., Sonuga-Barke, E. J., Beckett, C., Castle, J., Kreppner, J., Kumsta, R., Schlotz, W., Stevens, S. and Bell, C. A. (2010) 'Deprivation-specific psychological patterns: Effects of institutional deprivation', *Monographs of the Society for Research in Child Development*, 75(1), 1–252.

Ryan, C. E., Epstein, N. B., Keitner, G. I., Miller, I. W. and Bishop, D. S. (2005) *Evaluating and Treating Families: The McMaster Approach*, New York, NY: Brunner/Routledge.

Sackett, D. L. (1979) 'Bias in analytic research', *Journal of Chronic Diseases*, 32(1–2), 51–63.

Sackett, D. L. (2000) *Evidence-based Medicine: How to Practice and Teach EBM*, 2nd edn, Edinburgh; New York: Churchill Livingstone.

Sackett, D. L., Rosenberg, W. M. C., Gray, J. A. M., Haynes, R. B. and Richardson, W. S. (1996) 'Evidence based medicine: What it is and what it isn't', *British Medical Journal*, 312(7023), 71–72.

Salas, E. and Cannon-Bowers, J. A. (2001) 'The science of training: A decade of progress', *Annual Review of Psychology*, 52, 471–499.

Saleebey, D. (1996) 'The strengths perspective in social work practice: Extensions and cautions', *Social Work*, 41(3), 296–305.

Saleebey, D. (2000) 'Power in the people: Strengths and hope', *Advances in Social Work*, 1(2), 127–136.

Sanders, M. R. and Morawska, A. (2006) 'Towards a public health approach to parenting', *Psychologist*, 19(8), 476–479.

Sanders, M. R., Markie-Dadds, C., Tully, L. A. and Bor, W. (2000) 'The Triple P-Positive Parenting Program: A comparison of enhanced, standard, and self-directed behavioral family intervention for parents of children with early onset conduct problems', *Journal of Consulting and Clinical Psychology*, 68(4), 624–640.

Sanders, M. R. and Murphy-Brennan, M. (2010) 'The international dissemination of the Triple P-Positive Parenting Program', in J. R. Weisz and A. E. Kazdin (eds.) *Evidence-based Psychotherapies for Children and Adolescents*, 2nd edn, New York: Guilford Press, 519–537.

Sanders, M. R., Ralph, A., Sofronoff, K., Gardiner, P., Thompson, R., Dwyer, S. and Bidwell, K. (2008) 'Every family: A population approach to reducing behavioral and emotional problems in children making the transition to school', *Journal of Primary Prevention*, 29(3), 197–222.

Sanderson, I. (2002) 'Evaluation, policy learning and evidence-based policy making', *Public Administration*, 80(1), 1–22.

Satir, V. M. (1967) *Conjoint Family Therapy: A Guide to Theory and Technique*, Palo Alto, CA: Science and Behavior Books.

Satir, V. M. (1972) *Peoplemaking*, Palo Alto, CA: Science and Behavior Books.

Satir, V. M. (1982) 'The therapist and family therapy: Process model', in A. M. Horne and M. M. Ohlsen (eds.) *Family Counselling and Therapy*, Itasca, IL: F. E. Peacock.

Satir, V. M. and Baldwin, M. (1983) *Satir Step by Step: A Guide to Creating Change in Families*, Palo Alto, CA: Science and Behavior Books.

Satir, V. M., Banmen, J., Berber, J. and Gamori, M. (1991) *The Satir Model: Family Therapy and Beyond*, Palo Alto, CA: Science and Behavior Books.

Sawhill, I. V. and Baron, J. (2010) 'We need a new start for Head Start', *Education Week*, 29(23), 22–23.

Sayles, C. (2002) 'Transformational change: Based on the model of Virginia Satir', *Contemporary Family Therapy*, 24(1), 93–109.

Scarr, S., Weinberg, R. A., Levine, A. and Kagan, J. (1986) *Understanding Development*, San Diego: Harcourt Brace Jovanovich.

Schoppe, S. J., Mangelsdorf, S. C. and Frosch, C. A. (2001) 'Coparenting, family process, and family structure: Implications for preschoolers' externalizing behavior problems', *Journal of Family Psychology*, 15(3), 526–545.

Schoppe-Sullivan, S. J., Mangelsdorf, S. C., Frosch, C. A., and McHale, J. L. (2004) 'Associations between coparenting and marital behavior from infancy to the preschool years', *Journal of Family Psychology*, 18(1), 194–207.

Schoppe-Sullivan, S. J., Weldon, A. H., Claire Cook, J., Davis, E. F. and Buckley, C. K. (2009) 'Coparenting behavior moderates longitudinal relations between effortful control and preschool children's externalizing behavior', *Journal of Child Psychology and Psychiatry*, 50(6), 698–706.

Schore, A. N. (2001) 'Effects of a secure attachment relationship on right brain development, affect regulation, and infant mental health', *Infant Mental Health Journal*, 22(1–2), 7–66.

Schrag, R. D. A., Styfco, S. J. and Zigler, E. (2004) 'Familiar concept, new name: Social competence/ school readiness as the goal of Head Start', in E. Zigler and S. J. Styfco (eds.) *The Head Start Debates: Are We Failing the Children Most at Risk? 53 of America's Leading Experts Weigh In*, Baltimore, MD: Paul H. Brookes Publishing, 19–26.

Schumacher, R. (2003) *Family Support and Parent Involvement in Head Start: What do Head Start Program Performance Standards Require?* Online. Available HTTP: http://www.clasp.org/publications/HS_fam_supp.pdf (accessed 6 October 2005).

Schweinhart, L. J. (2002) 'How the High/Scope Perry Preschool study grew: A researcher's tale'. Online. Available HTTP: www.highscope.org/content.asp?ContentID=232 (accessed 30 October 2010).

Schweinhart, L. J., Barnes, H. and Weikart, D. P. (1993) *Significant Benefits: The High/Scope Perry Preschool Study through Age 27*, Monographs of the HighScope Educational Research Foundation, 10, Ypsilanti, MI: HighScope Press.

Schweinhart, L., Montie, J., Xiang, Z., Barnett, W., Belfield, C. and Nores, M. (2005) *Lifetime Effects: The High/Scope Perry Preschool Study through Age 40*, Monographs of the HighScope Educational Research Foundation, 14, Ypsilanti, MI: HighScope Press.

Scott, S. (2002) 'Parent training programmes', in M. Rutter and E. Taylor (eds.) *Child and Adolescent Psychiatry*, 4th edn, Oxford: Blackwell, 949–967.

Scott, S. (2010a) 'Nationwide dissemination of effective parenting interventions: Building a parenting academy for England', in J. Weisz and A. Kazdin (eds.) *Evidence-Based Psychotherapies for Children and Adolescents*, New York: Guilford Press, 500–518.

Scott, S. (2010b) 'National dissemination of effective parenting programs to improve child outcomes', *British Journal of Psychiatry*, 196(1), 1–3.

Scott, S., Carby, A. and Rendu, A. (under review) 'Impact of therapists' skill on effectiveness of parenting groups for child antisocial behaviour'.

Scott, S., Knapp, M., Henderson, J., and Maughan, B. (2001) 'Financial cost of social exclusion: Follow up study of antisocial children into adulthood', *British Medical Journal*, 323(7306), 191–194.

Scott, S., O'Connor, T. G., Futh, A., Matias, C., Price, J. and Doolan, M. (2010) 'Impact of a parenting program in a high-risk, multi-ethnic community: The PALS trial', *Journal of Child Psychology and Psychiatry*, 12, 1331–1341.

Scott, S., Sylva, K., Doolan, M., Price, J., Jacobs, B., Crook, C. and Landau, S. (2010) 'Randomised controlled trial of parent groups for child antisocial behaviour targeting multiple risk factors: the SPOKES project', *Journal of Child Psychology and Psychiatry*, 51(1), 48–57.

Sexton, T. L. (2007) 'The therapist as a moderator and mediator in successful therapeutic change', *Journal of Family Therapy*, 29(2), 104–108.

Sexton, T. L. and Alexander, J. F. (2003) 'Functional family therapy: A mature clinical model for working with at-risk adolescents and their families', in T. L. Sexton, G. R. Weeks and M. S. Robbins (eds.) *Handbook of Family Therapy: The Science and Practice of Working with Families and Couples*, New York: Brunner-Routledge, 323–350.

Sexton, T. L., Alexander, J. F. and Mease, A. L. (2004) 'Levels of evidence for the models and mechanisms of therapeutic change in family and couple therapy', in M. J. Lambert (ed.) *Bergin and Garfield's Handbook of Psychotherapy and Behaviour Change*, New York, NY: John Wiley & Sons, 590–646.

Sexton, T. L. and Kelley, S. D. (2010) 'Finding the common core: Evidence-based practices, clinically relevant evidence and core mechanisms of change', *Administration and Policy in Mental Health*, 37(81), 81–88.

Shadish, W. R., Cook, T. D. and Campbell, D. T. (2002) *Experimental and Quasi-Experimental Designs for Generalized Causal Inference*, Boston: Houghton Mifflin.

Shapiro, V. (2009) 'Reflections on the work of Professor Selma Fraiberg', *Clinical Social Work Journal*, 37(1), 45–55.

Shapiro, V. and Gisynski, M. (1989) 'Ghosts in the nursery revisited', *Child and Adolescent Social Work*, 6(1), 18–37.

Shaw, B. F., Elkin, I., Yamaguchi, J., Olmsted, M., Vallis, T. M., Dobson, K. S., Lowery, A., Sotsky, S. M., Watkins, J. T. and Imber, S. D. (1999) 'Therapist competence ratings in relation to clinical outcome in cognitive therapy of depression', *Journal of Consulting and Clinical Psychology*, 67(6), 837–846.

Sherman, L., Gottfredson, D., MacKenzie, D., Eck, K., Reuter, P. and Bushway, S. (1998) *Preventing Crime: What Works, What Doesn't, What's Promising, Research in Brief*, Washington, DC: U.S. Department of Justice, National Institute of Justice.

Shonkoff, J. P. and Phillips, D. (2000) *From Neurons to Neighbourhoods: The Science of Early Childhood Development*, Washington, DC: National Academy Press.

Sidebotham, P. (2000) 'Patterns of child abuse in early childhood, a cohort study of the "children of the nineties"', *Child Abuse Review*, 9(5), 311–320.

Sidebotham, P., Heron, J., and the ALSPAC Study Team (2006) 'Child maltreatment in the children of the nineties: A cohort study of risk factors', *Child Abuse and Neglect*, 30(5), 497–522.

Sieverding, J. A., Adler, N., Witt, S. and Ellen, J. (2005) 'The influence of parental monitoring on adolescent sexual initiation', *Archives of Pediatrics & Adolescent Medicine*, 159(8), 724–729.

Sieving, R. E., McNeely, C. S. and Blum, R. W. (2000) 'Maternal expectations, mother–child connectedness, and adolescent sexual debut', *Archives of Pediatrics & Adolescent Medicine*, 154(8), 809–816.

Skinner, B. F. (1953) *Science and Human Behavior*, New York, NY: Macmillan.

Skinner, B. F. (1972) *Beyond Freedom and Dignity*, New York, NY: Bantam.

Skinner, B. F. (1974) *About Behaviorism*, New York: Knopf.

Smith, D. K. and Chamberlain, P. (2010) 'Multidimensional treatment foster care for adolescents: Processes and outcomes', in J. R. Weisz and A. E. Kazdin (eds.) *Evidence-based Psychotherapies for Children and Adolescents*, 2nd edn, New York: Guilford Press, 243–276.

Snyder, J. (1995) 'Coercion: A two-level theory of antisocial behaviour', in W. T. O'Donohue and L. Krasner (eds.) *Theories of Behavior Therapy: Exploring Behavior Change*, Washington, DC: American Psychological Association, 313–348.

Snyder, J., Cramer, A., Afrank, J. and Patterson, G. R. (2005) 'The contributions of ineffective discipline and parental hostile attributions of child misbehavior to the development of conduct problems at home and school', *Developmental Psychology*, 41(1), 30–41.

Sobell, L. C. and Sobell, M. B. (1992) 'Timeline follow-back: A technique for assessing self-reported alcohol consumption', in R. Z. Litten and J. Allen (eds.) *Measuring Alcohol Consumption: Psychosocial and Biological Methods*, Totowa, NJ: Humana Press, 41–72.

Song, H., Kempermann, G., Overstreet Wadich, L., Zhao, C., Schinder, A. F. and Bischofberger, J. (2005) 'New neurons in the adult mammalian brain: Synaptogenesis and functional integration', *The Journal of Neuroscience*, 25(45), 10366–10368.

Sonuga-Barke, E., Daley, D. and Thompson, M. (2002) 'Does maternal AD/HD reduce the effectiveness of parent training for pre-school children's AD/HD?' *Journal of the American Academy of Child and Adolescent Psychiatry*, 41(6) 696–702.

Sonuga-Barke, E. J. S., Daley, D., Thompson, M., Laver-Bradbury, C. and Weeks, A. (2001) 'Parent-based therapies for preschool attention deficit/hyperactivity disorder: a randomized, controlled trial with a community sample', *Journal of the American Academy of Child and Adolescent Psychiatry*, 40(4) 402–408.

Sonuga-Barke, E. J. S., Thompson, M., Abikoff, H., Klein, R. and Brotman, L. M. (2006) 'Nonpharmacological interventions for preschoolers with ADHD: The case for specialized parent training', *Infants and Young Children*, 19(2), 142–153.

Spanier, G. B. (1976) 'Measuring dyadic adjustment: New scales for assessing the quality of marriage and similar dyads', *Journal of Marriage and the Family*, 38(1), 15–28.

Spoth, R., Clair, S., Greenberg, M., Redmond, C. and Shin, C. (2007) 'Toward dissemination of evidence-based family interventions: Maintenance of community-based partnership recruitment results and associated factors', *Journal of Family Psychology*, 21(2), 137–146.

Spoth, R., Clair, S., Shin, C. and Redmond, C. (2006) 'Long-term effects of universal prevention interventions on methamphetamine use among adolescents', *Archives of Pediatric Adolescence Medicine*, 160(9), 876–882.

Spoth, R. L., Redmond, C. and Shin, C. (2001) 'Randomized trial of brief family interventions for general populations: Adolescent substance use outcomes 4 years following baseline', *Journal of Consulting and Clinical Psychology*, 69(4), 627–642.

Spoth, R., Shin, C. and Randall, G. (2008) 'Increasing school success through partnership-based family competency training: Experimental study of long-term outcomes', *School Psychology Quarterly*, 23(1), 70.

Spoth, R., Trudeau, L., Shin, C. and Redmond, C. (2008) 'Long-term effects of universal preventive interventions on prescription drug misuse', *Addiction*, 103(7), 1160–1168.

Spouse, J. (2001) 'Bridging theory and practice in the supervisory relationship: A sociocultural perspective', *Journal of Advanced Nursing*, 33(4), 512–522.

Sroufe, L. A., Egeland, B., Carlson, E. A. and Collins, W. A. (2005) *The Development of the Person: The Minnesota Study of Risk and Adaptation from Birth to Adulthood*, New York: Guilford.

Staller, K. M. (2006) 'Railroads, runaways, and researchers – Returning evidence rhetoric to its practice base', *Qualitative Inquiry*, 12(3), 503–522.

Starfield, B. and Riley, A. (1998) 'Profiling health and illness in children and adolescents', in D. Drotar (ed.) *Quality of Life Assessment in Children and Adolescents with Chronic Health Conditions*, Mahwah, NJ: Lawrence Erlbaum, 85–104.

Stein, A., Woolley, H., Senior, R., Hertzmann, L., Lovel, M., Lee, J., Cooper, S., Wheatcroft, R., Challacombe, F., Patel, P., Nicol-Harper, R., Menzes, P., Schmidt, A., Juszczak, E. and Fairburn, C. G. (2006) 'Treating disturbances in the relationship between mothers with bulimic eating disorders and their infants: A randomized, controlled trial of video feedback', *American Journal of Psychiatry*, 163(5), 899–906.

Steinberg, L. (1986) 'Latchkey children and susceptibility to peer pressure: An ecological analysis', *Developmental Psychology*, 22(4), 433–439.

Steinberg, L. (1987) 'Impact of puberty on family relations: Effects of pubertal status and pubertal timing', *Developmental Psychology*, 23(3), 451–460.

Steinberg, L., Lamborn, S. D., Darling, N., Mounts, N. S. and Dornbusch, S. M. (1994) 'Over-time changes in adjustment and competence among adolescents from authoritative, authoritarian, indulgent, and neglectful families', *Child Development*, 65(3), 754–770.

Steinberg, L., Lamborn, S. D., Dornbusch, S. and Darling, N. (1992) 'Impact of parenting practices on adolescent achievement: Authoritative parenting, school involvement, and encouragement to succeed', *Child Development*, 63(5), 1266–1281.

Steinberg, L., Mounts, N. S., Lamborn, S. D. and Dornbusch, S. M. (1991) 'Authoritative parenting and adolescent adjustment across varied ecological niches', *Journal of Research on Adolescence*, 1, 19–36.

Steinberg, L. and Silverberg, S. B. (1986) 'The vicissitudes of autonomy in early adolescence', *Child Development*, 57(4), 841–851.

Steinberg, L. D. (1990) 'Interdependence in the family: Autonomy, conflict and harmony in the parent–adolescent relationship', in S. S. Feldman and G. R Elliott (eds.) *At the Threshold: The Developing Adolescent*, Cambridge, MA: Harvard University Press.

Steinberg, L. D. (2001) 'We know some things: Adolescent–parent relationships in retrospect and prospect', *Journal of Research on Adolescence*, 11(1), 1–19.

Steinhausen, H., Bösiger, R. and Metzke, C. (2006) 'Stability, correlates, and outcome of adolescent suicidal risk', *Journal of Child Psychology and Psychiatry*, 47(7), 713–722.

Stern, S. B., Alaggia, R., Watson, K. and Morton, T. R. (2008) 'Implementing an evidence-based parenting program with adherence in the real world of community practice', *Research on Social Work Practice*, 18(6), 543–554.

Stern, D. N., Beebe, B., Jaffe, J., and Bennett, S. (1977) 'The infant's stimulus world during social interaction: A study of caregiver behaviours with particular reference to repetition and timing', in H. R. Schaffer (ed.) *Studies in Mother–Infant Interaction*, London; New York: Academic Press, 177–202.

Stevens, S. S. (1946) 'On the theory of scales of measurement', *Science*, 103(2684), 677–680.

Stewart-Brown, S. (2008) 'Improving parenting: The why and the how', *Archives of Disease in Childhood*, 93(2), 102–104.

Stiles, J. (2008) *The Fundamentals of Human Brain Development. Integrating Nature and Nurture*, Cambridge, MA: Harvard University Press.

Straus, M. A. (1979) 'Measuring intrafamily conflict and violence: The Conflict Tactics Scale', *Journal of Marriage and the Family*, 41(1), 75–88.

Suchman, N., DeCoste, C., Castigliani, B. A., Legon, N. and Mayos, M. D. (2008) 'The mothers and toddlers program: Preliminary findings from an attachment-based parenting intervention for substance-abusing mothers', *Psychoanalytic Psychology*, 25(3), 499–517.

Suchman, N., Pajulo, M., DeCoste, C. and Mayes, L. (2006) 'Parenting interventions for drug-dependent mothers and their young children: The case for an attachment-based approach', *Family Relations*, 55(2), 211–226.

Sure Start (2002) *Sure Start: A Guide for Sixth Wave Programmes*, London: DfES *Sure Start* Unit.

Swanson, H. L. and Hoskyn, M. (2001) 'A meta-analysis of intervention research for adolescent students with learning disabilities', *Learning Disabilities Research and Practice*, 16(3), 109–119.

Sylva, K., Scott, S., Totsika, V., Ereky-Stevens, K. and Crook, C. (2008) 'Training parents to help their children read: A randomized control trial', *British Journal of Educational Psychology*, 78, 435–455.

Taylor, J., Lauder, W., Moy, M. and Corlett, J. (2009) 'Practitioner assessments of "good enough" parenting: Factorial survey', *Journal of Clinical Nursing*, 18(8), 1180–1189.

Taylor, T. K. and Biglan, A. (1998) 'Behavioral family interventions for improving child-rearing: A review of the literature for clinicians and policy makers', *Clinical Child and Family Psychology Review*, 1(1), 41–60.

Teicher, M. H., Dumont, N. L., Ito, Y., Vaituzis, C., Giedd, J. N. and Andersen, S. L. (2005) 'Childhood neglect is associated with reduced corpus callosum area', *Biological Psychiatry*, 56(2), 80–85.

Teicher, M. H., Ito, Y., Glod, C. A., Andersen, S. L., Dumont, N. and Ackerman, E. (1997) 'Preliminary evidence for abnormal cortical development in physically and sexually abused children using EEG coherence and MRI', *Annals of the New York Academy of Sciences*, 821(1), 160–175.

Teicher, M. H., Tomoda, A. and Andersen, S. L. (2006) 'Neurobiological consequences of early stress and childhood maltreatment', *Annals of the New York Academy of Science*, 1071(1), 313–323.

Thompson, M. J. J., Laver-Bradbury, C., Ayers, M., Le Poidevin, E., Mead, S., Dodds, C., Psychogiu, L., Paraskevi, B., Daley, D., Weeks, A., Miller, L., Brotman, L. M., Abikoff, H., Thompson, P.,

Sonuga-Barke, E. J. S. (2009) 'A small-scale randomized controlled trial of the revised New Forest parenting program for preschoolers with attention deficit hyperactivity disorder', *European Journal of Child and Adolescent Psychiatry*, 18(10), 605–616.

Tonigan, J. S. and Miller, W. R. (2002) 'The Inventory of Drug Use Consequences (InDUC): Test-retest stability and sensitivity to detect change', *Psychology of Addictive Behaviors*, 16(2), 165–168.

Toth, S. L., Maughan, A., Manly, J. T., Spagnola, M. and Cicchetti, D. (2002) 'The relative efficacy of two interventions in altering maltreated preschool children's representational models: Implications for attachment theory', *Development and Psychopathology*, 14(4), 877–908.

Trepka, C., Rees, A., Shapiro, D. A., Hardy, G. E. and Barkham, M. (2004) 'Therapist competence and outcome of cognitive therapy for depression', *Cognitive Therapy and Research*, 28(2), 143–157.

Tronick, E., Ricks, M. and Cohn, J. (1982) 'Maternal and infant affective exchange: Patterns of adaptation', in T. Field and A. Fogel (eds.) *Emotion and Early Interaction*, Hillsdale, NJ: Erlbaum, 83–100.

Tunnard, J. (2002) 'Matching needs and services: Emerging themes from its application in different social care settings', in H. Ward and W. Rose (eds.) *Approaches to Needs Assessment in Children's Services*, London: Jessica Kingsley, 99–126.

Tunstill, J., Meadows, P., Allnock, D., Akhurst, S. and Garbers, C. (2005) *Implementing Sure Start Local Programmes. An Integrated Overview of the First Four Years*, London: National Evaluation of Sure Start.

Tyson, K. (1995) *New Foundations for Scientific Social and Behavioural Research: The Heuristic Paradigm*, Boston, MA: Allyn and Bacon.

UK Cabinet Office (2000) *Wiring it Up: Whitehall's Management of Cross-cutting Policies and Services*, London: Stationery Office.

Upshur, R. E. G. (2006) 'Evidence-based medicine, reasoned medicine or both? Commentary on Jenicek, M. (2006) "The hard art of soft science"', *Journal of Evaluation in Clinical Practice*, 12(4), 420–422.

US Surgeon General (2001) *Youth Violence: A Report of the Surgeon General*, Rockville, MD: US Department of Health and Human Services.

Utting, D. (2009) *Assessing and Meeting the Need for Parenting Support Services: A Literature Review*, London: Family and Parenting Institute.

Uylings, H. B. M. (2001) 'The human cerebral cortex in development', in A. F. Kalverboer and A. Gramsbergen (eds) *Handbook of Brain and Behaviour in Human Development* (pp. 63–80), Amsterdam: Kluwer Academic.

Uylings, H. B. M. (2006) 'Development of the human cortex and the concept of "critical" or "sensitive" periods', *Language Learning*, 56, 59–90.

van der Horst, F. C. P., LeRoy, H. A. and van der Veer, R. (2008) '"When Strangers Meet": John Bowlby and Harry Harlow on attachment behavior', *Integrative Psychological and Behavioral Science*, 42(4), 370–388.

van der Horst, F. C. P., van der Veer, R. and van IJzendoorn, M. H. (2007) 'John Bowlby and ethology: An annotated interview with Robert Hinde', *Attachment & Human Development*, 9(4), 321–335.

Van Egeren, L. A. (2004) 'The development of the coparenting relationship over the transition to parenthood', *Infant Mental Health Journal*, 25(5), 453–477.

zan IJzendoorn, M. H. and Kroonenberg, P. M. (1988) 'Cross-cultural patterns of attachment: A meta-analysis of the strange situation', *Child Development*, 59(1), 147–156.

van IJzendoorn, M. H., Juffer, F. and Duyvesteyn, M. G. C. (1995) 'Breaking the intergenerational cycle of insecure attachment: A review of the effects of attachment-based interventions on maternal sensitivity and infant security', *Journal of Child Psychology and Psychiatry*, 36(2), 225–248.

Vazsonyi, A. T., Hibbert, J. R. and Snider, J. B. (2003) 'Exotic enterprise no more? Adolescent reports of family and parenting processes from youth in four countries', *Journal of Research on Adolescence*, 13(2), 129–160.

Velderman, M. K., Bakermans-Kranenburg, M. J., Juffer, F. and van Ijzendoorn, M. H. (2006) 'Effects of attachment-based interventions on maternal sensitivity and infant attachment: Differential susceptibility of highly reactive infants', *Journal of Family Psychology*, 20(2), 266–274.

Vinovskis, M. (2005) *The Birth of Head Start: Preschool Education Policies in the Kennedy and Johnson Administrations*, Chicago, IL: University of Chicago Press.

Waddell, C., McEwan, K., Shepherd, C. A., Offord, D. R. and Hua, J. M. (2005) 'A public health strategy to improve the mental health of Canadian children', *Canadian Journal of Psychiatry–Revue Canadienne de Psychiatrie*, 50(4), 226–233.

Wagner, M. M. and Clayton, S. L. (1999) 'The parents as teachers program: Results from two demonstrations', *Future of Children*, 9(1), 91–115.

Wakschlag, L. S., Chase-Lansdale, P. L. and Brooks-Gunn, J. (1996) 'Not just "ghosts in the nursery": Contemporaneous intergenerational relationships and parenting in young African-American families', *Child Development*, 67(5), 2131–2147.

Walker, L. J. and Taylor, J. H. (1991) 'Family interactions and the development of moral reasoning', *Child Development*, 62(2), 264–283.

Walker, L. J., Hennig, K. H. and Krettenauer, T. (2000) 'Parent and peer contexts for children's moral reasoning development', *Child Development*, 71(4), 1033–1048.

Waltz, J., Addis, M. E., Koerner, K. and Jacobson, N. S. (1993) 'Testing the integrity of a psychotherapy protocol: Assessment of adherence and competence', *Journal of Consulting and Clinical Psychology*, 61(4), 620–630.

Ward, E., King, M., Lloyd, M., Bower, P., Sibbald, B., Farrelly, S., Gabbay, M., Tarrier, N. and Addington-Hall, J. (2000) 'Randomised controlled trial of non-directive counselling, cognitive-behaviour therapy, and usual general practitioner care for patients with depression. I: Clinical effectiveness', *British Medical Journal*, 321(7273), 1383–1388.

Waters, E., Weinfield, N. S. and Hamilton, C. E. (2000) 'The stability of attachment security from infancy to adolescence and early adulthood: General discussion', *Child Development*, 71(3), 703–706.

Watzlawick, P., Weakland, J. H. and Fisch, R. (1974) *Change: Principles of Problem Formation and Problem Resolution*, New York, NY: Norton.

Webster-Stratton, C. (2004) 'Quality training, supervision, ongoing monitoring, and agency support: Key ingredients to implementing The Incredible Years programs with fidelity'. Online. Available: http://www.incredibleyears.com/library/items/quality-key-ingredients-fidelity-04.pdf (accessed 10 October 2010).

Webster-Stratton, C. and Hammond, M. (1999) 'Marital conflict management skills, parenting style, and early-onset conduct problems: Processes and pathways', *Journal of Child Psychology and Psychiatry and Allied Disciplines*, 40(6), 917–927.

Webster-Stratton, C., Rinaldi, J. and Reid, J. M. (2010) 'Long-term outcomes of Incredible Years parenting program: Predictors of adolescent adjustment', *Child and Adolescent Mental Health*. Online. Available HTTP: http://www.incredibleyears.com/Library/items/long-term-outcomes-of-iy-parenting-program_10.pdf (accessed 30 October 2010).

Weishaar, M. (2002) 'The life of Aaron T. Beck', in R. Leahy and E. T. Dowd (eds.) *Clinical Advances in Cognitive Psychotherapy*, New York, NY: Springer, 1–14.

Weiss, L. H. and Schwarz, J. C. (1996) 'The relationship between parenting types and older adolescents' personality, academic achievement, adjustment, and substance use', *Child Development*, 67(5), 2101–2114.

Weisz, J. R., Jensen, A. L. and McLeod, B. D. (2005) 'Development and dissemination of child and adolescent psychotherapies: Milestones, methods, and a new deployment-focused model', in E. D. Hibbs and P. S. Jensen (eds.) *Psychosocial Treatments for Child and Adolescent Disorders: Empirically Based Strategies for Clinical Practice*, Washington, DC: American Psychological Association, 9–39.

Weisz, J. R. and Kazdin, A. E. (2010) *Evidence-based Psychotherapies for Children and Adolescents*, 2nd edn, New York, NY: Guilford Press.

Weisz, J. R. and Kazdin, A. E. (2010) 'The present and future of evidence-based psychotherapies for children and adolescents', in J. R. Weisz and A. E. Kazdin (eds.) *Evidence-based Psychotherapies for Children and Adolescents*, 2nd edn, New York, NY: Guilford Press, 557–572.

Weisz, J. R., Weiss, B., Alicke, M. D. and Klotz, M. L. (1987) 'Effectiveness of psychotherapy with children and adolescents: A meta-analysis for clinicians', *Journal of Consulting and Clinical Psychology*, 55(4), 542–549.

Weisz, J. R., Weiss, B., Han, S. S., Granger, D. A. and Morton, T. (1995) 'Effects of psychotherapy with children and adolescents revisited: A meta-analysis of treatment outcome studies', *Psychological Bulletin*, 117(3), 450–468.

Welshman, J. (2010) 'From Head Start to *Sure Start*: Reflections on Policy Transfer', *Children & Society*, 24(2), 89–99.

Westen, D., Novotny, C. A. and Thompson-Brenner, H. (2004) 'The empirical status of empirically supported psychotherapies: Assumptions, findings, and reporting in controlled clinical trials', *Psychological Bulletin*, 130(4), 631–663.

Whitaker, D. J. and Miller, K. S. (2000) 'Parent–adolescent discussions about sex and condoms: Impact on peer influences of sexual risk behavior', *Journal of Adolescent Research*, 15(2), 251–273.

White, C., Warrener, M., Reeves, A. and La Valle, I. (2008) *Family Intervention Projects: An Evaluation of Their Design, Set-up and Early Outcomes*, Research Report No. 047, London: DCSF Publications.

Whitehurst, G. J., Arnold, D. S., Epstein, J. N., Angell, A. L., Smith, M. and Fischel, J. E. (1994) 'A picture book reading intervention in day-care and home for children from low-income families', *Developmental Psychology*, 30(5), 679–689.

Whitehurst, G. J., Epstein, J. N., Angell, A. L., Payne, A. C., Crone, D. A. and Fischel, J. E. (1994) 'Outcomes of an emergent literacy intervention in Head Start', *Journal of Educational Psychology*, 86(4), 542–555.

Whitehurst, G. J., Falco, F. L., Lonigan, C. J., Fischel, J. E., Debaryshe, B. D., Valdezmenchaca, M. C. and Caulfield, M. (1988) 'Accelerating language development through picture book reading', *Developmental Psychology*, 24(4), 552–559.

Whitehurst, G. J., Zevenbergen, A. A., Crone, D. A., Schultz, M. D., Velting, O. N. and Fischel, J. E. (1999) 'Outcomes of an emergent literacy intervention from Head Start through second grade', *Journal of Educational Psychology*, 91(2), 261–272.

Whittaker, K. A. and Cowley, S. (2010) 'An effective programme is not enough: A review of factors associated with poor attendance and engagement with parenting support programs', *Children in Society*. Online. Available HTTP: http://onlinelibrary.wiley.com/doi/10.1111/j.1099–0860.2010.00333.x/pdf (accessed 1 November 2010).

Whittle, S., Yap, M. B. H., Yucel, M., Fornito, A., Simmons, J. G., Barrett, A., Sheeber, L. and Allen, N. B. (2008) 'Prefrontal and amygdala volumes are related to adolescents' affective behaviors during parent–adolescent interactions', *Proceedings of the National Academy of Sciences USA*, 105(9), 3652–3657.

Whittle, S., Yap, M. B. H., Yucel, M., Sheeber, L., Simmons, J. H., Pantelis, C. and Allen, N. B. (2009) 'Maternal responses to adolescent positive affect are associated with adolescents' reward neuroanatomy', *Social Cognitive and affective Neurosciences*, 4(3), 247–256.

Winnicott, D. W. (1958) *Collected Papers: Through Paediatrics to Psycho-analysis*, London: Tavistock Publications.

Winnicott, D. W. (1960) 'The theory of the parent–infant relationship', in P. Buckley (ed.) *Essential Papers on Object Relations*, New York, NY: New York University Press, 233–253.

Winnicott, D. W. (2005) *Playing and Reality*, Abingdon: Routledge.

Winslow, E. B., Bonds, D., Wolchik, S., Sandler, I. and Braver, S. (2009) 'Predictors of enrollment and retention in a preventive parenting intervention for divorced families', *Journal of Primary Prevention*, 30(2), 151–172.

Wolchik, S. A., Sandler, I. N., Millsap, R. E., Plummer, B. A., Greene, S. M., Anderson, E. R., Dawson-McClure, S. R., Hipke, K. and Haine, R. A. (2002) 'Six-year follow-up of preventive interventions for children of divorce: A randomized controlled trial', *JAMA – Journal of the American Medical Association*, 288(15), 1874–1881.

Wolpe, J. (1958) *Psychotherapy by Reciprocal Inhibition*, Stanford, CA: Stanford University Press.

Womack, S. (2006) 'The Nanny State School for Good Parenting', *Telegraph*, 14 November.

Woodward, L., Fergusson, D. M. and Horwood, L. J. (2001) 'Risk factors and life processes associated with teenage pregnancy: Results of a prospective study from birth to 20 years', *Journal of Marriage and the Family*, 63(4), 1170–1184.

Youniss, J. and Smollar, J. (1985) *Adolescent Relations with Mothers, Fathers, and Friends*, Chicago: University of Chicago Press.

Zevenbergen, A. A. and Whitehurst, G. J. (2003) 'Dialogic reading: A shared picture book reading intervention for preschoolers', in A. V. Kleeck, S. A. Stahl and E. B. Bauer (eds.) *On Reading Books to Children: Parents and Teachers*, Mahwah, NJ: Erlbaum, 177–200.

Zigler, E. and Butterfield, E. C. (1968) 'Motivational aspects of changes in IQ test performance of culturally deprived nursery school children', *Child Development*, 39(1), 1–14.

Zigler, E. and Muenchow, S. (1992) *Head Start: The Inside Story of America's Most Successful Educational Experiment*, New York: Basic Books.

Zigler, E. and Styfco, S. J. (1994) 'Head Start: Criticisms in a constructive context', *American Psychologist*, 49(2), 127–132.

Zigler, E. and Styfco, S. J. (2004) *The Head Start Debates*, Baltimore, MD: Brookes Publishing Company.

Zigler, E. and Trickett, P. K. (1978) 'IQ, social competence, and evaluation of early-childhood intervention programs', *American Psychologist*, 33(9), 789–798.

Zubrick, S., Ward, K., Silburn, S., Lawrence, D., Williams, A., Blair, E., Robertson, D. and Sanders, M. (2005) 'Prevention of child behaviour problems through universal implementation of a group behavioural family intervention', *Prevention Science*, 6(4), 287–304.

Author index

needs assessments 206; parenting policies 3; parenting support 146, 237; *Preventing Mental, Emotional, and Behavioral Disorders among Young People* 9; research 8
Warrener, M. 19
Washington State 8
Waters, Everett 75
Watkins, J.T. 160
Watson, K. 158
Watzlawick, P. 130–1; reframing 137
Weakland, J.H. 130–1, 137
Webster-Stratton, C. 21b1.7, 92, 158, 159, 163, 197
Weeks, A. 72, 72b3.1
Weerth, C. de 67
Weikart, D.P. 4, 10b1.4, 12
Weinberg, R.A. 83
Weinfield, N.S. 75
Weishaar, M. 115
Weiss, B. 84, 162
Weiss, L.H. 84, 85
Weisz, J.R.: evidence based interventions 2, 238; external validity 43; *Incredible Years* 147; paraprofessionals 162; Parent Management Training-Oregon (PMTO) 82b3.4; randomized controlled trials (RCTs) 154; research 8
Weldon, A.H. 89, 91, 92
Wells, P.M.A. 105
Welshman, J. 12, 14, 19, 30
Westen, D. 155
Wewerke, S.S. 70
Wheatcroft, R. 76
Whitaker, C.J. 8, 160, 196–7
Whitaker, D.J. 2, 9, 85, 148, 196
White, C. 19
Whitehurst, G.J. 212b7.7

Whitley, M.K. 103, 145, 150, 152, 154
Whittaker, K.A. 148
Whittle, S. 71
Wienbruch, C. 67
Wilk, K.L. 70
Williams, A. 9b1.3
Williams, S.C.R. 68, 70
Wilson, A. 117
Windham, A. 6
Winnicott, D. 100–1, 125, 144
Winslow, E.B. 148
Witt, S. 85
Wolchik, S.A. 147b5.1, 148
Wollny, I. 234
Wolpe, J. 112, 122
Womack, S. 21
Wood, A. 153
Wood, D. 12, 14, 235
Woodward, L. 85
Woolley, H. 76

Xiang, Z. 4

Yamaguchi, J. 160
Yap, M.B.H. 71
Youniss, J. 86
Yurgelen-Todd, D.A. 71

Zahr, L.K. 171
Zeanah, C. 78
Zentall, S.R. 85
Zevenbergen, A.A. 212b7.7
Zhao, C. 68
Zigler, E. 4, 12, 30, 31b2.1, 32, 46
Zill, N. 31b2.1, 40
Zmich, D.E. 92
Zubrick, S. 9b1.3

Subject index